DRUG TRANSIT AND DISTRIBUTION, INTERCEPTION AND CONTROL

METHAMPHETAMINE: BACKGROUND, CONTROLS AND ISSUES

DRUG TRANSIT AND DISTRIBUTION, INTERCEPTION AND CONTROL

Additional books in this series can be found on Nova's website under the Series tab.

Additional E-books in this series can be found on Nova's website under the E-books tab.

DRUG TRANSIT AND DISTRIBUTION, INTERCEPTION AND CONTROL

METHAMPHETAMINE: BACKGROUND, CONTROLS AND ISSUES

ANDREA S. SANDOVAL
EDITOR

Nova Science Publishers, Inc.
New York

For permission to use material from this book please contact us:
Telephone 631-231-7269; Fax 631-231-8175
Web Site: http://www.novapublishers.com

LIBRARY OF CONGRESS CATALOGING-IN-PUBLICATION DATA
Methamphetamine : background, controls and issues / editor, Andrea S. Sandoval.
p. cm.
Includes index.
ISBN 978-1-60692-548-5 (hardcover)
1. Methamphetamine abuse--United States. 2. Methamphetamine--United States. I. Sandoval, Andrea S.
RC568.A45M487 2010
362.29'9--dc22
2010027292

Published by Nova Science Publishers, Inc. ✣ New York

CONTENTS

PREFACE

This book examines methamphetamines, which have risen to the top of the American drug-policy agenda. For most of its history, it was regarded in law and public opinion as a secondary or regional concern, different from and less damaging than the drugs — heroin, cocaine, and marijuana — that have defined the focus of national drug policy. More recently, however, as the production, trafficking, and use of methamphetamine have spread, a gathering consensus has come to regard it as one of the most dangerous substances available in illegal markets.

Chapter 1 - Methamphetamine has risen to the top of the American drug-policy agenda. For most of its history, it was regarded in law and public opinion as a secondary or regional concern, different from and less damaging than the drugs — heroin, cocaine, and marijuana — that have defined the focus of national drug policy. More recently, however, as the production, trafficking, and use of methamphetamine have spread, a gathering consensus has come to regard it as one of the most dangerous substances available in illegal markets. Methamphetamine's dangers, including the devastating impact of the drug on child welfare and health care systems in blighted communities, the risk of fires and explosions and the environmental contamination resulting from illicit manufacture of the drug, and the rapid increase in foreign suppliers of the drug are likely to keep this drug problem at the forefront of the congressional agenda.

Existing evidence of the pattern of methamphetamine abuse and the effectiveness of alternative responses to its abuse are in some cases highly imperfect, and policymaking in this field remains an exercise in decision making under uncertainty. There is, however, little doubt that methamphetamine use has risen significantly since the early 1990s. Indeed, this trend arguably is the most important change in drug consumption patterns since the crack cocaine epidemic of the late 1 980s and early 1990s. The prospect of increased methamphetamine use is a major concern for the future.

During the 109th Congress, more than 25 bills were introduced to address the methamphetamine problem, including its implications for public health, child welfare, crime and public safety, border security, and international relations. Of these proposals, Title VII of H.R. 3199, the *PATRIOT Act Renewal Act of 2005* (P.L. 109-177), was signed into law on March 9, 2006. The new law establishes measures to control the availability of methamphetamine precursor chemicals used for the illicit manufacturing of methamphetamine by drug trafficking organizations and amateur producers. The law limits the amount of cold and sinus medicine that can be purchased by consumers and requires that retailers maintain a registry of purchasers and secure their drug inventories. Among other provisions, P.L. 109-177 provides for limits on imports of methamphetamine precursor chemicals and requires the Departments of Justice and State to work with Mexico to effectively disrupt the smuggling of illicit methamphetamine across the U.S.-Mexico border.

This chapter begins with a brief overview of the history of methamphetamine use, followed by an analysis of the available prevalence data on the drug's use. The final section of the report provides a few overall conclusions that can be inferred from over two decades of congressional action to control illicit methamphetamine use, manufacture, and distribution. Appendices include a description of past congressional action and a brief description of three case studies analyzing the impact and effectiveness of past congressional efforts to regulate and control methamphetamine and its precursor chemicals.

Chapter 2 - Illicit methamphetamine (MA) production and use are longstanding and severe problems in some states. In recent years, concerns were raised that this drug problem was spreading nationwide, and MA issues became an important federal concern. During the 110th Congress, legislation was introduced on a broad range of issues related to MA abuse, illicit manufacture, treatment, and drug trafficking offenses. For example, S. 1276, the Methamphetamine Production Prevention Act of 2008 (P.L. 110-415), further specified the procedures retailers must follow for tracking the retail purchases of over- the-counter (OTC) medications containing MA precursor chemicals. H.R. 1199, the Drug-Endangered Children Act of 2007 (P.L. 110-345), extended the authority of the Drug-Endangered Children grant program through FY2009. Some of the MA legislation would have built on provisions enacted in the Combat Methamphetamine Epidemic Act (CMEA, P.L. 109-177), which were designed to control and limit the availability of MA and its precursor chemicals. MA abuse has implications for public health, child welfare, crime and public safety, and international relations. This chapter provides a brief overview of MA abuse, its illicit domestic manufacture, federal responses, and anti-MA legislation introduced in the 110th Congress.

Chapter 3 - Methamphetamine production and distribution are undergoing significant strategic shifts, resulting in new challenges to law enforcement and public health agencies. Law enforcement pressure and strong precursor chemical sales restrictions have achieved marked success in decreasing domestic methamphetamine production. Mexican DTOs, however, have exploited the vacuum created by rapidly expanding their control over methamphetamine distribution—even to eastern states—as users and distributors who previously produced the drug have sought new, consistent sources. These Mexican methamphetamine distribution groups (supported by increased methamphetamine production in Mexico) are often more difficult for local law enforcement agencies to identify, investigate, and dismantle because they typically are much more organized and experienced than local independent producers and distributors. Moreover, these Mexican criminal groups typically produce and distribute ice methamphetamine that usually is smoked, potentially resulting in a more rapid onset of addiction to the drug. These numerous factors contribute to the significant threat posed to the United States by the trafficking and abuse of methamphetamine. In fact, according to National Drug Threat Survey (NDTS) 2006 data, 38.8 percent of state and local law enforcement officials nationwide report methamphetamine as the greatest drug threat to their areas, a higher percentage than that for any other drug.

Chapter 4 - This chapter is edited and excerpted memorandum for the Secretary of State.

Chapter 5 - This chapter highlights good news for America: a nationwide drop in methamphetamine laboratory incidents. This is a pattern observed, to varying degrees, in nearly every State. In 2004, there were approximately 17,750 methamphetamine laboratory incident seizures by law enforcement in the United States. In 2005, this number was 12,500 – a decline of more than 30%. Although 2006 numbers are not yet final, early 2006 data suggests that the decline is continuing at about the same pace.

The primary reason for this positive trend is the enactment of various State laws, starting with Oklahoma in April 2004, which implemented restrictions on transactions involving products containing certain chemicals (primarily, ephedrine and pseudoephedrine) that can be used to make methamphetamine. By early 2006, more than 40 States had implemented some type of new restriction on retail transactions involving these products. Then, on September 30, 2006, the Combat Methamphetamine Epidemic Act of 2005 (CMEA) went fully into effect. The law set a nationwide baseline standard for how to legally sell these products, which include some popular over-the-counter cold medications.

Although the CMEA is effective nationwide, the State laws, which vary widely in content, are concurrently in effect. The most notable provisions of the Federal law are also addressed by many of the State laws: where products containing these chemicals can be sold, how and where the products must be stored, what amount may be purchased or sold in a single transaction or in a month, and whether purchasers must show identification and sign a logbook. If the State law is less strict than the Federal CMEA on a certain issue, then compliance with the State provision is insufficient, and the Federal law, as a practical matter, is controlling. Conversely, if the State law is stricter on a certain issue than the Federal CMEA, then the State law, as a practical matter, is the controlling standard on that point. (In both cases, of course, retailers and others subject to the laws must show compliance with both.) Unsurprisingly, some States are a hybrid of the two situations, with the State law more lenient in some respects and stricter in others.

This chapter attempts to describe the various restrictions in all 50 States and compare them to the Federal CMEA standard implemented in September 2006.[1] It is not intended as a legal guide, and should not be used by retailers or others to gauge their own compliance. This chapter attempts to measure the impact of the various State laws in light of the declines in methamphetamine production in the State, and it also notes changes in positive drug tests for amphetamine in the workplace. In some States, enactment of the law was followed by a swift and sudden decline in methamphetamine laboratory incidents – sometimes, by as much as 75% or more. In some other States, however, the decline was less dramatic. This chapter may be helpful to State policymakers interested in understanding the effect of various types of restrictions on the sale of these chemicals, or in considering further restrictions at the State level.

Results of workplace drug testing for amphetamines (which include methamphetamine) are included for the first five months of 2006, compared to the same time period in 2005 and previous years back to, and including, 2000. Although the State methamphetamine precursor control laws were generally aimed at curbing methamphetamine production primarily (and use secondarily), workplace drug-testing information is provided in the hope that it will be additionally helpful data for State policymakers interested in understanding the extent of drug use in their State.

The Combat Methamphetamine Epidemic Act, in effect for exactly two months at the time of this chapter's release, is based on these successful State approaches for curbing methamphetamine production. The Bush Administration is committed to the CMEA's full implementation, and looks forward to aggressively pursuing further declines in methamphetamine production in the United States.

Chapter 6 - This chapter is edited and excerpted testimony at the hearing before the Committee on Finance on September 12, 2006.

Chapter 7 - This chapter is edited and excerpted testimony of Karen P. Tandy before the Subcommittee on International Economic Policy, Export and Trade Promotion on June 21, 2006.

Chapter 8 - This chapter is edited and excerpted testimony of Anne W. Patterson before the Subcommittee on International Economic Policy Export and Trade Promotion on June 21, 2006.

Chapter 9 - This chapter is edited and excerpted testimony of the Honorable John P. Walters before the Subcommittee on International Economic Policy, Export and Trade Promotion on June 21, 2006.

Chapter 10 - This chapter is edited and excerpted remarks prepared for Michael B. Mukasey at the National Methamphetamine Chemicals Initiative Conference on May 7, 2008.

In: Methamphetamine: Background, Controls and Issues ISBN: 978-1-60692-548-5
Editor: Andrea S. Sandoval

Chapter 1

METHAMPHETAMINE: BACKGROUND, PREVALENCE, AND FEDERAL DRUG CONTROL POLICIES

Celinda Franco

SUMMARY

Methamphetamine has risen to the top of the American drug-policy agenda. For most of its history, it was regarded in law and public opinion as a secondary or regional concern, different from and less damaging than the drugs — heroin, cocaine, and marijuana — that have defined the focus of national drug policy. More recently, however, as the production, trafficking, and use of methamphetamine have spread, a gathering consensus has come to regard it as one of the most dangerous substances available in illegal markets. Methamphetamine's dangers, including the devastating impact of the drug on child welfare and health care systems in blighted communities, the risk of fires and explosions and the environmental contamination resulting from illicit manufacture of the drug, and the rapid increase in foreign suppliers of the drug are likely to keep this drug problem at the forefront of the congressional agenda.

Existing evidence of the pattern of methamphetamine abuse and the effectiveness of alternative responses to its abuse are in some cases highly imperfect, and policymaking in this field remains an exercise in decision making under uncertainty. There is, however, little doubt that methamphetamine use has risen significantly since the early 1990s. Indeed, this trend arguably is the most important change in drug consumption patterns since the crack cocaine epidemic of the late 1 980s and early 1990s. The prospect of increased methamphetamine use is a major concern for the future.

During the 109th Congress, more than 25 bills were introduced to address the methamphetamine problem, including its implications for public health, child welfare, crime and public safety, border security, and international relations. Of these proposals, Title VII of H.R. 3199, the *PATRIOT Act Renewal Act of 2005* (P.L. 109-177), was signed into law on March 9, 2006. The new law establishes measures to control the availability of methamphetamine precursor chemicals used for the illicit manufacturing of methamphetamine by drug trafficking organizations and amateur producers. The law limits the amount of cold and sinus medicine that can be purchased by consumers and requires that retailers maintain a registry of purchasers and secure their drug inventories. Among other provisions, P.L. 109-177 provides for limits on imports of methamphetamine precursor chemicals and requires the Departments of Justice and State to work with Mexico to effectively disrupt the smuggling of illicit methamphetamine across the U.S.-Mexico border.

This chapter begins with a brief overview of the history of methamphetamine use, followed by an analysis of the available prevalence data on the drug's use. The final section of the report provides a few overall conclusions that can be inferred from over two decades of congressional action to control illicit methamphetamine use, manufacture, and distribution. Appendices include a description of past congressional action and a brief description of three case studies analyzing the impact and effectiveness of past congressional efforts to regulate and control methamphetamine and its precursor chemicals.

INTRODUCTION: THE ISSUE BEFORE CONGRESS

Methamphetamine has risen to the top of the American drug-policy agenda. For most of its history, it was regarded in law and public opinion as a secondary or regional concern, different from and less damaging than the drugs — heroin, cocaine, and marijuana — that have defined the focus of national drug policy. The issue before Congress is how to effectively disrupt the illicit manufacture, trafficking, and use of methamphetamine that has spread eastward from the traditional center of the drug's use in the Pacific west. As historical drug-policy priorities have been revised to reflect methamphetamine's devastating impact on children of users, user health, risk to the user's community, and the environmental damage caused by the drug's manufacture, a comprehensive range of methamphetamine-related issues has come before Congress. Legislation was enacted in the 109th Congress that addresses various aspects of the problem.

During the 109th Congress, the *Combat Methamphetamine Epidemic Act* (CMEA) was enacted as part of the reauthorization of the PATRIOT Act (P.L. 109- 177). Signed into law on March 9, 2006, P.L. 109-177 establishes measures designed to further criminalize and control the illicit use of methamphetamine by limiting the availability of certain precursor chemicals used in the illicit manufacturing of methamphetamine by drug trafficking organizations and amateur domestic producers. The new law restricts the amount of over-the-counter (OTC) cold and sinus medicine that consumers can purchase and requires retailers to maintain a registry of purchasers and secure these drug inventories. P.L. 109-177 also sets limits on imports of methamphetamine precursor chemicals and requires the Departments of Justice and State to work with Mexico to disrupt the smuggling of illicit methamphetamine across the U.S.-Mexico border. (For additional information on the provisions of the law, see Appendix A.)

In addition to the enactment of the CMEA, two other new laws have been enacted to address a number of methamphetamine-related issues that are beyond the scope of this chapter. P.L. 109-288 (H.R. 3525), enacted on September 28, 2006, authorizes the Secretary of Health and Human Services to make competitive grants to regional partnerships that provide programs and services designed to address concerns related to children in foster care due to a parent's or caretaker's methamphetamine or other substance abuse.[1] P.L. 109-347 (H.R. 4954), enacted on October 13, 2006, requires the Customs and Border Patrol (CBP) agency to track and report the seizure of methamphetamine and methamphetamine precursor chemicals as part of the agency's annual performance plan with respect to the interdiction of illegal drugs entering the United States.

In addition to what was enacted, a number of bills were introduced in the 109th Congress that would have addressed the methamphetamine problem through such measures as providing grants for technology to detect the smuggling of methamphetamine and its precursor chemicals, and grants for mentoring, after- school, and educational enrichment programs for children whose parents are methamphetamine addicts. The broad range of legislation that was introduced indicates Congress's perception of the far-reaching implications of the methamphetamine problem in the United States. The problem of methamphetamine abuse and its clandestine manufacture is not new, reaching back over 50 years. What makes methamphetamine a uniquely worrisome illicit drug for Congress is that it has easily adapted to changing federal prohibitions and continued to flourish.[2] Moreover, the chemicals from which methamphetamine is synthesized are produced and used for legitimate medical purposes and cannot be eliminated or eradicated.

This chapter begins with a brief overview of the background and history of methamphetamine use and abuse, followed by the sources of the drug in the country today. The report then provides an analysis of trends in illicit methamphetamine use, prevalence and geographic shift. The final section of the report provides a few conclusions that can be inferred from two decades of efforts to control illicit methamphetamine use and production. Two appendices follow that provide an overview of congressional efforts to address the problem, including a summary of the relevant provisions of the recently enacted law, P.L. 109-177, and an analysis of past congressional efforts to control methamphetamine.

BACKGROUND

Methamphetamine was first synthesized in 1893 by the Japanese chemist Nagayoshi Nagai,[3] but its medical uses were identified only in the 1930s.[4] Methamphetamine was marketed by Burroughs Wellcome and Co. as a pharmaceutical drug under the trade name Methedrine beginning in 1940 and by Abbott Laboratories under the trade name Desoxyn® beginning in 1943. Originally used as a nasal decongestant and bronchiodialator, between 1932 and 1949 many other medical uses for methamphetamine and amphetamines became accepted, including treatment of schizophrenia, tobacco smoking, heart block, radiation sickness, and morphine and codeine addiction.

Chemistry of Methamphetamine

Methamphetamine, an easily manufactured drug of the amphetamine group, is a powerful and addictive central nervous system (CNS) stimulant with long-lasting effects. The precursor drug ephedrine, from which methamphetamine can be produced, occurs naturally in plants of the genus *Ephedra*, and natural amphetamines are present in several plant species. Unlike heroin, cocaine, and marijuana, which are derived from botanical materials produced by large workforces dispersed over vast territories, methamphetamine is synthesized from chemicals produced in discrete factories around the world. Today, methamphetamine is produced synthetically, using either synthetically produced ephedrine or other synthetic products, such as pseudoephedrine and phenylpropanolamine, chemicals contained in OTC cold and sinus medications.

History of Methamphetamine Use and Regulation

Amphetamines were used by combatants in the Spanish Civil War (1936-39) and the Second Sino- Japanese War (China and Japan, 1937-45), and both amphetamine and methamphetamine came into wide use during World War II, when Japan, Germany, and the United States distributed the drugs to troops in order to increase their endurance and performance.[5] It has been estimated that 200 million amphetamine or methamphetamine tablets were supplied to U.S. troops over the course of the war.[6] In Japan, methamphetamine was also widely distributed to wartime factory workers. After the war, surplus methamphetamine stocks were dumped on the market in Japan, leading to the first major methamphetamine epidemic (1945-1957).[7]

Amphetamines were widely available in the United States without a prescription until 1951, and amphetamine-containing inhalers were available over the counter until 1959. Stimulants were widely used by long-haul truckers on transcontinental trips and students for staying awake to study.[8] The drugs were also widely used by construction workers and other blue-collar workers, shift workers, housewives, and office workers to help them stay awake or give them an extra "edge" in their endeavors. Amphetamines were popular diet pills for anyone interested in losing weight, particularly among women. In the 1 950s, methamphetamine was considered to be a promising therapy for depression.

Methamphetamine use has a lengthy history in the United States. Medical use of methamphetamine began in the 193 0s, when it was manufactured as a bronchial dilator, and soon after prescribed for a variety of conditions, including narcolepsy, attention deficit disorder, obesity, and fatigue. By the 1950s, methamphetamine was readily available legally and widely used. In the 1 960s, a liquid form of methamphetamine gained popularity as a treatment for heroin addiction, which quickly developed into a new abuse pattern involving injecting methamphetamine. During this period, the black market for amphetamine and methamphetamine consisted of diverted supplies from pharmaceutical companies, distributors, and physicians.

In response to the growing abuse of amphetamine and methamphetamine, restrictions were placed on the availability of Desoxyn® and Methedrine in the pharmaceutical market in late 1962. These restrictions led to the emergence of the first illicit methamphetamine laboratories generally operated by motorcycle gangs, first in the San Francisco area and later more widely in the western states. These illicit "biker" laboratories synthesized methamphetamine using phenyl-2-propanone (P-2-P) and methylamine as precursor chemicals, yielding a mixture of two isomers (levo- and dextro-methamphetamine).[9] The resulting substance was commonly referred to as "crank,"[10] which was a less potent form of methamphetamine than the pharmaceutical product. This illicit form of methamphetamine was manufactured and distributed by motorcycle gangs (also referred to as "outlaw biker gangs") beginning in the mid-1960s, and its use quickly spread along the Pacific Coast.

As the dangers associated with the use of amphetamine and methamphetamine became better understood, further restrictions were placed on how much could be legally produced and distributed. As a part of the Controlled Substances Act of 1970, methamphetamine was classified as a Schedule II drug. The response to further federal regulation of these pharmaceuticals fueled the illicit production of "crank," and its use spread beyond white- and blue-collar workers to include college students, young professionals, minorities, and women.[11] By the 1980s, increased law enforcement efforts to target the motorcycle gang subculture and its dominance of the illicit methamphetamine supply led underground chemists to seek other methods of illicitly manufacturing methamphetamine. The laws designed to crack down on biker gangs selling methamphetamine inadvertently resulted in the development of a new, easier method of manufacturing illicit methamphetamine that changed the production and distribution of the drug.[12] The new method of manufacturing illicit methamphetamine was the simpler, ephedrine reduction-based method first popularized in Southern California, primarily centered in San Diego. Use of the "reduction" method made it not only simpler to manufacture methamphetamine, but inadvertently led to the production of the significantly more potent form of methamphetamine in use today.[13] (See **Appendix A** for a more detailed description of the federal legislative history of methamphetamine regulation.)

Current Uses of Methamphetamine

Today, methamphetamine is medically used to treat a limited number of health conditions. These can include the treatment of narcolepsy; attention deficit disorder; attention deficit/hyperactivity disorder (ADD/ADHD); depression, as an adjunct to antidepressant medication; post- stroke patients with cognitive impairment; and obesity.[14] However, medical use of methamphetamine is very limited, and alternative drugs are most often used to treat the conditions that methamphetamine is currently approved to treat.

There are four forms of illicit methamphetamine: tablet, powder, base, and crystal. Methamphetamine tablets usually contain a combination of methamphetamine hydrochloride and caffeine. Methamphetamine tablets can be taken orally, or after being crushed, the tablets can be smoked or taken intravenously. Methamphetamine powder is crystalline hydrochloride salt and is water-soluble, and can be taken orally, smoked, snorted, or injected, but in the United States it is usually snorted or injected.[15] Methamphetamine "base," also known as "wax," is a damp, sticky, waxy or oily form of powder or paste of high purity that is thought to result when the illicit methamphetamine producer does not have the skill to produce the hydrochloride salt methamphetamine.[16] It can be ingested orally or taken intravenously. Crystal methamphetamine is methamphetamine hydrochloride powder that has been re-crystallized using isopropyl alcohol or water and looks like pieces of cracked ice or glass. This form of methamphetamine is usually smoked, but can also be injected, snorted, or taken orally. The street name for crystal methamphetamine is "ice," and it is generally characterized by a level of purity greater than 80%.[17]

The estimated level of past-year methamphetamine use in the United States in 2004 was approximately 0.6 % of the population, significantly lower than use of some other illicit drugs: marijuana (10.6%), prescription pain relievers used non- medically (4.7%), cocaine (2.4%), tranquilizers (2.1%), and hallucinogens (1.6%). [18] Among National Survey on Drug Use and Health (NSDUH) estimates of *past month* illicit drug use in 2005, methamphetamine falls behind a number of other illicitly used substances at 0.2% of those persons over age 12: marijuana and hashish (6.0%), prescription pain relievers used non-medically (1.9%), cocaine (1.0%), tranquilizers (0.7%), and hallucinogens (0.4%).[19] It is also important to note that methamphetamine past month use among those over age 12, although less than many other illicit substances, is equal to Ecstacy (0.2%) and twice that of heroin (0.1%) reported by NSDUH.[20]

Sources of Illicit Methamphetamine

According to the Drug Enforcement Administration (DEA), most illicit methamphetamine consumed in the United States is produced in clandestine 'super' labs in Mexico and California operated by Mexican drug trafficking organizations (DTOs). DEA estimates that more than 80% of methamphetamine available illicitly is supplied by Mexican DTOs.

The Office of National Drug Policy's (ONDCP) *National Drug Threat Assessment 2007*, concluded that Mexican DTOs have expanded their control over methamphetamine distribution in the U.S. This development is the result of greatly reduced domestic methamphetamine production by amateur cooks in response to more tightly controlled precursor chemicals, first by state law in certain areas,[21] followed in 2006 by federal law. The consolidation of methamphetamine production and distribution by Mexican DTOs means that these considerably stronger and expanded and more highly organized groups are producing and marketing a higher purity methamphetamine.

The remainder of the U.S. market is supplied by small, makeshift, amateur clandestine methamphetamine laboratories.[22] Methamphetamine is relatively easy and cheap to manufacture in small quantities by individuals with little knowledge of chemistry or laboratory skills and equipment. Clandestine methamphetamine labs are dangerous because the volatile chemicals used in the drug's manufacture make these laboratories vulnerable to fire and explosion,[23] as well as environmental contamination.[24] Clandestine methamphetamine labs have been seized in numerous settings, hidden from view but often in areas dangerous to children, such as sleeping areas, kitchens and eating areas where food is prepared and stored, garages, vehicles, hotel and motel rooms, storage lockers, mobile homes, apartments, ranches, campgrounds, rural and urban dwellings, abandoned dumps, restrooms, houseboats, and other locations. Amateur laboratories spread eastward along with the drug's use, cropping up in states that had not previously had a significant methamphetamine problem. Concerns over the public health and environmental problems caused by the proliferation of amateur laboratories also contributed to the sense of urgency behind recent anti-methamphetamine legislation considered at the federal and state levels.

Amateur laboratories are distinct from super labs in their size and productivity, as well as in their sources of the precursor chemicals, the chemicals used to manufacture methamphetamine. Amateur laboratories generally rely on supplies of retail OTC cold and sinus medicines as the principle source of precursor chemicals that can be extracted from these products and synthesized into methamphetamine. In contrast, super labs are dependent on huge quantities[25] of the pure precursor chemicals pseudoephedrine and ephedrine. These precursor chemicals used by Mexican DTOs are generally purchased in ton-quantities[26] from chemical companies in Europe, Asia, and the Far East, and then smuggled into Mexico where the methamphetamine is manufactured and smuggled across the border for distribution in the United States. Domestic super labs typically rely on large quantities of precursor chemicals being smuggled into the United States from Canada or Mexico, and most of these domestic laboratories tend to be located in California, or occasionally in other western states.

Dangers of Methamphetamine

Illicitly used, methamphetamine can be administered orally, nasally, by injection, and, in the powder form that resembles granulated crystals, often referred to as "ice," by smoking. Methamphetamine can cause convulsions, stroke, cardiac arrhythmia, and hyperthermia.[27] Chronic abuse can lead to irreversible brain and heart damage, memory loss, psychotic behavior including paranoid ideation, visual and auditory hallucinations, and rages and violence.[28] Withdrawal from the drug can induce paranoia, depression, anxiety, and fatigue.

The attendant dangers of manufacturing the drug in clandestine laboratories include heightened risk of fires, explosions, and environmental damage,[29] due to the toxic and volatile chemicals used in synthesizing methamphetamine. Concerns about these dangers from methamphetamine manufacture increased as the number of these laboratory sites proliferated and spread across western and midwestern urban and rural communities. Similarly, the profound effects of methamphetamine abuse on the users' health, children, families, as well as their communities, quickly strained resources for substance abuse treatment; foster care systems; and state, local, and tribal law enforcement efforts to control access to the drug.[30] Individuals, particularly children, living in direct or indirect contact with the toxic fumes produced as the drug is "cooked," can be subject to problems associated with exposure to toxic chemicals and drug residues produced or left behind by the manufacturing process.[31] Exposure to these residues can result in respiratory illnesses and central nervous system (CNS) disorders.

Those living near a clandestine methamphetamine laboratory site can also be at risk of the fires and explosions of clandestine laboratories due to the volatile and toxic nature of the chemicals used in the drug's manufacture, as can law enforcement officers and first responders who are called to the scene of a clandestine laboratory. The manufacture of each pound of methamphetamine produces five to seven pounds of toxic waste products.[32] Because there are no federal standards for clandestine methamphetamine laboratory clean-up, many state and local entities are left to manage the issue of methamphetamine contamination as they see fit.

Laboratory Seizures.[33]

In 1993, DEA reported total federal, state, and local seizures of 218 clandestine methamphetamine laboratories. By 1999, federal, state, and local law enforcement reportedly seized over 9,000 laboratories/lab incidents; by 2002, 16,212 laboratories/lab incidents were seized. In 2004, a total of 17,170 clandestine labs were reported by the DEA; in 2005, the number of laboratory seizures had dropped to 12,484, a one-year decrease of 27%.[34] Between 2004 and 2005, the number of clandestine laboratory seizures decreased by 42%, from 10,015 in 2004 to 5,846 in 2005.[35] According to DEA's El Paso Intelligence Center (EPIC), preliminary 2006 data indicate that the number of clandestine methamphetamine laboratories has continued to drop further.

Methamphetamine labs also have been discovered on federal lands across the country, in such areas as near or in caves, camping and recreational areas, and in abandoned mines.[36] The number of reported methamphetamine laboratory seizures on Department of Interior lands increased from 28 in 2001, to 41 in 2002, to 83 in 2003. During 2002, 187 laboratories were seized on National Forest System lands; the number decreased to 56 seizures in 2003.[37]

Trends in Illicit Methamphetamine Use

Historically, methamphetamine was a problem largely in the Pacific West, particularly in Hawaii and California. However, during the 1 990s, the use of methamphetamine grew and began to spread, first into the northwestern states, and, by 2000, its use had spread to the Midwest and South and to a much lesser degree to the Northeast and Mid-Atlantic region.[38] For policymakers, it is important to understand the depth and pervasiveness of the methamphetamine problem in order to craft legislative responses that can effectively address the issues. Drug-use surveys and other data sources can help to inform these discussions.

Is There a Methamphetamine Epidemic?

During recent congressional deliberations on the latest round of antimethamphetamine legislation, questions were raised about whether the methamphetamine problem was truly a *national* drug priority. Critics of U.S. drug policy argued that national drug data from the NSDUH did not support the urgency of claims that a methamphetamine "epidemic" was spreading across the nation.[39] The response of congressional policymakers to anecdotal stories that methamphetamine use was spiraling out of control in their home districts was considered by some critics to be another "drug panic" fueled, in part, by sensational media coverage. To consider the question, "is there a methamphetamine epidemic in the country?" first, one would need to specify the period in question. Second, one would need to consider the definition of "epidemic" that would be applied. Finally, it would be important to consider how accurately the available drug-use data capture these developments nationally and whether these data could be used for estimating drug-use patterns in local or regional areas.

If the question of a methamphetamine epidemic were posed today, there are several lines of evidence indicating that the national prevalence of methamphetamine use increased dramatically between 1994-2004.

Table 1. Methamphetamine Use Among Persons Aged 12 or Older, 2002-2005 (in thousands)

Use	2002	2003	2004	2005
Lifetime Use	12,383	12,303	11,726	10,357
Age 12-17	366	328	299	296
Age 18-25	1,756	1,650	1,688	1,682
26 years of age or older	10,261	10,325	9,739	8,379
Use in Last Year	1,541	1,315	1,440	1,297
Age 12-17	226	174	163	170
Age 18-25	525	506	516	482
26 years of age or older	790	636	761	645
New Users in Last Year	299	260	318	192
Use in the Last Month	597	607	583	512
Age 12-17	63	69	57	66
Age 18-25	160	185	186	194
26 years of age or older	375	353	340	252
Dependent Use in Last Month	164	250	346	257
Stimulant is Primary Drug of Abuse	63	92	130	103
Other Illicit Drug is Primary Drug of Abuse	101	158	216	154

Source: DHHS, Substance Abuse and Mental Health Administration (SAMHSA), NSDUH 2002- 2005.

Since 2004, however, national survey data indicate that the number of methamphetamine lifetime users and first time users is declining nationally after peaking in, or around, 2004. However, the latest NSDUH data for 2005 do not support a national epidemic because the survey estimates that methamphetamine use has declined since 2004. Limitations of the NSDUH sample[40] and other survey and administrative data sets make it difficult to extrapolate methamphetamine use for small and rural communities. As a result, NSDUH and other national drug-use data sets may not adequately track drug trends in these communities, particularly in the case of methamphetamine use. Evidence from clandestine laboratory seizures, although not a typical indicator of drug use, do indicate that there was a noteable proliferation of amateur methamphetamine laboratories spread from states in the West, moving into the Midwest and southeastern states between 1999 and 2004. Other drug-use indicators reflect increases in methamphetamine-related emergency department visits and substance abuse treatment rates spreading into states in the Midwest and South. Reports from state and local law enforcement agencies in certain regions that methamphetamine use continues to be the most significant drug problem further corroborates the variability of the problem.

National Prevalence Estimates

Since 1994, national estimates of selfreported methamphetamine use, as reflected in NSDUH,[41] indicate that among individuals age 12 or older there has been a significant increase among those reporting use of methamphetamine in their lifetimes, more than doubling over the 10- year period from just over 2% of the general population in 1994 to 4.9% in 2004.42 Over the shorter term, those reporting having ever used methamphetamine in their lifetimes dropped by 16.4% between 2002 and 2005, from 12.4 million to 10.4 million individuals (see Table 1). Similarly, the number of persons reporting methamphetamine use in the last year dropped by 6.7%, from 1.5 million in 2002 to 1.4 million in 2004. During the 2002-2004 period, the proportion of NSDUH respondents over age 12 that reported lifetime use of methamphetamine has remained a relatively constant proportion of the general population over age 12 compared with the growth over the previous 10-year period.

Better indicators of drug prevalence provided by data in Table 1 are in the category *use in the last month* and *dependent use in the last month* because these respondents are reporting more current or ongoing use of methamphetamine. Among respondents age 12-17 years of age, methamphetamine *use in the last month* increased by 4.3% between 2004 and 2005. Among respondents age 18-25, reported *use in the last month* rates increased by 15.6% from 2002 to 2003, remained relatively stable between 2003 and 2004 rising by only 0.5%, and increased again by 5.8% between 2004 and 2005. Moreover, among respondents over age 12 reporting *dependent use in the last month*, between 2002 and 2005 the increases were more notable: an increase of almost 56.7%; an increase of 63.5% for those reporting dependence on a stimulant as their primary drug of abuse.

Additional corroboration of the slight downward trend in self-reported national estimates of *lifetime* use of methamphetamine use is indicated in two other sources of national drug use data, Monitoring the Future (MTF)[43] and the Youth Risk Behavioral Surveillance System (YRBSS).[44] These two surveys of youths indicate declining self-reported methamphetamine use among junior high and high school students. The MTF survey indicates a significant decrease in lifetime use of over 40% for 12th graders between 1999 and 2005, after a significant one-year drop between 2004 and 2005 from 6.2% to 4.5% (see Table 2). The YRBSS reports a decline of over 16% among students in all grades who used methamphetamine one or more times during their lives between 1999 and 2003, with the largest decline among 12th graders.

Other drug-use data sources measure national trends in methamphetamine by tracking instances of drug users using the health care system for substance abuse treatment or in a drug-related emergency department visit. Unlike the national estimates based on self-reported methamphetamine use such as NSDUH, MTF, and YRBSS, two often-cited healthcare administrative data sets indicate that methamphetamine use has been on the rise since the 1 990s. The Treatment Episode Data Set (TED S)[45] reports that treatment admissions in cases where the primary drug dependence is methamphetamine/amphetamine[46] have risen from 1% of all treatment admissions in 1992, to 7.4% in 2002.[47] Similarly, methamphetamine-related emergency room visits captured by the Drug Abuse Warning Network (DAWN)[48] indicate that methamphetamine/amphetamine-related emergency department (ED) mentions,[49] while fluctuating since 1995, have been on the rise since 1999, increasing by almost 70% by 2002. Between 1999 and 2002, ED mentions rose from 10,447 to 1 7,696.[50]

National estimates of methamphetamine prevalence do not uniformly indicate that methamphetamine's use has been increasing, and the rate of growth varies among the drug-use surveys and datasets. Among some of the drug-use surveys, namely TEDS and DAWN, there is evidence indicating that, in the case of methamphetamine, national prevalence estimates may mask important regional changes in the drug's use, described above. Based on NSDUH data, some critics of federal drug policy argue that the prevalence of methamphetamine does not warrant the kind of congressional attention the problem received at the federal level in the last couple of years. Indeed, some argue, methamphetamine use in the last month among persons aged 12 or older ranks far below other illicit drug use with only 0.2% of the total population over age 12 reporting such use (see **Table 3**), the same percentage that used Ecstacy and twice as many as used heroin, OxyContin, and sedatives. Yet, there is general agreement that the illicit use of heroin, OxyContin, and sedatives is a serious concern that should be addressed by anti-drug policies without the drug's abuse being of "epidemic" proportions.

Table 2. Prevalence of Lifetime Methamphetamine Use Among High School Seniors, 1999-2005 (percent)

Year	Methamphetamine
1999	8.2
2000	7.9
2001	6.9
2002	6.7
2003	6.2
2004	6.2
2005	4.5

Source: Monitoring the Future, U.S. Department of Health and Human Services, 1999-2005.

Table 3. Past Month Use of Drugs Measured by the National Survey on Drug Use and Health, 2005, Ranked by Percent of Persons Aged 12 or Older Using the Substance

Rank	Drug	Percent
1	Any Illicit Drug	8.1
2	Marijuana and Hashish	6.0
3	Illicit Drug other than Marijuana	3.7
4	Nonmedical Use of Psychotherapeutics	2.6
5	Pain Relievers (incl. OxyContin)	1.9
6	Cocaine (incl. Crack)	1.0
7	Tranquilizers	0.7
8	Stimulants (incl. **Methamphetamine**)	0.4
9	Hallucinogens (incl. LSD, PCP, Ecstasy)	0.4
10	Inhalants	0.3
10	Crack	0.3
11	Ecstasy	0.2
11	**Methamphetamine**	0.2
12	Heroin	0.1
12	OxyContin	0.1
12	Sedatives	0.1
13	LSD	0.0
13	PCP	0.0

Source: SAMHSA, Office of Applied Studies, NSDUH, 2005.

Evidence for a Geographic Spread or Shift

The methamphetamine problem, perhaps more than most other illicit drug problems, has tended to be more regional and cyclical in nature, which may partially explain some of the stability in the national prevalence estimates. National drug-use surveys, such as NSDUH, could fail to report certain important localized variations in drug use, particularly when acute drug problems occur in smaller cities or rural areas and regions with lower populations.[51] Most experts agree that, to a large extent, the recent congressional action on anti-methamphetamine legislation was spearheaded by Members from Midwestern states. While national estimates of methamphetamine prevalence provide some mixed indications of the drug's use, illicit methamphetamine use has become more geographically widespread than it has been in previous decades.

In 2001, DAWN rates for methamphetamine/amphetamine ED visits remained concentrated in the Midwest and western cities surveyed. By 2002, rates per 100,000 population were growing the most dramatically in DAWN-surveyed cities in the South and Northeast.[52] The metropolitan areas reporting the highest rates (visits per 100,000 population) in 2002 were San Francisco (91), San Diego (68), Phoenix (65), Seattle (46), and Los Angeles (39).[53] For the Northeast cities, Boston had the highest rate (15 per 100,000 population), followed by Newark (9 per 100,000 population). Although there were significant *percentage* increases in the rates of ED visits for some cities in the Northeast and South, between 2001 and 2002 rates increased in Boston from 11 to 15 (+45%), Buffalo from 2 to 4 (+100%), Newark from 14 to 23 (+64%), New Orleans from 11 to 16 (+45%), and St. Louis from 12 to 24 (+100%), these rates remained significantly lower than the rates for most cities in the West.[54]

According to the National Institute on Drug Abuse's Community Epidemiology Work Group (CEWG),[55] in 2004 and 2005 methamphetamine indicators remained high in West Coast areas and parts of the Southwest, as well as in Hawaii.[56] In addition, regional differences were indicated by the report's finding that in one midwestern CEWG area, St. Louis, Missouri, methamphetamine use grew, with ED admissions increasing by 15% between 2004 and 2005.[57] The National Drug Intelligence Center (NDIC)[58] reports that methamphetamine is widely available throughout the Pacific, Southwest, and West Central regions of the United States, and is increasingly available in the Great Lakes and Southeast regions.[59] Data from the Arrestee Drug Abuse Monitoring (ADAM)[60] program survey sites, during 2002, lend further support to the finding that the greatest concentration of methamphetamine use is in the Western region of the country.[61] In 2002, out of 36 sites, the highest percentages of adult male arrestees testing positive for methamphetamine when arrested were located in Honolulu (44. 8%), Sacramento (3 3.5%), San Diego (31.7%), and Phoenix (31 .2%).[62] For female arrestees, out of 23 sites, the highest percentages of adult female arrestees testing positive for methamphetamine were located in Honolulu (50%), San Jose (42.8%), Phoenix (41.7%), Salt Lake City (37.7%), and San Diego (36.8%).[63]

In 2002, TEDS reported that methamphetamine admission rates for substance abuse treatment were highest in the West, although there was significant variation in certain states.[64] According to the report, 21 states had admission rates over the national average and 12 states had admission rates that were twice the national average. The 12 states with rates twice the national average accounted for 15% or more of total national admissions. Several states with large rural populations, including Arkansas, Oklahoma, Idaho, Utah, Iowa, and Nebraska, all reported that 20% or more of their substance abuse admissions in 2003 cited methamphetamine as the primary drug of abuse. Similarly, DAWN data on "methamphetamine ED mentions" changed regionally between 1995 and 2002. Areas with relatively high methamphetamine mentions in 1995 experienced significant drops in their ED mentions by 2002, including Denver (-43%), Dallas, TX (-51.7%), and San Francisco (-34.3%). In contrast, in areas where methamphetamine use was more recent, certain cities experienced dramatic increases in ED mentions, such as in Minneapolis (+243%), Miami (+200%), and New Orleans (+174%).[65]

Evidence of the geographic spread of methamphetamine use from the West to Midwest and Southeast states is also apparent from data on clandestine laboratory seizures. According to DEA's El Paso Intelligence Center (EPIC), reports by state and local law enforcement of seizures of clandestine methamphetamine laboratories rose dramatically in number between 1999 (7,438) peaking in 2003 (17,356), and began to slow in 2004.[66] Not only did the number of clandestine methamphetamine laboratories increase dramatically during the period, but some western states also experienced declines in laboratory seizures. California laboratory seizures went from 2,579 in 1999 (35% of all seizures) to 470 in 2005 (4% of all laboratory seizures); Washington state began in 1999 with 599 reported methamphetamine seizures (8% of all seizures), peaked in 2001 with 1,480 seizures (almost 11% of all seizures), and by 2005 reported 532 seizures (just over 4% of all seizures). In the Midwest, Missouri went from 439 laboratory seizures in 1999, to 2,176 in 2005.[67]

National Epidemic, Regional Drug Problem, or the Latest Drug Panic?

In the case of national methamphetamine prevalence estimates, there are some limitations on how quickly and reliably the drug-use data sources reflect changes in patterns of use. Until the resurgence of methamphetamine use in the mid- 1990s, the low reported incidence of methamphetamine use, compared to the use of drugs such as marijuana or cocaine, hampered the development of state drug-use estimates from national estimates. As a result, until recently, these drug-use surveys and treatment admission datasets reported methamphetamine as part of a more general category of "stimulants (non-cocaine)."[68] This combined reporting has made it difficult to track national methamphetamine trends over time. In addition, the small sample size of survey respondents reporting methamphetamine use makes it difficult to estimate state-level prevalence data on the drug's use for any single year.[69] Moreover, such data limitations, in turn, complicate capturing regional or state variations in methamphetamine prevalence.[70] In the case of recent trends in methamphetamine use, the most recent national prevalence estimates for 2005 do not show significant changes in regional variations and geographic shifts in the drug's use.

Webster's Ninth Collegiate Dictionary defines an "epidemic"as an occurrence "affecting or tending to affect many individuals within a population, community, or region at the same time." In the public health literature, epidemic is a term often used in a non-biological sense, referring to widespread and growing societal problems, such as drug addiction. The *Columbia Electronic Encyclopedia*[71] defines "epidemic" as the appearance of new cases of a disease, during a given period, "at a rate that substantially exceeds what is expected based on recent experience." As such, defining an epidemic can be subjective, depending on what is "expected" or the recent experience of a given population. Because what is meant by epidemic can vary based on subjective judgements of what is "expected" or considered normal, the incidence of a few cases of a disease could be considered an "epidemic"in one area, while in another area where many cases of the same disease are common a few more cases would not be considered an epidemic.

Whether or not the prominence of methamphetamine on the congressional antidrug agenda was due to an actual drug "epidemic" or instead the result of a geographic shift in the drug's prevalence is, in part, a question of semantics. Clearly, there are states that have been experiencing epidemic levels of methamphetamine use for decades without provoking a national sense of crisis and prominence on the congressional agenda. In these states with historically high methamphetamine prevalence, recent trends continue to indicate continued growth in the drug's use but at a less dramatic pace than that seen in certain Midwestern states where methamphetamine use was less common and rose quickly. Understandably, there are some who would argue that the characterization of a geographic shift or spreading of the abuse of methamphetamine as an "epidemic" was an overstatement of the drug problem. The media's use of graphic images of methamphetamine abuse and manufacture - photos of men and women whose faces have been ravaged by the drug's use or the sensational damage to houses or other structures from explosions and fires resulting from highly flammable and volatile chemicals used in the manufacture of methamphetamine by clandestine laboratories - could have contributed to an exaggerated public perception of the problem. In any case, the spread of the methamphetamine problem across a number of states in the Midwest and South, although not numerically significant on a national scale, was enough to trigger a national response.

Federal Branch Law Enforcement Programs and Policies

Federal approaches to illicit drug use take one of three basic forms: (1) demand reduction (prevention and treatment), (2) domestic law enforcement, and (3) interdiction.[72] Many law enforcement efforts at all levels of government rely on arrest and incarceration, drug seizures, and production interruptions at the drug's major sources. The sources of methamphetamine manufacture are unique because the drug can be synthesized from precursor chemicals that are produced for medical purposes and available in bulk for DTOs from certain chemical manufacturers around the globe. Many of the other chemicals used in the synthesis of the drug are chemicals found in household products that are not easy to regulate.

Illicit methamphetamine production is particularly sensitive to law enforcement efforts to limit access to its chemical precursors because, without ephedrine and pseudoephedrine, methamphetamine simply cannot be readily synthesized. In addition, the manufacture of methamphetamine' s precursors is a capital-intensive, difficult chemical process that requires exacting laboratory techniques and equipment that does not lend itself to illicit manufacture. As a result, these methamphetamine precursors are only manufactured in bulk by a handful of chemical companies around the world. Therefore, new federal restrictions on methamphetamine's precursor chemicals can have a significant impact on the availability and abuse of illicit methamphetamine. Federal and state laws have been developed to regulate the precursor chemicals used, including ephedrine and pseudoephedrine OTC products, as well as anhydrous ammonia, an agricultural product that is used in some methods of synthesizing methamphetamine.

Drug Enforcement Agency (DEA)

DEA is the principal federal agency tasked with enforcing federal drug control laws. Defendants arrested by DEA agents within the United States and its territories are tracked by the DEA Defendant Statistical System. Not all suspects arrested by DEA agents are federally prosecuted; many suspects are transferred to state or local jurisdictions for prosecution instead of being transferred to the U.S. Marshals Service for federal prosecution.[73]

DEA employs several methods to combat the proliferation of methamphetamine. In FY2005, DEA made 5,870 methamphetamine arrests and seized 2,491 kilograms of the drug. Through DEA's *Operation Three Hour Tour*, high-level Columbian and Mexican drug traffickers in the U.S. were targeted resulting in the dismantling of three major transportation cells and 27 distribution groups and the seizing of 155 pounds of methamphetamine.[74]

In addition, DEA works closely with state and local law enforcement in partnership on investigations and operation, dismantling and removing toxic wastes from clandestine laboratories, and regulating precursor chemicals. DEA commits more than $145 million per year to address the methamphetamine problem.[75] DEA's clandestine methamphetamine laboratory efforts can include training for police officers and sheriff's deputies on best practices for responding to methamphetaminerelated situations, providing containers for transporting toxic waste from laboratory sites, and removing hazardous materials.

DEA is also involved in establishing methamphetamine enforcement teams with Mexican counterparts to investigate and target Mexican methamphetamine drug trafficking organizations. DEA and the Customs and Border Protection Services work together to target suspicious cargo that may be related to methamphetamine trafficking organizations.[76] In addition, DEA and Mexican counterparts are working to share intelligence, establish collaboration, and implement joint strategies to address the methamphetamine problem on both sides of the U.S. - Mexico border.[77]

COPS Methamphetamine Initiative

The "Meth Hot Spots" program under the Community Oriented Policing Services (COPS) program is a grant program that *specifically* provides funding for a broad range of initiatives designed to assist state and local law enforcement to undertake anti-methamphetamine initiatives. For FY2006, the Meth Hot Spots program received appropriations of $63.6 million. Since 1998, the COPS program has provided over $350 million nationwide to address the methamphetamine problem.[78] The COPS Methamphetamine Initiative supports law enforcement, training, and lab cleanup activities targeting areas of greatest need for assistance combating methamphetamine production, distribution, and use. The program provides grants for community policing approaches to methamphetamine reduction, as well as grants for state and local innovative strategies focused on combating the methamphetamine problem.

The grants have been used by communities for many purposes, including developing law enforcement and businesses and/or community partnerships to educate and enforce anti-methamphetamine plans; drug-free workplace initiatives; media campaigns to increase public awareness; database development; substance abuse treatment; drug use surveys; clandestine lab seizures; law enforcement training; and community policing strategies.

Other DOJ Grant Programs

Additional DOJ grant programs provide assistance for a broad range of programs and initiatives which *can* include anti-methamphetamine efforts. Table 4 reports DOJ funding for grants awarded to state and local programs related to antimethamphetamine initiatives across the country.[79] Cumulatively, for the period FY2000 - FY2005, 470 grants were provided, totaling $263.8 million.

Drug Courts

Drug courts offer an alternative to incarceration that includes mandatory substance abuse treatment with intensive supervision and monitoring. Enacted by the *Violent Crime Control and Law Enforcement Act of 1994* (P.L. 103-322), drug courts are designed to allow judges to monitor drug treatment of defendants as a means of ending their use of illicit drugs. Drug courts are considered to be an important component of the national anti-drug abuse strategy, and while not designed to address the illicit methamphetamine abuse problem, drug courts in several states have used the drug court model for methamphetamine offenders.[80]

Other Federal Responses to Illicit Methamphetamine

Many agencies and bureaus within DOJ are involved in addressing the issue of illicit methamphetamine. In addition to DEA's efforts to control the supply of illicit methamphetamine, DEA collaborates with the Federal Bureau of Investigation (FBI) and numerous task forces, as well as the Organized Crime Drug Enforcement Task Force (OCDETF) and the High Intensity Drug Trafficking Areas (HIDTA) program. In addition and jointly with other federal, state and local law enforcement agencies, DEA targets drug traffickers both domestically and internationally to stem the flow of methamphetamine in the United States.

Table 4. DOJ Grant Awards Relating to Methamphetamine Initiatives, FY2000 - FY2005.

Fiscal Year	2000	2001	2002	2003	2004	2005
Total Grant Amount (in millions)	$12.6	$32.5	$52.5	$62.9	$55.0	$48.3
Total Number of Grants	23	44	118	101	97	87

Source: DOJ, Bureau of Justice Assistance, totals as of October 19, 2005.

LEGISLATIVE ISSUES

Numerous bills were introduced during the 109th Congress to address the issues of curbing illicit methamphetamine use, trafficking, and production. While most policy makers agree that methamphetamine is a devastating drug that negatively affects entire communities, they do not agree on which approach is best for confronting this problem. However, interest in responding to the methamphetamine problem fostered agreement on the provisions enacted in the *Combat Methamphetamine Epidemic Act* (CMEA) in Title VII of the *USA PATRIOT Act Reauthorization and Improvement Act* (P.L. 109-177).

The CMEA was signed into law on March 9, 2006. As enacted, P.L. 109-177 establishes measures to control the availability of methamphetamine precursor chemicals used for the illicit manufacturing of methamphetamine by drug trafficking organizations and amateur producers through restrictions on the amount of over-the- counter (OTC) cold and sinus medicine that could be purchased by consumers in a month, and the requirements that retailers maintain a registry of purchasers and secure their drug inventories. Grants to states for programs designed to provide substance abuse treatment for parenting mothers while keeping them with their children are provided under the new law. Among other provisions, P.L. 109-177 sets limits on imports of methamphetamine precursor chemicals and requires the Departments of Justice and State to work with Mexico to disrupt the smuggling of illicit methamphetamine across the U.S.-Mexico border.

In addition to the enactment of the CMEA, two new laws were enacted and several bills were introduced in the 109th Congress to address a number of methamphetamine-related issues that are beyond the scope of this chapter. For example, P.L. 109-288 (H.R. 3525), enacted on September 28, 2006, authorizes the Secretary of Health and Human Services (DHHS) to make competitive grants to regional partnerships to provide programs and services designed to increase the wellbeing, permanency of outcomes, and enhance the safety of children who are in foster care as a result of a parent's or caretaker's methamphetamine or other substance abuse.[81] P.L. 109-347 (H.R. 4954), enacted on October 13, 2006, requires the Customs and Border Patrol (CBP) agency to track and report the seizure of methamphetamine and methamphetamine precursor chemicals as part of the agency's annual performance plan with respect to the interdiction of illegal drugs entering the United States.

For Congress, oversight of the recently enacted regulations of the CMEA could be a major concern in the overall effort to control illicit methamphetamine use. The regulation of retail sales of OTC cold and sinus medications containing precursor chemicals could be a strategy that Congress may want to monitor to determine whether federal regulations are effectively limiting the diversion of these chemicals for the illicit manufacture of methamphetamine. In exercising its oversight role, Congress may also want to explore how the enhanced federal criminal penalties are being applied to defendants convicted and sentenced under the new law. Similarly, Congress may be interested in overseeing and evaluating the funding and implementation of the new grant program enacted in P.L. 109-177 for children and parenting mothers undergoing substance abuse treatment for methamphetamine addiction. In addition, Congress may be interested in monitoring the Departments of Justice and State's efforts to reduce the smuggling of methamphetamine or its precursor chemicals across the United States - Mexico border. CBP's efforts to track and report seizures of the drug and its precursors, as provided under P.L. 109-347, may also be of critical interest to Congress as it monitors efforts to control the illicit supply of methamphetamine. Grants for regional partnerships to help children in foster care because their parent or caretaker's substance abuse (P.L. 109-288) could also inform Congress on the effectiveness of this type of discretionary grant program and shape future legislative responses.

Reports that cheap, high purity methamphetamine smuggled into the United States from Mexico quickly supplanted much of the drug formerly manufactured in small amateur laboratories indicate that methamphetamine continues to be a drug of concern. As such, monitoring CBP's efforts to track and report methamphetamine seizures at the U.S. - Mexico border may also be an oversight issue of concern to Congress. Congress may also want to monitor DEA and CBP efforts to coordinate and share information on interdiction of methamphetamine and its precursor chemicals with the Mexican government's anti-drug forces. Evidence that the demand for methamphetamine in the United States continues to make smuggling a lucrative undertaking suggests that the drug's use will continue despite continued law enforcement and interdiction efforts. Congress may want to consider other approaches that encompass demand reduction (treatment and prevention measures) to reduce the illicit use of methamphetamine. Finally, to monitor and evaluate the effectiveness of federal drug regulations, Congress may want to consider a significant improvement and expansion of drug-use surveys and drug-related administrative data sets, along with drug interdiction data collection.

Summary and Conclusion

The illicit use of methamphetamine is seen as a serious problem in the United States. The severity of the problem varies in communities across the country and in some states methamphetamine has been a serious problem for decades. There is evidence that methamphetamine use has been moving eastward into new regions of the country, into both rural and urban communities, often with devastating results. Methamphetamine is not a new 'drug of abuse' but its low price, long-lasting effects, high purity, ease of manufacture, and ready supply from Mexican drug trafficking organizations raise concerns that methamphetamine use may continue to be difficult to control.

Legislation considered and recently enacted by Congress relies on interdiction and law enforcement efforts as the primary means of controlling the availability of methamphetamine. Past experience suggests that such approaches can succeed, and there is reason to believe that the most recently enacted law (P.L. 109-177) can significantly reduce the availability of illicit methamphetamine. In the past, when precursor chemicals became difficult to obtain, methamphetamine prices rose, the drug's purity declined, and fewer addicts were able to maintain their methamphetamine habit. As a result, some methamphetamine addicts entered treatment, substituted other drugs to ease withdrawal, or just quit.

The anti-methamphetamine provisions of P.L. 109-177 placed restrictions on the availability of retail OTC cold and sinus medicines to eliminate access to methamphetamine precursor chemicals for amateur labs, reducing the attendant dangers of clandestine labs. States that passed such restrictions on OTC precursors experienced significant declines in the number of clandestine laboratory seizures. Numerous reports from state and local law enforcement indicate that the Mexican drug trafficking organizations that already supply most of the drug that is used in the United States have been able to quickly step in and supply methamphetamine markets that formerly relied on amateur produced methamphetamine, providing a purer, more addictive product. As a result, the restrictions on OTC medications may not have as great an impact on the overall methamphetamine problem. The new law, however, may help eliminate more informal clandestine laboratories by replacing the state patchwork of laws with a federal floor restricting retail sales of methamphetamine precursors. Simultaneously, communities will be spared the attendant dangers of fires and explosions from amateur methamphetamine labs, making it less likely that children would be exposed to toxic fumes and other dangers from methamphetamine manufacture.

The methamphetamine market has been profoundly affected by past attempts to regulate precursor chemicals, albeit temporarily (see Appendix B). However, new laws are immediately scrutinized by drug traffickers for any weaknesses or loopholes that can be exploited. As described in Appendices A and B, the history of methamphetamine regulation points to the temporary impact of federal interventions in the face of an ever-evolving drug market fed by international drug organizations.

When methamphetamine precursors were unregulated in Canada, DTOs exploited that source, smuggling methamphetamine or precursors into the United States until the Canadian government began regulating pseudoephedrine and other precursor chemicals in 2003. Drug traffickers then shifted methamphetamine production to Mexico, readily supplied with the necessary methamphetamine precursor chemicals by other international chemical companies willing and able to provide ton-quantities. Recent press accounts indicate that the Mexican government has announced that it has begun taking steps to limit imports of methamphetamine precursor chemicals to correspond to legitimate domestic demands. Such a move by Mexico could begin to reduce access to methamphetamine precursors by drug trafficking organizations.[82] The effectiveness and durability of these Mexican policies are difficult to gauge, and it is particularly important to remember that methamphetamine precursors are manufactured outside of Mexico, and could be made into methamphetamine and smuggled into the U.S. via other routes. A singular focus on Mexico as the source country of illegal methamphetamine could be shortsighted.

Drug traffickers and drug markets are highly adaptable, responding quickly to changing laws, by stockpiling chemicals or adopting new production methods, or switching chemical suppliers in order to continue their illicit, highly profitable, enterprises. Such a flexible and dynamic market requires that federal drug policy be equally adaptive and as well informed as possible. Better data on all aspects of drug use and drug markets could help with the formulation of more responsive and successful federal policies. Current drug use surveys and datasets could be expanded and funded at higher levels to improve the quality and reliability of the information available to Congress and policymakers.

Supply-side interventions alone will not eliminate the illicit methamphetamine drug problem. Efforts to prevent the use of methamphetamine offer an opportunity to target prevention efforts in areas where methamphetamine use has not already taken hold, especially in the Mid-Atlantic and Northeast regions of the country. Illicit drug use generally is cyclical in nature. Just as patterns of illicit drug use vary over time, there are critical points during a drug epidemic when prevention and treatment interventions can be most effective.[83] Drug research indicates that certain interventions work better at different points in a drug "epidemic," or cycle. While it is difficult to know the optimum time in which to intensify a drug control intervention,[84] once methamphetamine is readily available in an area it is much more difficult to prevent its illicit use. Public education and awareness initiatives could be effective methods for preventing the spread of methamphetamine use. In addition, efforts could be increased to treat addiction using the latest research findings to provide effective therapies and social services to support the recovery process.[85] Although research indicates that methamphetamine addiction may require longer treatment periods and methods, its treatment can be just as successful as that of other drugs. Limited treatment funds at all levels of government suggest that treatment interventions for methamphetamine addiction should be based on what research indicates is effective. Both prevention and treatment strategies could result in fewer methamphetamine users entering the criminal justice system and taxing law enforcement resources and penal institutions.

Appendix A. Federal Legislative History of Methamphetamine Controls

Federal policy on illicit methamphetamine has evolved in a complex historical environment of the legal and illegal use of stimulants. Thus, the complicated relationship between the legitimate production and uses of methamphetamine precursor chemicals and the illicit abuse of methamphetamine continues today. This appendix briefly summarizes the major federal anti-drug laws that attempt to control the availability of and demand for illicit methamphetamine. It also provides the current federal penalties for possession of methamphetamine.

Drug Abuse Control Amendments of 1965

The *Drug Abuse Control Amendments of 1965* (DACA, P.L. 89-74) included the first federal effort to establish special controls on stimulant drugs, namely amphetamine, by bringing the drug or any of its optical isomers under federal regulation. The law required that any drug containing any amount of amphetamine be more tightly regulated by requiring that it could only be legally obtained by physician's prescription. This law marked the first time that manufacturers, suppliers, distributors, and others involved in producing stimulant drugs were subject to registration and regulation under the Federal Food, Drug and Cosmetic Act.

Controlled Substances Act of 1970

Methamphetamine first became a Schedule II[86] drug under the *Controlled Substances Act of 1970* (CSA, P.L. 91-51 3).[87] Since its enactment, the scope of the CSA has been expanded to include regulation of chemicals used in the illicit production of methamphetamine and other illicit drugs.[88] Initially, only injectable methamphetamine was classified as a Schedule II drug; all other amphetamines were classified as Schedule III drugs. In 1971, all amphetamines, including all forms of methamphetamine, were reclassified under Schedule II.

Chemical Diversion and Trafficking Act of 1988

The *Chemical Diversion and Trafficking Act of 1988* (CDTA, P.L. 100-690) regulated bulk ephedrine and pseudoephedrine, the precursor chemicals from which methamphetamine is synthesized. This was the first major federal attempt at controlling methamphetamine precursor chemicals. The law required record keeping, reporting requirements, and import/export notification requirements for bulk, pure (single entity) ephedrine and pseudoephedrine products. However, the requirements for bulk methamphetamine precursor chemicals in P.L. 100-690, did not apply to OTC tablets or capsules containing ephedrine and pseudoephedrine.

Domestic Chemical Diversion Control Act of 1993

The *Domestic Chemical Diversion Control Act of 1993* (DCDCA, P.L. 103-200) removed the record-keeping and reporting exemption for pure (single entity) ephedrine products. The new law was enacted in 1993, went into effect in April 1994, but federal regulations implementing the law were not issued until August 1995. The law required distributors, importers, and exporters of List I chemicals[89] to register with DEA, and gave DEA the power to revoke a company's registration without proof of criminal intent.

Comprehensive Methamphetamine Control Act of 1996

The *Comprehensive Methamphetamine Control Act of 1996* (MCA, P.L. 104-237), broadened federal regulation of listed chemicals to include those found in OTC cold and sinus medicines. Under the MCA, the methamphetamine precursor chemicals containing ephedrine, pseudoephedrine, or phenylpropanolamine were added to Schedule II of the CSA, broadening existing restrictions on these precursor chemicals used to produce illicit methamphetamine. Other provisions of the MCA also increased penalties for the trafficking and manufacturing of methamphetamine and methamphetamine-related listed chemicals.[90]

Methamphetamine Trafficking Penalty Enhancement Act of 1998

The *Methamphetamine Trafficking Penalty Enhancement Act of 1998* (P.L. 105-277) lowered the quantity thresholds of methamphetamine necessary to trigger mandatory minimum drug trafficking penalties. The law cut in half the quantities of methamphetamine mixture and pure methamphetamine substance necessary to trigger the five- and ten-year mandatory minimum prison sentences for individuals convicted of certain methamphetamine offenses.[91]

Methamphetamine Anti-Proliferation Act of 2000.

The *Methamphetamine Anti-Proliferation Act of 2000* (MAPA, P.L. 106-3 96) included provisions to address the problem of diversion of OTC drug products containing methamphetamine precursor chemicals from retail and mail order sources to the illicit production of methamphetamine. MAPA established thresholds for single purchases of OTC medicines containing ephedrine, pseudoephedrine and phenylpropanolamine (PPA) at 9 grams per day. P.L. 106-396 added the requirement that the products be packaged in containers of not more than 3 grams of precursor base chemical. Products packaged in "blister packaging" were provided a 'safe harbor' exemption from the threshold limits set by MAPA. The act also strengthened sentencing guidelines and provided training for federal and state law enforcement officers on methamphetamine investigations and the handling of the chemicals used in clandestine methamphetamine labs. It also put in place controls on the distribution of the chemical ingredients used in methamphetamine production and expanded substance abuse prevention efforts.

Combating Methamphetamine Epidemic Act of 2005

The *USA PATRIOT Improvement and Reauthorization Act* (P.L. 109-177), signed into law on March 9, 2006, included provisions to regulate the domestic and international commerce in methamphetamine precursor chemicals and increased penalties for methamphetamine offenses.[92] In addition, the new law contained provisions to expand environmental regulations related to toxic chemical dumping by clandestine methamphetamine labs, and provide grant programs for drug-endangered children and adults afflicted by methamphetamine abuse and addiction.

Specifically, P.L. 109-177 establishes a new set of controls for the methamphetamine precursor chemicals, ephedrine, pseudoephedrine, and phenylpropanolamine,[93] that are designed to control illicit diversion. The following limits apply to retail sales of OTC products containing methamphetamine precursor chemicals:

- drugstores, convenience stores, grocery stores, news stands, mobile retailers (i.e., lunch wagons, street vendors) and other retailer limits on sales of these OTC products to 3.6 grams of the precursor base per customer per day (previously limited to 9 grams per transaction) (21 U.S.C. 830(d), 802(46), 802(47);
- limits mobile retail sales to 7.5 grams of precursor base per customer per month (21 U.S.C 830(e)(1)(A);
- requires that products containing methamphetamine precursor chemicals be kept "behind the counter" and, for mobile retailers, that the products be secured under lock and key (21 U.S.C. 830(e)(1)(A));
- with the exception of sales of less than 60 milligrams (two 30 mg doses) or less, retailers are required to maintain a logbook that must be kept for at least two years, recording the time and date of sale, the name and quantity of the product sold, and the name and address of each purchaser (21 U.S.C. 830(e)(1)(A));

purchasers are required to present a government-issued photo identification, sign the logbook for the sale providing their name, address, and the date and time of the sale (21 U.S.C. 830(e)(1)(A));

requires that retailer's logbooks include a warning that false statements will be punishable under 18 U.S.C. 1001 with a term of imprisonment of up to five years and/or a fine of not more than $250,000 for an individual offender, or $500,000 in cases involving an organization (21 U.S.C. 830(e)(1)(A), 830(e)(1)(D));

requires the Attorney General to promulgate regulations to protect the privacy of the logbook entries, except for access by federal, state, and local law enforcement;

requires that retailers train their employees on the methamphetamine precursor products statutory and regulatory provisions of the law (21 U.S.C. 830(e)(1)(A), (B));

provides retailers civil immunity for disclosure of logbook information to law enforcement, unless the disclosure constitutes gross negligence or intentional, wanton, or willful misconduct (21 U.S.C. 830(e)(1)(E)); and

requires retailers to take measures against possible employee theft or diversion of OTC products containing methamphetamine precursor chemicals, and preempts any state law that prohibits employers from asking prospective employees about their past methamphetamine precursor or controlled substance convictions (21 U.S.C. 830(e)(1)(G)).

These provisions went into effect on September 30, 2006, with the exception of the per day, per customer, 3.6 gram limit on retail sales of products containing methamphetamine precursor chemicals which went into effect 30 days after enactment. Mail order retailers of such products are required to confirm the identities of their customers, in addition to limiting sales of these products to 7.5 grams per customer, per month. The Attorney General is permitted to waive the 3.6 gram limit on retail sales and the 7.5 gram monthly limit on mail order or mobile retail sales if the AG determines that an OTC product containing methamphetamine precursor chemicals cannot be used in the manufacture of illicit methamphetamine.

Current Federal Penalties for Methamphetamine Possession

Concern about the illicit production and abuse of methamphetamine were behind recent efforts in the 109th Congress to enact the *Combating Methamphetamine Epidemic Act of 2005*, which was enacted in P.L. 109-177 on March 9, 2006. The new law, among other things, amends penalties for possession and distribution of methamphetamine under the Controlled Substances Act (CSA).

The CSA, as recently amended, provides penalties for methamphetamine offenses according to the amount of the drug in the offender's possession upon arrest.

For a first offense, if the individual possesses 5-49 grams of pure methamphetamine or 50-499 grams of a mixture containing methamphetamine, the penalty would be not less than five years and not more than 40 years imprisonment; if death or serious injury occurred, from 20 years or up to life imprisonment. Fines could amount to $2 million if the case involved an individual offender, and up to $5 million if the case involved the conviction of more than one offender.

For a second offense, the penalty for possessing 5-49 grams would be from 10 years to life imprisonment; if death or serious injury occurred, life imprisonment. Fines could amount to $4 million for an individual offender or up to $10 million if the case involved multiple offenders.

For 50 grams or more of pure methamphetamine, or 500 grams or more of a mixture containing methamphetamine, for a first offense the penalty would be from 10 years to life imprisonment; if death or serious injury occurred, from 20 years to life imprisonment. Fines could amount to $4 million if the case involved an individual offender, $10 million if multiple offenders were convicted.

For a second offense, the penalty would be from 20 years to life imprisonment; if death or serious injury occurred, life imprisonment. Fines could amount to $8 million if the case involved an individual offender, $20 million if multiple offenders were convicted.

Appendix B. What Works? Case Studies of the Effectiveness of Federal Laws to Control Methamphetamine

Experts in the area of drug policy have long debated how effectively the federal war on drugs has controlled drug abuse in the U.S. The orientation of U.S. anti-drug policies relies heavily on supply-side controls whose efficacy is frequently questioned as the primary anti-drug strategy.[94] Some federal anti-drug policies have had unintended consequences. For example, researchers of drug policy often note that abuse of amphetamines led to federal law that banned the substance, which unintentionally fostered demand for an alternative stimulant, which in turn led to the development of increased use of methamphetamine. By the late 1 960s, the increased illicit use of methamphetamine led to the enactment of federal measures to restrict the availability of phenylpropanolamine (PPA), a precursor chemical widely used at the time to manufacture one form of illicit methamphetamine (crank). Federal controls restricting the availability of PPA significantly disrupted the illicit production and distribution of *crank* (*levo-dextro*-methamphetamine) by biker gangs. This drove underground chemists, eager to meet the demand for an alternative stimulant in the illicit drug market, to seek a substitute for PPA. Thus, PPA's chemical cousins, ephedrine and pseudoephedrine, came to be the key ingredients of a new and improved form of the stimulant — the most potent and addictive form of methamphetamine (*dextro*-methamphetamine), and a form of the drug that could be easily synthesized. Inadvertently, tighter regulation of PPA was the catalyst behind the development of the form of illicit methamphetamine abused and manufactured today.

The following section considers three case studies that attempt to discern whether or not the enactment of certain federal laws had an effect on the supply of methamphetamine.

An analysis by Carlos Dobkin and Nancy Nicosia[95] looks at the impact of two large interventions that occurred in May 1995. The first was the implementation of the *Domestic Chemical Diversion Control Act of 1993* (DCDCA (P.L. 103-200)), and the second was a large DEA drug bust. Taken together the two interventions were of unprecedented scale. The DEA drug bust shut down two significant methamphetamine precursor suppliers whose production potential was 24 metric tons of methamphetamine in 1994: (1) Clifton

Pharmaceuticals - producing 25 metric tons of methamphetamine precursors, and (2) Xpressive Looks International - 500 cases and a distribution network that was responsible for supplying 830 million tablets of methamphetamine.

For the federal government's strategy of disrupting the supply of methamphetamine and methamphetamine precursor chemicals, these 2 cases were impressive successes. Although the federal policy resulted in a dramatic reduction in the availability of methamphetamine, the effects were temporary. Dobkin and Nicosia's analysis indicates that the impact of the two DEA interventions was made possible by the enactment and implementation of methamphetamine precursor controls in the DCDCA. Their analysis further shows that DEA's actions eliminated a huge share of the available methamphetamine precursor supply in California, an amount equal to 70% of the ONDCP's estimated national methamphetamine consumption of 34.1 metric tons in 1994. The passage of the DCDCA in 1993, which went into effect in April 1994, was followed by final regulations implementing the new law in August 1995. The DCDCA eliminated the exemption of single entity (pure) ephedrine products, so products containing ephedrine were subject to record keeping and import/export notification requirements like those required of transactions of bulk ephedrine and pseudoephedrine.[96] The DCDCA also permitted DEA to deny or revoke a company's registration without proof of criminal intent. The implementation of these two new provisions of the law was essential to disrupting the market for methamphetamine precursor chemicals at that point in time.

According to Dobkin and Nicosia, these two companies were supplying more than 50% of the precursors used nationally to produce methamphetamine. DEA's actions eliminated two very large ephedrine and pseudoephedrine suppliers operating in California at that time.[97] As a result, DEA's efforts caused a significant reduction in the national precursor supply which triggered an increase in price, from $30 to $100 per gram, and caused purity of methamphetamine to drop from 90% to less than 20% over the five month period that followed. Dobkin and Nicosia's work showed that the provisions of the DCDCA enabled DEA to disrupt the supply of methamphetamine precursor chemicals, and as a result the supply, purity, and price of methamphetamine were profoundly affected. However, while the immediate effect was profound, it was also temporary, and the analysis found that prices recovered within four months, while purity of methamphetamine took much longer to return to previous levels, almost 20 months to climb back to 85%.[98]

Dobkin and Nicosia also analyzed data from the ADAM/DUF survey[99] in relation to the DEA drug busts in May 1995 as an alternative measure of the effectiveness of the DCDCA regulations. Their analysis focused on exploring the relationship between methamphetamine use and crime by looking at the ADAM/DUF data for the period 1993-1996. They found that methamphetamine use among arrestees in three California cities (San Diego, Los Angeles, and San Jose) declined by 55%. Felony drug arrests, unlike some other crime trends including reported property crime and violent crime, declined by 50% after the DEA intervention, and misdemeanor drug arrests decreased by 25%.

The success of disrupting chemical inputs needed for manufacturing methamphetamine, their analysis concluded, was evident in the drug-use indicators of hospital admissions, drug treatment admissions, arrestee drug use, and drug arrests. These indicators of methamphetamine prevalence also tracked closely with changes in the purity of methamphetamine following the DEA intervention event, but do not track as well with changes in the price of methamphetamine after the event. Their analysis also concluded that even a large-scale disruption only reduced adverse health effects and drug crime temporarily.

In a similar analysis, Cunningham and Liu looked at the effects on hospital admissions of three federal policies that regulated ephedrine and pseudoephedrine in 1989, 1995, and 1997.[100] The federal interventions included (1) the 1989 implementation of the *Chemical Diversion and Trafficking Act of 1988*, which regulated bulk quantities of ephedrine and pseudoephedrine; (2) the 1995 implementation of the *Domestic Chemical Diversion Control Act of 1993*, which regulated the distribution of products that contained ephedrine as the only active medicinal ingredient; and (3) the 1997 implementation of the *Comprehensive Methamphetamine Control Act of 1996*, which regulated products that included pseudoephedrine, with or without other active ingredients, and the distribution of products that included ephedrine in combination with other active medicinal ingredients. Each of the federal interventions built on the previous regulation, often closing loopholes that were newly exploited by drug trafficking organizations (DTOs). These federal interventions focused on responding to large-scale methamphetamine producers, until passage of the *Comprehensive Methamphetamine Control Act* of 1996, which focused on the distribution of sinus and cold medicines.[101]

Cunningham and Liu's analysis looked at methamphetamine related hospital admissions and how they were affected by all three precursor regulations in California. They also looked at the impact of three of these regulations in the late 1990s in Arizona and Nevada, both of which border California. Using an autoregressive-integrated moving average time-series analysis they found that after seven years of steady increases in methamphetamine related admissions in California, the number of methamphetamine admissions began to decline for about two years following the intervention in 1989 (P.L. 100-690).[102] What followed was a resurgence in methamphetamine admissions that continued until August 1995, a month after the regulation of single ingredient ephedrine took effect.

A report from the Office of National Drug Control Policy (ONDCP) on the price and purity of illicit drugs adds support to the findings of Dobkin and Nicosia, and Cunningham and Liu.[103] Using the DEA's System to Retrieve Information from Drug Evidence (STRIDE)[104] data base, the study provided estimates of the price and purity of methamphetamine through the second quarter of 2003.[105] Acknowledging illicit drug pricing variations across cities, the ONDCP report showed that methamphetamine prices from 1981 to 2003 rose overall, but that there were three very large price spikes in the years following three precursor control regulations in 1989, 1995, and 1997. In addition, the report found that purity trends for methamphetamine did not move the way that might be expected for other drugs. Unlike other illicit drugs, the analysis found that methamphetamine prices and purity were very volatile and did not exhibit the same trends. This analysis also found that the spikes in price and purity of methamphetamine were related to the regulation of precursor chemicals introduced in 1989, 1995, and 1997.[106]

The analyses described above indicate that legislative changes aimed at regulating the methamphetamine precursor chemicals had a significant effect on the supply, price and purity of illicit methamphetamine in the short term. The findings of Dobkins and Nicosia, and Cunningham and Liu also found that the changes brought on by new, more restrictive federal law only worked temporarily, as illicit suppliers found alternative ways to circumvent the regulations or develop alternative suppliers of precursor chemicals. Thus, what these analyses show is that preventive legal strategies developed by Congress over the past 17 years have steadily strengthened restrictions on the distribution of pseudoephedrine/ephedrine-containing products. However, these analyses also point out that these changes in federal law only brought about temporary changes. Federal drug policy and regulation work effectively and may benefit by being adaptive and responsive to the adaptive changes that suppliers of illicit methamphetamine, and other illicit drugs, willingly undergo to supply the demand for illicit drugs in the United States.

End Notes

[1] For more information on the impact of methamphetamine abuse and child welfare issues see, CRS Congressional Distribution Memorandum, *Child Welfare and Methamphetamine Abuse: Issues and Resources*, by Meredith Peterson, June 7, 2006. For information on the methamphetamine provisions of P.L. 109-288, see CRS Report RL33354, *The Promoting of Safe and Stable Families Program: Reauthorization in the 109th Congress*, by Emilie Stoltzfus.

[2] For information on two case studies analyzing the impact of past federal laws to control methamphetamine, see **Appendix B**.

[3] Charles W. Meredith, MD, Craig Jaffe, MD, Kathleen Ang-Lee, MD, and Andrew J. Saxon, MD, *Implications of Chronic Methamphetamine Use: A Literature Review*, Harvard Review of Psychiatry, May/Jun. 2005, p. 142.

[4] U.S. Department of Justice, Drug Enforcement Agency, National Drug Intelligence Center, *Drugs of Abuse*, 2005 Edition, p. 34.

[5] Douglas M. Anglin, Cynthia Burke, Brian Perrochet, Ewa Stamper, Samia Dawud-Noursi, "History of the Methamphetamine Problem," *Journal of Psychoactive Drugs*, vol. 32, no. 2 (Apr.-June 2000), p. 137.

[6] Advisory Council on the Misuse of Drugs, *Methylamphetamine Review*, 2005.

[7] Douglas M. Anglin, et. al., *History of Methamphetamine Problem*, p. 137; Michael S. Vaughn, Frank F.Y. Huang and Christine Rose Ramirez, "Drug Abuse and Anti-Drug Policy in Japan," *British Journal of Criminology*, vol. 35, no. 4 (Autumn 1995), pp. 497-498.

[8] Errol Yudko, Harold V. Hall, and Sandra B. McPherson, *Methamphetamine Use: Clinical and Forensic Aspects*, 2003, p. 6.

[9] The illicit manufacture of methamphetamine by biker gangs led to scheduling of the drug under the Controlled Substances Act of 1970, as a Schedule II drug (discussed below).

[10] The use of the term "crank" in this chapter refers to the weaker form of illicit methamphetamine, also known as methamphetamine sulfate, that was largely manufactured and distributed by West Coast motorcycle gangs.

[11] Many added "crank" to their coffee, often referred to as "biker's coffee."

[12] Errol Yudko, et. al., *Methamphetamine Use: Clinical and Forensic Aspects*, p. 6.

[13] Generally, the two most commonly used methods for reducing ephedrine, pseudoephedrine, or phenylpropanolamine (PPA) in order to manufacture illicit methamphetamine are (1) reduction of the chemical precursors by boiling them with hydroiodic acid and red phosphorus, or (2) reduction using lithium (from batteries) and ammonia.

[14] U.S. Department of Health and Human Services, National Toxicology Program, Center For the Evaluation of Risks to Human Reproduction, *NTP-CERHR Expert Panel Report on the Reproductive and Developmental Toxicity of Amphetamine and Methamphetamine*, "Chapter 1.0 Chemistry, Use and Human Exposure," Mar. 2005, p. 11.

[15] Jane Carlisle Maxwell, "Emerging Research on Methamphetamine," *Current Opinion in Psychiatry*, vol. 18, p. 235.

[16] Methamphetamine base has also been found in Australia. See, National Drug and Alcohol Research Centre, *Methamphetamine: Forms and Use Patterns*, University of New South Wales, 2006, available at [http://ndarc.med.unsw.edu.au/NDARCWeb.nsf/resourcesNDLERF_Methamphetamine/$file/NDLERF+ICE+FORMS+AND+USE.pdf], accessed on Jan. 10, 2007.

[17] U.S. Department of Justice, National Drug Intelligence Center, *National Methamphetamine Threat Assessment 2007*, Nov. 2006, p. 17.

[18] Center for Substance Abuse Research (CESAR), University of Maryland, College Park, October 3, 2005, Vol. 14, Issue 40, available at [http://www.cesar.umd.edu], accessed on Jan. 10, 2007.

[19] U.S. Department of Health and Human Services, Substance Abuse and Mental Health Services Administration, Office of Applied Studies, NSDUH, 2005, p. 229.

[20] Ibid.

[21] According to the National Alliance For Model State Drug Laws, the following states restrict sales of products containing ephedrine and pseudoephedrine on the basis of quantity purchased only: Arizona, California, North

Dakota, Oklahoma, Oregon, Utah, and Washington. The following states restrict sales on the basis of quantity purchased, packaging, and display/offer: Alabama, Arkansas, Illinois, Iowa, and Missouri. Nevada restricts sales of products containing ephedrine and/or pseudoephedrine on the basis of packaging.

[22] These amateur labs are also commonly referred to as "mom-and-pop" labs, "Beavis and Butthead" labs, "kitchen" labs, or "box" labs. Because each of these labs produces five to seven pounds of toxic hazardous waste for each pound of methamphetamine produced, they are also often referred to as "small toxic labs."

[23] As many as 15% of all methamphetamine labs are discovered as a result of explosions or fire. See, U.S. D.O.J., Office of Justice Programs, Office of Victims of Crime, "Children at Clandestine Meth Labs: Helping Meth's Youngest Victims," by Karen Swetlow, *OVC Bulletin*, June 2003, p. 4.

[24] For a discussion of legislation related to methamphetamine laboratory remediation, see CRS Report RL32959, *Methamphetamine Lab Clean-Up and Remediation Issues*, by Michael Simpson.

[25] The amounts of precursor chemical used by super laboratories are so large that they are often reported in tons rather than in pounds.

[26] Super laboratories are typically sites capable of producing over 10 pounds of methamphetamine during a production cycle.

[27] U.S. Department of Health and Human Services (DHHS), National Institutes of Health (NIH), National Institute on Drug Abuse (NIDA), "Methamphetamine Abuse and Addiction," *Research Report Series*, NIH Publication No. 06-42 10, Revised September 2006, p. 4.

[28] Ibid.

[29] Dan Hannan, *Occupational Hazards: Meth Labs Understanding Exposure Hazards and Associated Problems*, June 2005, p. 24.

[30] Dana Hunt, Sarah Kuck, Linda Truitt, "Methamphetamine Use: Lessons Learned," Abt Associates, Inc., for U.S. DHHS, NIJ, Feb. 2006, p. 34.

[31] U.S. DOJ, NDIC, Chemical Precursor Committee, "Children at Risk," *Information Bulletin*, July 2002, p. 2.; Scott, Michael S., Clandestine Drug Labs: Problem-Oriented Guides for Police Services, U. S. DOJ, Office of Community Oriented Policing Services (COPS), Apr. 2002, no. 16, page 3.

[32] U.S. DOJ, NDIC, "Methamphetamine Identification and Hazzards," p. 2, available at [http://www.usdoj.gov/ndic/pubs7/7341/7341p.pdf], accessed on: Jan. 10, 2007.

[33] DEA's National Clandestine Laboratory Seizure (NCLS) database includes the reported total number of laboratory seizures of (1) chemicals and glassware used for manufacturing methamphetamine, (2) dumpsites of toxic waste products from the methamphetamine production process, (3) and laboratories where methamphetamine was actively being produced. The data includes information reported to DEA from state and local law enforcement, as well as lab seizures by DEA. The El Paso Intelligence Center (EPIC), created by the DEA in 1974, administers the database and relies on state and local law enforcement agencies to voluntarily report their statistics for inclusion in its NCLS database. However, only three states — California, Missouri, and Oklahoma — have mandatory reporting requirements of their statistics. Chemical dump sites or equipment used in the manufacture of methamphetamine found in isolation are sometimes referred to as a "lab incident." For more information on EPIC and the NCLS database, see [http://www.usdoj .gov/oig/reports/COPS/a06 1 6/exec.htm], accessed on Jan. 10, 2007.

[34] U.S. DOJ, DEA, available at [http://www.dea.gov/concern/map_lab_seizures.html], accessed on Jan. 10, 2007.

[35] U.S. Department of Justice, National Drug Intelligence Center, *National Drug Threat Assessment 2007*, Product No. 2006-Q03 17-003, October 2006, p. i.

[36] Office of National Drug Control Policy, "Methamphetamine - Facts and Figures," at [http://www.whitehousedrugpolicy.gov/drugfact/methamphetamine/index.html], accessed on Jan. 10, 2007.

[37] Ibid.

[38] U.S . DOJ, OJP, NIJ, *Meth Matters: Report on Methamphetamine Users in Five Western Cities*, by Susan Pennell, Joe Ellett, Cynthia Rienick, and Jackie Grimes, April 1999, p. 4.;

[39] Jack Shafer, "Meth Madness at *Newsweek*," *Slate Magazine*, Aug. 3, 2005, available at [http://www.slate.com/id/2123838], accessed on Jan. 10, 2007.

[40] Extrapolating prevalence estimates from a sample survey can be complicated by many factors, including sample size (the sample is not large enough to provide reliable year-by- year annual state estimates of prevalence), differences in the sample population (persons over age 12 vs. adults age 18 and over) and survey administration (i.e., in school vs. in home, over-the-phone interviews vs. in-person interviews), and comparisons among data sources need to be made with caution. Although it is not always appropriate to compare prevalence estimates across different surveys for a single year, it is possible to compare trends across years in a single survey. Trend lines from different surveys can indicate increases or decreases in prevalence over time, and as such are useful for substance abuse policy development and service provision. A potential source of bias in any survey is the understatement or overstatement of actual behaviors and there is always the possibility that individuals might underreport behavior that they perceive as sensitive or unacceptable, while some respondents might exaggerate or boast about certain behaviors. The validity of self-reported data depends on the honesty, memory, and understanding of the respondents.

[41] The NSDUH survey is a household survey that samples the civilian noninstitutionalized population age 12 and older about drug use. Individuals are asked about illicit drug, tobacco, and alcohol use in their lifetime, the last year, the last month, and in the last month as a dependent user. The 2005 sample included 68,308 persons. More detailed information is available at [http://webapp.icpsr.umich.edu/cocoon accessed on Jan. 10, 2007.

[42] U.S. Department of Justice, National Institute of Justice, *Methamphetamine Use: Lessons Learned*, by Dana Hunt, Sarah Kuck, and Linda Truitt, February 2006, p. iii.

[43] MTF is an annual survey of students in the 8th, 10th, and 12th grades about their history of illicit substance use. In 2005, 49,300 students in 402 public and private schools were included in the sample.

[44] Youth Risk Behavior Surveillance System (YRBSS) is conducted by the Center for Disease Control and Prevention (CDC) and measures the prevalence of six priority health risk behavior categories, including drug use. YRBSS is a national school-based survey that in 2005 included a sample of 13,953 students in grades 9 through 12.

[45] TEDS is an administrative data set collected by SAMHSA that is comprised of almost 2 million admissions reported by more than 10,000 facilities providing substance abuse treatment.

[46] Since some states do not distinguish between methamphetamine and amphetamine admissions for substance abuse treatment, reporting a single total, SAMHSA estimates that methamphetamine admissions account for 80% of all amphetamine admissions.

[47] Hunt, Dana, Sarah Kuck, Linda Truitt, *Methamphetamine Use: Lessons Learned*, prepared for the Department of Justice on a grant from the Office of Justice Programs, February 2006, p. 11.

[48] DAWN collects information on drug-related episodes from over 1,000 hospital emergency departments (EDs) in 21 cities across the country. Although DAWN does not monitor drug use directly, it does measure the consequences of drug use that results in ED visits.

[49] An emergency department *mention* refers to patient visits in which the patient is treated for a drug abuse-related medical problem.

[50] Hunt, Dana, Sarah Kuck, Linda Truitt, *Methamphetamine Use: Lessons Learned*, on grant from U.S. DOJ, OJP, Feb. 2006, p. iii.

[51] Sally Satel, "Much Ado About Meth?,"American Enterprise Institute for Public Policy Research, Nov. 4, 2005, at [http://www.aei.org/inlcude/pub_print.asp?pubID=234 14], accessed on: Jan. 10, 2007, accessed on Nov. 6, 2005.

[52] U.S. DHHS, Office of Applied Statistics, SAMHSA, DAWN, "Amphetamine and Methamphetamine Emergency Department Visits, 1995-2002," *The DAWN Report*, July 2002, [http : //dawninfo . samhsa. gov/old_dawn/ pubs_94_02/shortreports/files/ DAWN _tdr _amphetamine.pdf], accessed on January 24, 2007.

[53] Ibid.

[54] Ibid.

[55] CEWG is a network of researchers from major metropolitan areas around the country and internationally providing community-level surveillance on drug abuse at the National Institute on Drug Abuse (NIDA).

[56] According to CEWG, the areas where methamphetamine use remains high are: Atlanta, Denver, Honolulu, Los Angeles, Phoenix, Seattle, San Diego, and Texas.

[57] U.S. DHHS, NIH, CEWG, *Epidemiologic Trends in Drug Use*, (Advance Report), June 2006, p. 11, available at [http://www.drugabuse.gov/PDF/CEWG/AdvReport606.pdf], accessed on Jan. 17, 2007.

[58] NDIC was established in 1993 as a component of DOJ charged with monitoring strategic domestic counterdrug intelligence.

[59] U.S. DEA, National Drug Intelligence Center, *National Drug Threat Assessment, 2005.* [60] The ADAM program is a bioassay survey collecting urine samples and self-reported drug use information from booked adult and juvenile arrestees in 35 urban areas across the country.

[60] The ADAM program is a bioassay survey collecting urine samples and self-reported drug use information from booked adult and juvenile arrestees in 35 urban areas across the country.

[61] Missouri Department of Mental Health, Missouri Division of Alcohol and Drug Abuse, *Methamphetamine in Missouri 2004*, April 2004, p. 6, available at [http://mimh200.mimh.edu/mimhweb/pie/reports/meth2004.pdf], accessed on Jan. 17, 2007.

[62] Ibid.

[63] Ibid.

[64] U.S. Department of Health and Human Services, SAMHSA, Office of Applied Statistics, *Treatment Episode Data Set 1994-2004*, July 2006.

[65] Hunt, Dana, Sarah Kuck, Linda Truitt, *Methamphetamine Use: Lessons Learned*, prepared for the Department of Justice on a grant from the Office of Justice, February 2006, p. 15.

[66] For detailed maps of all methamphetamine clandestine laboratory seizure incidents, see [http://www.dea.gov/ concern/map_lab_seizures], accessed on Jan. 15, 2007.

[67] U.S. DOJ, DEA, *Maps of Methamphetamine Lab Incidents*, available at [http://www.usdoj.gov/dea/concern/map _lab_seizures.html], accessed on Jan. 15, 2007.

[68] The category of stimulants often included amphetamines, as well as the illicit use of legal pharmaceutical substances such as Ritalin, Adderall, and appetite suppressants.

[69] SAMHSA provides periodic state-level methamphetamine prevalence estimates using three-year average NSDUH data to strengthen the reliability of the available state data, available at [http://www.oas.samhsa .gov/methTabs.htm], accessed on December 20, 2006.

[70] U.S. Department of Justice, National Institute of Justice, *Methamphetamine Use: Lessons Learned*, by Dana Hunt, Sarah Kuck, and Linda Truitt, February 2006, p. 6.

[71] The Columbia Electronic Encyclopedia, Sixth Edition Copyright © 2003, Columbia University Press, available at [http://www.cc.columbia.edu/cu/cup/], accessed on Jan. 10, 2007.

[72] Throughout the federal government there are programs that provide grants, activities, and services related to the prevention, education, and treatment of methamphetamine, as well as for assisting localities with clandestine lab remediation. These programs are beyond the scope of this chapter, which focuses on DOJ programs related to the enforcement of federal drug laws.

[73] U.S. DOJ, OJP, Bureau of Justice Statistics, *Compendium of Federal Statistics, 2003*, October 5, 2005, p. 17, available at [http://www.ojp.usdoj .gov/bj s/pub/pdf/cfj s03 .pdf], accessed on Jan. 15, 2007.

[74] U.S. DOJ, DOJ Public Affairs, *Fact Sheet: The Department of Justice's Efforts to Combat Methamphetamine*, Jun. 16, 2006, at [http://www.dea.gov/pubs/pressrel/pr06 1 6006p.html], accessed on Jan. 10, 2007.

[75] Ibid.

[76] U.S. DOJ, DEA, Joseph T. Rannazzisi, Deputy Assistant Administrator, Office of Diversion Control, Congressional testimony before House Government Reform Committee, Subcommittee on Criminal Justice, Drug Policy and Human Resources, June 16, 2006, available at [http://www.usdoj .gov/dea/pubs/cngrtest/ct06 1 606p.html], accessed on Jan. 10, 2007.

[77] U.S. DOJ, DEA Public Affairs, News Release, "DEA: Meth Superlab Discovered by Mexican Authorities," available at [http://www.ojp.usdoj .gov/bj s/pub/pdf/cfj s03 .pdf], accessed on Jan. 17, 2007.

[78] U.S. DOJ, Office of Community Oriented Policing Services, *COPS Fact Sheet: Methamphetamine Initiative*, Sept.2004, available at [http://www.cops.usdoj .gov] , accessed on Jan. 10, 2007.

[79] The amounts provided in **Table 4** exclude grants under the COPS Methamphetamine Initiative.

[80] U.S. Department of Justice, Office of Justice Programs, Bureau of Justice Assistance, *Drug Courts: An Effective Strategy for Communities Facing Methamphetamine*, BJA Bulletin, May 2005, p. 2. Available at [http://www.ojp.usdoj .gov/BJA], accessed on Jan. 10, 2007.

[81] For information, see CRS Report RL3354, *The Promoting Safe and Stable Families Program: Reauthorization in the 109th Congress,* by Emilie Stoltzfus.

[82] U.S. — Mexico relations are beyond the scope of this chapter. For more information, see CRS Report RL3 2724, *Mexico — U.S. Relations: Issues for the 109th Congress*, by K. Larry Storrs.

[83] Doris A. Behrens, Jonathan P. Caulkins, Gernot Tragler, Gustav Feichtinger, "Optimal Control of Drug Epidemics: Prevent and Treat — But Not at the Same Time?" *Management Science*, Mar. 2000, vol. 46, no. 3, March 2000, p. 333.

[84] Ibid, p. 346.

[85] U.S. DHHS, NIH, NIDA, "Methamphetamine Abuse and Addiction," *Research Report Series*, NIH no. 06-42 10, Sept. 2006, p. 7.

[86] See 21 C.F.R §1308.12.

[87] Schedule II drugs are those with a recognized medical use but a high potential for abuse and a high incidence of physical or psychological dependence. These are available only by prescription, and distribution is carefully controlled and monitored by the DEA. In addition to methamphetamine and amphetamine, Schedule II drugs include, among others, cocaine; methylphenidate (Ritalin); most pure opioid agonists such as Demerol, fentanyl, opium, oxycodone, morphine, methadone; and short-acting barbiturates such as secobarbital.

[88] For more information on regulation of pseudoephedrine in OTC medications see, CRS Report RS22 177, *The Legal Regulation of Over-the-Counter Cold Medication*, by Jody Feder.

[89] In addition to regulating illegal drugs, the CSA also regulates certain chemicals that, although they may have legitimate medical purposes, can be used in the illicit production of illegal drugs. List I chemicals are defined as those that are used in the manufacture of controlled substances and are important to the manufacture of the substances. See, DEA, U.S. Chemical Control at [http://www.usdoj .gov/dea/concern/chemical], accessed on Jan. 10, 2007.

[90] In 2000, the Food and Drug Administration (FDA) issued a health advisory on the use of OTC and prescription products containing phenylpropanolamine hydrochloride because its use increased the risk of hemorrhagic stroke. While many drug manufacturers voluntarily reformulated their products to remove phenylpropanolamine, some products using the chemical remain on the market.

[91] For the Sentencing Commission's implementation of the law see, U.S. Sentencing Commission, *Methamphetamine*, Final Report, Nov. 1999, at [http://www.ussc.gov/publicat/ methreport.pdf], accessed on Jan. 10, 2007.

[92] For a legal analysis of the provisions of P.L. 109-177, see CRS Report RL33332, *USA PATRIOT Improvement and Reauthorization Act of 2005: A Legal Analysis*, by Brian T. Yeh and Charles Doyle.

[93] P.L. 109-177 defines the methamphetamine precursors as "scheduled listed chemical products" and as such can be marketed or distributed lawfully as a nonprescription drug under the federal Food, Drug and Cosmetic Act (21 U.S.C. 802(45)).

[94] Reuter, Peter, "The Limits of Drug Control," American Foreign Service Association, January 2002, at [http://www.afsa.org/fsj/jan02/reuter.cfm], accessed on: Jan. 10, 2007.

[95] Dobkin, Carlos and Nancy Nicosia, "The War on Drugs: Methamphetamine, Public Health and Crime," (forthcoming), and Carlos Dobkin, "The Impact of Methamphetamine Abuse on Health and Crime," unpublished paper, Jan. 18, 2005.

[96] Dobkin and Nicosia, p. 8.

[97] Dobkin and Nicosia, "The War on Drugs: Methamphetamine, Public Health and Crime," p. 2.

[98] Ibid., p. 21.

[99] They note that the ADAM/DUF data are a "selected sample rather than a census," acknowledging that the data cannot be extrapolated to indicate any broader trends in the population, but is only representative of the specific sample of arrestees.

[100] James K. Cunningham and Lon-Mu Liu, "Impacts of Federal Ephedrine and Pseudoephedrine Regulations on Methamphetamine-Related Hospital Admissions," *Society for the Study of Addiction to Alcohol and Other Drugs*, vol. 98, no. 9 (September 2003), pp. 1229-1237.

[101] Ibid., p. 1230.

[102] Ibid., p. 1231.

[103] ONDCP, *The Price and Purity of Illicit Drugs: 1981 Through the Second Quarter of 2003*, November 2003, p. 13.

[104] STRIDE is a forensic database containing information obtained by DEA from seizures, purchases, and other drug acquisition activities. DEA uses STRIDE for inventory control of drug acquisitions by DEA, as well as for scientific data collected regarding the quality and quantity of the drugs for use in the judicial process.

[105] ONDCP, *The Price and Purity of Illicit Drugs*, p. 1.

[106] Ibid., p. 14.

In: Methamphetamine: Background, Controls and Issues ISBN: 978-1-60692-548-5
Editor: Andrea S. Sandoval

Chapter 2

METHAMPHETAMINE: LEGISLATION AND ISSUES IN THE 110TH CONGRESS

Celinda Franco

SUMMARY

Illicit methamphetamine (MA) production and use are longstanding and severe problems in some states. In recent years, concerns were raised that this drug problem was spreading nationwide, and MA issues became an important federal concern. During the 110th Congress, legislation was introduced on a broad range of issues related to MA abuse, illicit manufacture, treatment, and drug trafficking offenses. For example, S. 1276, the Methamphetamine Production Prevention Act of 2008 (P.L. 110-415), further specified the procedures retailers must follow for tracking the retail purchases of over- the-counter (OTC) medications containing MA precursor chemicals. H.R. 1199, the Drug-Endangered Children Act of 2007 (P.L. 110-345), extended the authority of the Drug-Endangered Children grant program through FY2009. Some of the MA legislation would have built on provisions enacted in the Combat Methamphetamine Epidemic Act (CMEA, P.L. 109-177), which were designed to control and limit the availability of MA and its precursor chemicals. MA abuse has implications for public health, child welfare, crime and public safety, and international relations. This chapter provides a brief overview of MA abuse, its illicit domestic manufacture, federal responses, and anti-MA legislation introduced in the 110th Congress.

BACKGROUND

Methamphetamine (MA), a drug of the amphetamine group, is a powerful and addictive central nervous system stimulant. Originally used as a nasal decongestant and bronchiodialator, MA has been marketed under the trade names Methedrine® and Desoxyn® since the 1940s. MA is currently used to treat a limited number of medical conditions, including narcolepsy, attention deficit disorder/attention deficit/hyperactivity disorder

(ADD/ADHD), and obesity. MA can be administered orally, nasally, by injection, and, in the powder form that resembles granulated crystals, often referred to as "ice," by smoking.[1] MA use can cause convulsions, stroke, cardiac arrhythmia, and hyperthermia. Chronic use can lead to irreversible brain and heart damage, psychotic behavior including paranoid ideation, visual and auditory hallucinations, rages and violence. Withdrawal from MA can induce long-term depression, anxiety, and fatigue.

Illicit MA manufacture and abuse are longstanding and severe problems in some states and regions of the country, particularly in the West, Midwest, and Southeast. Over the past 30 years, Congress has passed legislation designed to address the problem of illicit MA abuse and its manufacture in clandestine labs, including legislation to regulate MA precursor chemicals, enhance penalties for drug trafficking, and increase funding for MA-specific law enforcement programs. Congress continues to be concerned about the abuse and illicit manufacture of MA.

According to the 2007 National Survey on Drug Use and Health (NSDUH), there were approximately 529,000 current users of MA aged 12 or older (0.2% of the population), compared with the 2006 estimate of 731,000 current MA users (0.3% of the populations).[2] Reported MA use among young adults aged 18 to 25 decreased from 0.6% to 0.4% between 2006 and 2007. Table 1 provides the latest NSDUH data available on the number of past-month MA users who met the criteria for illicit drug *dependence* or *abuse*. The number MA users reporting dependence or abuse increased from 250,000 users in 2003 to 257,000 in 2005, although there was a marked spike in the number reporting *dependence or abuse* of MA in 2004. Of those persons reporting *dependent use in the last month* in 2005, 103,000, or 20%, reported using stimulants (most often MA) as their primary substance of abuse.

Sources of Illicit Methamphetamine

According to the Drug Enforcement Agency (DEA), most illicit MA available in the United States is produced in laboratories located in Mexico or California, which is then distributed across the country using existing drug trafficking routes. DEA estimates that around 80% of all MA consumed in the United States is smuggled into the country from Mexico.[3]

Clandestine "Super" Laboratories

As noted above, most illicit MA available in the United States is produced in large clandestine laboratories in Mexico and California.[4] In these large labs, known as "super labs,"[5] MA is produced by persons linked to established drug trafficking organizations (DTOs). These super labs most often obtain the precursor chemicals they need to manufacture illicit MA in wholesale quantities on the international market. According to DEA, much of the MA precursor chemical, pseudoephedrine, is either purchased by DTOs from one of seven chemical companies in Europe, Asia, and the Far East and smuggled into Mexico and the United States, or diverted from legitimate sources.

Small Clandestine Labs

The small domestic amateur labs, commonly referred to as "box" or "mom-and-pop" labs, can be set up in home kitchens, motel rooms, or other similar spaces, and produce MA with pseudoephedrine and other ingredients available at retail stores. These small labs produce illicit MA using one of several relatively simple methods that are readily available on the Internet and other sources. The methods most commonly used to manufacture MA in amateur labs rely on the precursor chemicals, ephedrine, pseudoephedrine, or phenylpropanolamine, which are commonly found in over-the-counter (OTC) cold and sinus medicines available from any drug store.[6] In combination with common household and agricultural products, such as acetone, hydrochloric acid, sodium hydroxide, ether, anhydrous ammonia, cat litter, antifreeze, and drain cleaner, precursor chemicals are synthesized into MA.

FEDERAL ENFORCEMENT PROGRAMS[7]

Many agencies and bureaus within DOJ are involved in addressing the issue of illicit MA. Chief among them is the DEA. Through collaborations with the Federal Bureau of Investigation (FBI), and numerous task forces, including the Organized Crime Drug Enforcement Task Force (OCDETF) and the High Intensity Drug Trafficking Areas (HIDTA), and collaborations with other federal, state, and local law enforcement, DEA targets drug traffickers across the country and internationally to stem the flow of illegal drugs in the United States. According to DEA, the total amount of MA interdicted at the U.S.-Mexico border in 2002 had increased by more than 17% since 1999.[8]

Table 1. Use of MA among Persons Aged 12 or Older, 2003-2006 (in thousands)

Use	2003	2004	2005	2006
Lifetime Use	15,139	14,512	12,663	14,206
Use in Last Year	1,602	1,808	1,603	1,889
New Users in Last Year	260	318	192	259
Use in Past Month	726	706	628	731
Dependent Use in Last Month	250	346	257	N/A
Stimulant is Primary Drug of Abuse	92	130	103	N/A
Other Illicit Drug is Primary Drug of Abuse	158	216	154	N/A

Source: U.S. Department of Health and Human Services, Substance Abuse and Mental Health Services Administration, Office of Applied Studies, National Survey of Drug Use and Health, 2003-2006.

The "Meth Hot Spots" program under the Community Oriented Policing Services (COPS)[9] program is a grant program that *specifically* provides funding for a broad range of initiatives designed to assist state and local law enforcement in undertaking anti-MA initiatives. Between 1998 and 2007, the COPS program has provided more than $448 million nationwide to address the MA problem.[10] For FY2007, approximately $47 million was available for COPS Methamphetamine initiative.[11] The Consolidated Appropriations Act,

2008 (P.L. 110-161), included funding of almost $61.2 million for the Meth Hot Spots program.[12]

The Combat Methamphetamine Epidemic Act (P.L. 109-177)

During the 109th Congress, passage of the USA PATRIOT Improvement and Reauthorization Act of 2005, included Title VII, the Combat Methamphetamine Epidemic Act (P.L. 109-177), legislation designed to curb MA use, trafficking, and production. Signed into law on March 9, 2006, Title VII of P.L. 109-177 included provisions to limit the diversion of MA precursor chemicals, domestically and internationally, increase MA- related criminal penalties, expand measures related to illicit MA laboratory clean up, and create a grant program to prevent and treat MA abuse among parenting women. The law

- limits OTC retail purchases of cold and sinus medications containing MA-precursor chemicals13 to 3.6 grams a day; limits mail order purchases of similar OTC medications to 7.5 grams a month;
- requires that retailers of OTC medications containing MA-precursors be kept behind the counter, and that purchasers of more than 60 mg (two dosage units) of pseudoephedrine must show a form of government- issued photo identification and sign a registry for such purchases;
- requires that the Attorney General (AG) establish production and import quotas for MA-precursor chemicals; impose criminal sanctions for violations of these quotas; expands the AG's authority to regulate controlled substance imports;
- provides additional criminal penalty enhancements equal to a consecutive term of up to 15 years imprisonment for individuals convicted of smuggling MA using dedicated commuter lanes at border crossings and further makes such persons permanently ineligible from using such lanes; a maximum fine of not less than $500,000 for manufacturing a controlled substance on federal property; reductions in the threshold amounts of MA required to trigger prosecution as an MA "drug kingpin"; additional term of imprisonment of up to 20 years in cases where the manufacture or trafficking in MA is carried out where children are present or reside;
- requires mandatory drug testing and sanctions for drug court participantsand authorizes appropriations of $70 million for drug court grants;
- reauthorizes the COPS Meth Hot Spots program, authorizingappropriations of $99 million for each of the fiscal years 2006-2010;
- authorizes appropriations of $20 million for FY2006 and FY2007 for grants to states for drug-endangered children programs; and
- authorizes such sums as may be necessary for a competitive grant program for state, local, and tribal governments to provide services for MA use by pregnant and parenting women offenders.

LEGISLATION IN THE 110TH CONGRESS

Legislation to address the ongoing problem of illicit use and manufacture of MA was considered and enacted during the 110th Congress. H.R. 1199, the Drug-Endangered Children Act of 2007 (P.L. 110-345), passed by the House and Senate on September 24, 2008, extended the authority of the Drug-Endangered Children grant program through FY2009. Four bills, S. 85, S. 267, H.R. 545, and S. 2087, would have clarified that territories and Indian tribes were eligible to receive MA-related grants for drug- endangered children and for addressing MA use by pregnant and parenting women offenders provided under CMEA. These bills were not enacted, although Congress did enact similar amendments under the Consolidated Appropriations Act, 2008 (P.L. 110- 161), to include territories and Indian tribes among those entities eligible to receive such grants.

H.R. 405, S. 884, S. 1367, H.R. 3130, H.R. 3749, and H.R. 6901 would have amended the Public Health Service Act to provide residential family treatment programs for pregnant and parenting women, including treatment for MA addiction and MA treatment alternatives to incarceration for non-violent offenders.[14] H.R. 3186 and S. 1906 would have established a program to investigate oral health problems associated with MA use, known as "meth mouth," while H.R. 3187 and S. 1907 would have focused on similar oral health problems among prison inmates. H.R. 3433 would have required a survey of research on MA treatment and recommend additional research avenues.

H.R. 365 (P.L. 110-143) provided for a research program for remediation of clandestine MA laboratories,[15] similar to those included in S. 635. P.L. 110-143 also provided for the establishment of voluntary guidelines for the remediation of MA laboratory sites; established a research program to support the development, assessment, and revision of these guidelines; and authorized appropriations of $2.5 million to fund research on the residual toxic effects of MA laboratories, and research on developing new MA site detection technologies, such as field test kits and other methods of detecting these toxic sites. H.R. 955 would have, among other things, authorized funding for environmental cleanup of lands contaminated by hazardous substances associated with the illicit manufacture of MA, and provided grants for state and local governments to cleanup and dispose of hazardous MA by-products. S. 2100 would have required that federal forfeiture funds be used, in part, to pay for MA laboratory cleanup.

S. 4, Improving America's Security Act of 2007 (P.L. 110-53), included provisions to establish a "Rural Policing Institute" as part of the Federal Law Enforcement Training Center (based in Glynco, Georgia) where, among other things, programs for rural law enforcement agencies would include training on addressing MA addiction and distribution. H.R. 1028, S. 560, and H.R. 1697 included similar provisions. S. 368 and H.R. 1700 would have amended the COPS program to authorize, among other things, the AG to establish and implement innovative programs to reduce and prevent the illegal manufacturing, distribution, and use of MA.

S. 132 would have lowered the threshold for possession of MA required to constitute violation under current law (21 U.S.C. §848) and triggering prosecution as a "continuing criminal enterprise," as well as increasing penalties and fines for violations involving MA or its salts, isomers, or salts of isomers. H.R. 3143 and S. 2137 would have lowered the criminal thresholds for classifying an offender as an MA "kingpin" and increased the penalty enhancements for such crimes, as well as establishing a multi-jurisdictional MA task forces of federal, state, local law enforcement. H.R. 1118 would have enhanced criminal penalties for drug trafficking offenses relating to the manufacture and distribution of large amounts of MA. Similarly, H.R. 2425 would have enhanced penalties for marketing MA and other drugs to minors, while S. 1211 would have enhanced penalties for marketing *all* controlled substance to minors. H.R. 246 and S. 1178 would have required the AG to conduct a study evaluating whether there is a connection between the commission of MA-related crimes and identity theft crimes.

S. 1276, the Methamphetamine Production Prevention Act of 2008 (P.L. 110-415), as amended and passed by the Senate and the House on September 29, 2008, specified the procedures and identification requirements for tracking the retail purchases of over-the-counter (OTC) medications containing MA precursor chemicals. S. 1276 required that retailers obtain and record identifying information from prospective purchasers of certain types of OTC medications, further specified how paper or electronic signatures are to be collected, and required that retailers retain this information for at least two years. H.R. 2747 and S. 2237 also would have established a grant program to support the use of electronic logbooks for collecting and maintaining records of MA-precursor transactions to aid in the control of MA precursor chemicals. S. 2071 and H.R. 5619 would have required the self-certification of all "persons" selling MA precursor chemicals from behind the counter in retail stores.

End Notes

[1] U.S. Department of Justice, Drug Enforcement Agency, *Methamphetamine and Amphetamines*, Fact Sheet, at [http://www.dea.gov/concern/meth_factsheet.html].

[2] U.S. Department of Health and Human Services, Substance Abuse and Mental Health Services Administration, Office of Applied Statistics, *2007 National Survey on Drug Use and Health Report*, September 4, 2008.

[3] Ibid.

[4] U.S. DOJ, DEA, Methamphetamine Brief, available online at [http://www.usdoj.gov/dea/ concern/ meth_factsheet.html].

[5] A "super lab" is one that is capable of producing 10 pounds or more of MA per production cycle.

[6] For example, pseudoephedrine is an active ingredient in products like Sudafed, Actifed, NyQuil, and Claritin-D.

[7] Other federal programs providing prevention and treatment of MA use, and assisting localities with clandestine lab remediation, are beyond the scope of this chapter.

[8] DEA Resources, For Law Enforcement Officers, Intelligence Reports, Federal-Wide Drug Seizures, available at [http://www.usdoj .gov/dea/].

[9] For more information on the COPS program, see CRS Report RL33308, *The Community Oriented Policing Serives (COPS): Background, Legislation and Issues*, by Nathan James.

[10] U.S. Department of Justice, Office of Community Oriented Policing Services, *COPS Fact Sheet: Methamphetamine Initiative*, August 2007, available at [http://www.cops.usdoj .gov].

[11] Ibid.

[12] Other DOJ grant programs under the Office of Justice Programs provide assistance for a broad range of state and local law enforcement programs and initiatives which *can* include anti-MA efforts.

[13] MA precursors include pseudoephedrine, ephedrine, and phenylpropanolamine.

[14] For more information, see CRS Report RL33354, *The Promoting Safe and Stable Families Act: Reauthorization in the 109th Congress*, by Emilie Stoltzfus.

[15] For more information, see CRS Report RL32959, *Methamphetamine Lab Clean-Up and Remediation Issues*, by Michael M. Simpson.

In: Methamphetamine: Background, Controls and Issues ISBN: 978-1-60692-548-5
Editor: Andrea S. Sandoval

Chapter 3

NATIONAL METHAMPHETAMINE THREAT ASSESSMENT 2007

United States Department of Justice

STRATEGIC FINDINGS

Sharp decreases in domestic methamphetamine production since 2003 have been offset by increased production in Mexico for U.S. distribution by Mexican drug trafficking organizations (DTOs).

Recent strong chemical control efforts in Mexico may be challenging Mexican DTOs' ability to maintain their current high level of methamphetamine production.

Mexican DTOs and criminal groups are expanding their position relative to methamphetamine distribution, particularly ice methamphetamine, including in the eastern United States.

OVERVIEW

Methamphetamine production and distribution are undergoing significant strategic shifts, resulting in new challenges to law enforcement and public health agencies. Law enforcement pressure and strong precursor chemical sales restrictions have achieved marked success in decreasing domestic methamphetamine production. Mexican DTOs, however, have exploited the vacuum created by rapidly expanding their control over methamphetamine distribution—even to eastern states—as users and distributors who previously produced the drug have sought new, consistent sources. These Mexican methamphetamine distribution groups (supported by increased methamphetamine production in Mexico) are often more difficult for local law enforcement agencies to identify, investigate, and dismantle because they typically are much more organized and experienced than local independent producers and distributors. Moreover, these Mexican criminal groups typically produce and distribute ice methamphetamine that usually is smoked, potentially resulting in a more rapid onset of addiction to the drug. These numerous factors contribute to the significant threat posed to the United States by the trafficking and abuse of methamphetamine. In fact, according to National Drug Threat Survey (NDTS) 2006 data, 38.8 percent of state and local law enforcement officials nationwide report methamphetamine as the greatest drug threat to their areas, a higher percentage than that for any other drug.

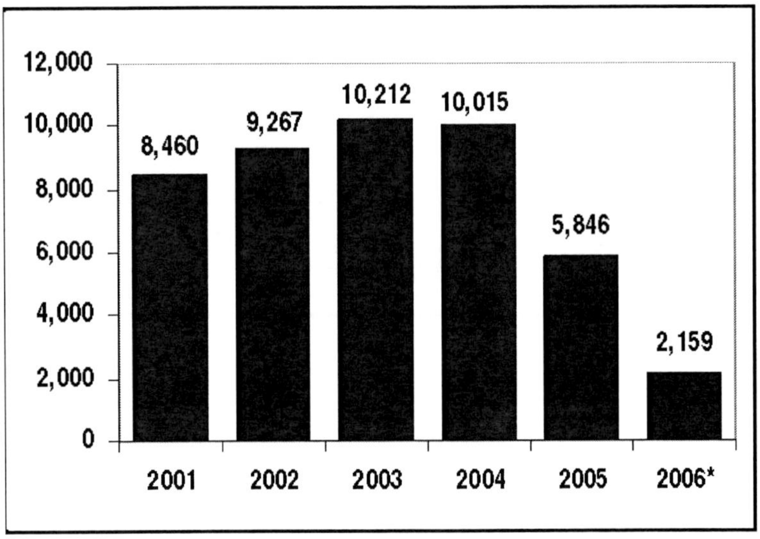

Source: National Clandestine Laboratory Seizure System (Run date— September 13, 2006).
*Data for 2006 are incomplete.

Figure 1. Reported methamphetamine laboratory seizures, 2001–2006.

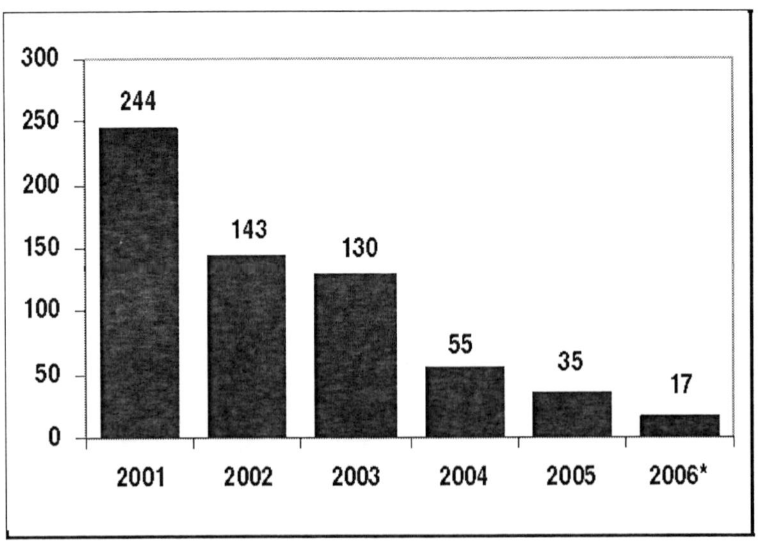

Source: National Clandestine Laboratory Seizure System (Run date— September 13, 2006).
*Data for 2006 are incomplete.

Figure 2. Reported methamphetamine superlab seizures, 2001–2006.

State-level precursor chemical controls have contributed to a sharp decrease in domestic methamphetamine production: Since April 2004, 44 states have restricted retail sales of ephedrine and pseudoephedrine products to varying degrees, complementing already strong federal controls over wholesale precursor chemical sales. Retail sales restrictions—supported by sustained law enforcement pressure—have limited the amount of pseudoephedrine available to small-scale methamphetamine producers, resulting in a sharp decrease in the prevalence of small methamphetamine laboratories nationally. In fact, El Paso Intelligence Center (EPIC) National Clandestine Laboratory Seizure System (NCLSS) data show that the overall number of reported methamphetamine laboratory seizures nationwide decreased 43 percent from 10,212 in 2003 to 5,846 in 2005 (see Figure 1 on page 2). Preliminary data indicate that this trend has continued in 2006, and the number of laboratory seizures will quite likely decrease further as more states implement similar restrictions—six more states and the District of Columbia are considering retail sales restrictions.

Precursor chemical restrictions and law enforcement pressure have forced most California superlabs to relocate: Restrictions on pseudoephedrine imports from Canada to the United States in 2003 resulted in an immediate and significant decrease in the number of reported domestic superlab (capable of producing 10 or more pounds of methamphetamine per production cycle) seizures (see Figure 2). Many of these laboratories— primarily operated by Mexican criminal groups— have relocated to Mexico, where bulk quantities of ephedrine and pseudoephedrine are more available. However, some Mexican criminal groups have remained in the United States to produce methamphetamine in superlabs, particularly in California, which accounted for 29 of 35 reported superlab seizures in 2005. Of the criminal groups that have remained in the United States, many have relocated their superlab operations to very remote rural areas, usually in the Central Valley region of California, in an attempt to decrease the risk of detection from sustained, intense law enforcement pressure. Although Mexican criminal groups have long produced methamphetamine on farms and in rural areas of California, this practice has increased since 2002 as law enforcement pressure and public awareness have increased in more populated areas. In fact, NCLSS data show that superlab seizures in urban areas are now somewhat rare, accounting for only 6 of 29 superlab seizures in California in 2005. By relocating most superlab operations to rural areas with less law enforcement presence, Mexican criminal groups have been able to maintain significant methamphetamine production in California.

Methamphetamine production in Mexico has increased sharply; however, chemical restrictions may render current production levels difficult to sustain: There are no widely accepted estimates regarding the amount of methamphetamine produced in Mexico; however, ample law enforcement reporting and drug seizure data at the U.S.–Mexico border indicate a significant increase in methamphetamine production in Mexico since 2003. In fact, Customs and Border Protection (CBP) data show that seizures of methamphetamine (both ice and powder) along the Southwest Border increased from 2,706 pounds in fiscal year (FY) 2003, to 3,017 pounds in FY2004, to 4,346 pounds in FY 2005, and reached 1,988 pounds through the first 6 months of FY2006. Further production increases are unlikely in the near term, however, and sustaining the current high level of production in Mexico has become more difficult, since the government of Mexico recently reduced ephedrine and pseudoephedrine imports 40.8 percent from 224 metric tons in 2004 to 132.5 metric tons in 2005 (with a goal of 70 metric tons for 2006). Attempts to defeat the increasing chemical restrictions in Mexico will quite likely include routing chemical shipments through transit countries, particularly in Central and South America, for subsequent smuggling into Mexico.

Methamphetamine distribution by Mexican criminal groups is expanding to sustain markets previously supplied by local production, particularly in midwestern and eastern states: As methamphetamine production in small-scale laboratories has decreased nationally since 2004, Mexican criminal groups have expanded direct distribution of Mexico-produced methamphetamine, even in many smaller communities. For example, in midwestern states such as Iowa, Missouri, Illinois, and Ohio, where methamphetamine laboratory seizures have decreased significantly— in some states by more than 55 percent—Mexican criminal groups have gained control over most distribution of the drug in these states. In fact, the Midwest High Intensity Drug Trafficking Area (HIDTA) reports that in cities such as Des Moines and Sioux City, Iowa, where methamphetamine production and distribution previously were controlled by local independent traffickers, Mexican criminal groups, primarily distributing ice methamphetamine, have supplanted independent traffickers. Law enforcement reporting confirms a similar trend throughout much of the Great Lakes, Mid-Atlantic, Florida/Caribbean, Southeast, and West Central Organized Crime Drug Enforcement Task Force (OCDETF) Regions (see Figure 6 on page 5). These groups pose an increased challenge to local law enforcement because they are often Mexico-based, well-organized, and experienced drug distributors who have been successful in blending into somewhat insular Hispanic communities or among Hispanic workers employed in the agricultural, landscaping, construction, and meat packing industries. The ability of Mexican criminal groups to continue the expansion of methamphetamine distribution into more communities in the eastern United States appears to be limited only by their capability to further expand methamphetamine production in Mexico.

Increased ice availability is most likely contributing to increased methamphetamine addiction: Since 2001 the availability of Mexico-produced ice methamphetamine—a form of methamphetamine that typically is smoked—has increased sharply in most U.S. methamphetamine markets. For example, CBP data show that seizures of ice methamphetamine along the Southwest Border increased from 260 pounds in FY2003, to 1,034 pounds in FY2004, and 1,423 pounds in FY2005. According to the National Institute on Drug Abuse (NIDA), smoking methamphetamine may result in more rapid addiction to the drug than snorting or injection because smoking causes a nearly instantaneous, intense, and longer-lasting high. Although casual use of methamphetamine appears to be stable (see Appendix B, Tables 1 and 2), national-level data show a rise in the number of methamphetamine-related treatment admissions and methamphetamine-dependent individuals nationwide (see Figure 3 and Figure 4 on page 3), particularly since ice availability began to increase.[1] In fact, even prior to the current influx of ice methamphetamine, users were increasingly choosing smoking as their primary mode of administration (see Figure 5). Increased rates of smoking ice methamphetamine, leading to increased rates of addiction, will further strain the resources of public health agencies, particularly drug treatment facilities in smaller communities.

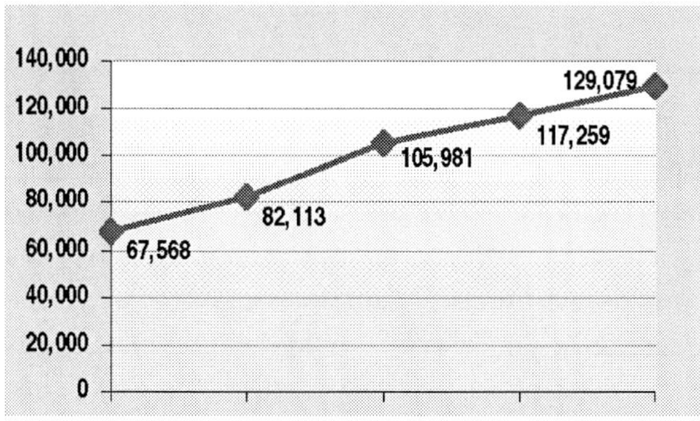

Source: Treatment Episode Data Set.

Figure 3. Primary methamphetamine admissions, 2000–2004.

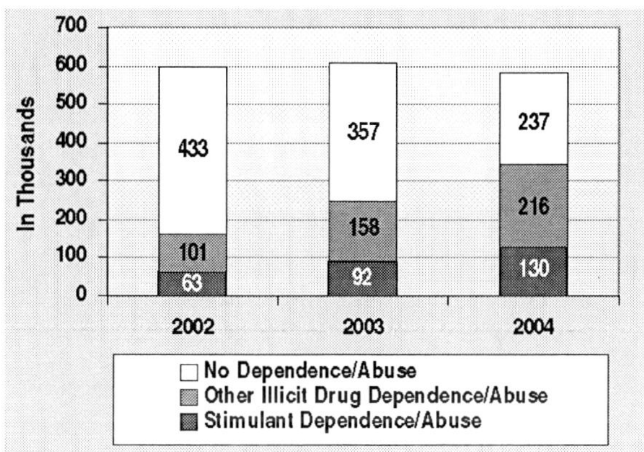

Source: National Survey on Drug Use and Health.

Figure 4. Estimated number of methamphetamine users dependent on or abusing illicit drugs or stimulants, 2002–2004.

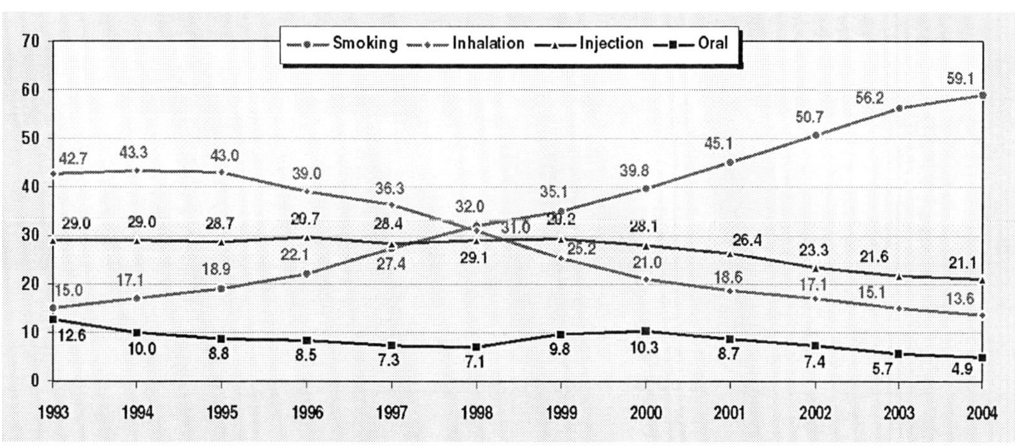

Source: Treatment Episode Data Set.

Figure 5. Percentage of primary methamphetamine or amphetamine admissions, by route of administration, 1 993–2004.

INTELLIGENCE GAPS

The extent of precursor chemical diversion and trafficking from sources of supply in Asia is unclear. Intelligence and law enforcement reporting confirms the shipment of wholesale (multiton) quantities of ephedrine and pseudoephedrine —often repackaged with vague labeling and disguised as legitimate business transactions—to Mexico from source areas in Asia, particularly Hong Kong. However, there are relatively few data available to measure such activity, thereby impeding a full and accurate assessment of the situation.

There are no generally accepted methamphetamine production estimates or comprehensive laboratory seizure data for most foreign countries. This lack of data limits the accuracy of analysis regarding foreign production in areas of particular interest such as Mexico, Canada, and Asia.

OCDETF REGIONAL METHAMPHETAMINE SUMMARIES

The following regional summaries provide strategic overviews of the methamphetamine situation in each of the nine OCDETF regions, highlighting significant trends and law enforcement concerns relating to the trafficking and abuse of the drug. The summaries were prepared through detailed analysis of recent law enforcement reporting, information obtained through interviews with law enforcement and public health officials, OCDETF case files, and currently available statistical data.

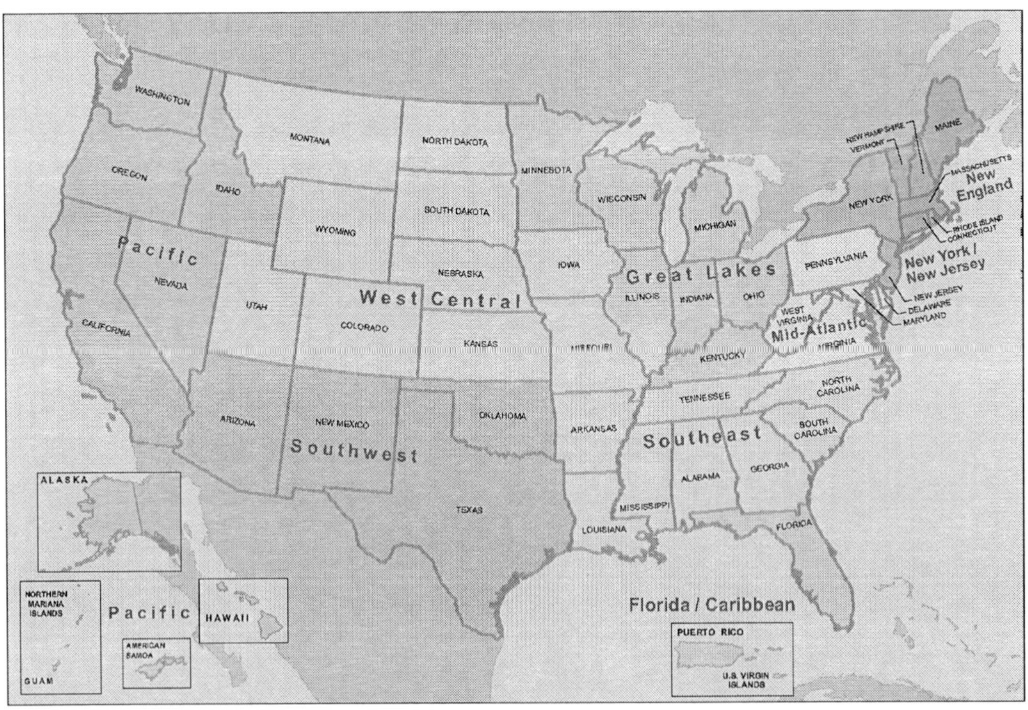

Figure 6. Nine OCDETF regions.

Florida/Caribbean OCDETF Region

Ice availability rising, driven by Mexican DTOs

Methamphetamine is a significant and increasing problem throughout Florida. Mexican DTOs, which have long been the primary suppliers of methamphetamine available in the region, are increasingly supplying large quantities of ice methamphetamine to distributors in Florida. As a result, ice has become the predominant form of methamphetamine sold in Florida. As availability of the drug has risen, abuse has spread from rural areas of the state to a number of cities, including Orlando and Tampa. Methamphetamine is rare in Puerto Rico and the U.S. Virgin Islands, and no clandestine laboratories were seized there in the last 4 years.

Precursor laws causing drop in local laboratories

State precursor laws enacted in June 2005 have strongly contributed to a decline in local methamphetamine production in Florida. Statewide, laboratory seizures increased from 301 in 2004 to 337 in 2005 but dropped to 49 through September 2006. Nonetheless, many producers in Florida are circumventing the new precursor laws by making multiple purchases of ephedrine and pseudoephedrine under the threshold amount at different stores. Because the Florida law only limits the amount of ephedrine or pseudoephedrine that can be purchased per visit and does not establish a mechanism to track the identity and purchase history of buyers, producers who live in or near metropolitan areas and have access to many businesses that sell ephedrine and pseudoephedrine products can simply drive from store to store to purchase precursor chemicals. Some major retail stores have begun to independently track the identity and purchase history of buyers in an attempt to limit access to these chemicals to legitimate users. If the current situation with regard to tightening domestic precursor chemical controls and increasing availability of Mexico-produced methamphetamine remains unchanged, domestic methamphetamine production will most likely decline further.

Great Lakes OCDETF Region

Methamphetamine production continues to cause health and environmental concerns

Methamphetamine production levels have increased significantly in the Great Lakes Region over the past 5 years, and although several indicators suggest the onset of a downward trend, such production continues to jeopardize the safety of citizens and drain law enforcement resources. According to NCLSS data, the number of reported methamphetamine laboratory seizures skyrocketed in the Great Lakes Region from 2001 (1,316) to 2004 (2,954) before decreasing in 2005 (2,698) and again through September 2006 (637). Law enforcement officials attribute the decrease in 2005 to a combination of factors, including the rising availability of Mexico-produced ice methamphetamine, aggressive law enforcement efforts, public awareness campaigns, and precursor chemical control legislation. Nonetheless, methamphetamine production levels at small-capacity laboratories (those that produce 2 ounces or less per cycle), usually operated by Caucasian local independent dealers and outlaw motorcycle gangs (OMG)s, remain high in many areas in the Great Lakes Region, including Ohio and southwest Michigan, and continue to adversely affect law enforcement, citizens, and the environment. NCLSS data indicate that federal, state, and local law enforcement agencies in the Great Lakes Region spent over $4.7 million on methamphetamine laboratory cleanup costs in 2005, up from $3.3 million in 2004.

Methamphetamine distribution and abuse have increased in the region

The availability and abuse of methamphetamine (both powder and ice) are increasing and pose one of the most significant challenges for law enforcement officials in the Great Lakes Region, including in Chicago, which historically has had limited problems associated with distribution and abuse of the drug. Federal- wide Drug Seizure System (FDSS) data indicate that the amount of methamphetamine reported seized by federal law enforcement officials in the Great Lakes Region increased overall from 2001 (147 kg) to 2005 (465 kg). In addition, Treatment Episode Data Set (TEDS) data indicate that the number of admissions for methamphetamine abuse to publicly funded treatment facilities in the Great Lakes Region more than tripled from 2000 (3,535) to 2004 (12,259). The increases in the total amount of methamphetamine seized and in the number of methamphetamine-related treatment admissions are primarily due to rising availability of Mexico- produced ice methamphetamine.

Mexican traffickers transport significant quantities of ice methamphetamine to the region; some is destined for other regions

Mexican drug traffickers are the primary methamphetamine transporters to and through the Great Lakes Region, typically transporting significant quantities of the drug in private and commercial vehicles from Mexico and southwestern states to stash houses in Chicago, Illinois; Cleveland and Cincinnati, Ohio; Detroit, Michigan; Indianapolis, Indiana; and Minneapolis-St. Paul, Minnesota. From these cities, significant quantities of these drugs are further transported to smaller drug markets in and outside the Great Lakes Region. For instance, law enforcement reporting indicates that Mexican DTOs transport significant quantities of ice methamphetamine through Chicago and Detroit for distribution in the West Central, New York/New Jersey, and Southeast Regions.

Ice methamphetamine is now available in areas that previously had no methamphetamine threat

Mexican DTOs, the primary wholesale and midlevel distributors of methamphetamine in the Great Lakes Region, have developed new markets for Mexico-produced Ice methamphetamine in areas where methamphetamine was previously unavailable. Since the late 1990s Mexican DTOs have expanded their cocaine and marijuana distribution activities to include methamphetamine in some larger drug markets in the Great Lakes Region such as Cincinnati, Cleveland, Columbus, and Toledo, Ohio, and Minneapolis.

Mid-Atlantic OCDETF Region

Methamphetamine threat increasing as Mexico-produced ice is entering region

The methamphetamine threat in the Mid-Atlantic region (MAR) is moderate but increasing in some areas. Overall methamphetamine availability in the region is low but increasing, particularly in the Shenandoah Valley of Virginia and the northwestern counties and Pocono Mountains area of Pennsylvania. In 2005 the number of methamphetamine laboratories seized in the MAR dropped; however, increasing amounts of ice methamphetamine transported into the region by Mexican DTOs has kept availability of the drug stable.

Recent state-level precursor chemical controls have contributed to a sharp decrease in domestic methamphetamine production in the region

Precursor legislation enacted in several Mid- Atlantic states has been instrumental in combating local methamphetamine production. Since April 2004 four states—Delaware, Pennsylvania, Virginia, and West Virginia—have restricted retail sales of ephedrine and pseudoephedrine products to varying degrees, complementing already strong federal controls over wholesale precursor chemical sales. Retail sales restrictions—supported by sustained law enforcement pressure and rising public awareness—have greatly limited the amount of pseudoephedrine available to small-scale methamphetamine producers in the region, resulting in a sharp decrease in the prevalence of small methamphetamine laboratories. In fact, NCLSS data show that the overall number of reported methamphetamine laboratory seizures in the Mid-Atlantic Region decreased from 233 in 2004 to 177 in 2005. Preliminary data indicate that this trend has continued for 2006 and will very likely decrease further, since Maryland and the District of Columbia have proposed the implementation of similar restrictions.

Methamphetamine demand low but increasing among some segments

The overall demand for methamphetamine in the MAR is relatively low, far less than the demand for cocaine and comparable to the demand for heroin; however, methamphetamine demand is increasing in the region among certain groups. Amphetamine-related admissions to publicly funded treatment facilities in the MAR (95 percent of which are methamphetamine-related) have increased substantially over the past several years. However, treatment providers report that high methamphetamine availability in specific locations such as northern Virginia is attracting new adolescent abusers. Lower- to middle-income, blue-collar Caucasians have traditionally been the major abusers of methamphetamine in the MAR. Abuse of ice appears to be rising among teenagers and young adults as well as gay males involved in the club scene.

Mexican DTOs dominant methamphetamine transporters

Local Mexican wholesale distributors transport multipound quantities of methamphetamine into the region from superlab production sites in Mexico and transshipment locations in the Southwest Region, northern and central California, Nevada, North Carolina, and Georgia. Most methamphetamine is transported by private and rented vehicles with hidden compartments. Ounce and pound quantities of methamphetamine also are shipped on a regular basis by mail and parcel delivery services from California and other western states to recipients in northern Delaware and eastern Pennsylvania. OMGs such as Outlaws, Pagan's, and Warlocks; Asian DTOs; and long-distance truck drivers also transport gram to ounce quantities of methamphetamine into the region, occasionally in pill form from Canada. Members of the gay community transport ice methamphetamine into the urban areas of the MAR (most notably the District of Columbia) from sources in New York City. Other primary destinations for methamphetamine shipments in the MAR include cities and towns in West

Virginia, the suburbs of the District of Columbia, and the Tidewater and Richmond areas of Virginia.

Hispanic street gangs prominent in midlevel and retail sales

Mexican DTOs and Hispanic street gangs control much of the midlevel and retail distribution in cities and towns; however, Caucasian independent dealers have been the predominant retail dealers in the rural areas, where much of the drug is distributed and consumed. Lower- to middle-income, blue-collar Caucasians are the traditional street-level purchasers and abusers of powder methamphetamine. However, Mexico-produced ice is increasingly being abused by young adults and teenagers at parties, raves, and nightclubs and by members of the gay community at private residences and alternative lifestyle establishments.

New England OCDETF Region

Methamphetamine threat low but increasing; ice rarely available

Methamphetamine is an emerging drug threat in New England, with increasing clandestine laboratory seizures occurring in Connecticut, Maine, and New Hampshire. Treatment admissions are low and stable, but providers are concerned because methamphetamine abuse is expanding among the general population. Pound and kilogram quantities of methamphetamine increasingly have been seized by law enforcement officials, signaling a rise in the midlevel distribution of the drug in the region. The drug is most prevalent in Connecticut, Massachusetts, and New Hampshire. Powder methamphetamine is the type most commonly sold in the region; New England is one of the few areas of the nation where ice is rarely encountered.

Local production up; state legislation restricting precursor availability

Methamphetamine production levels in the New England Region (NER) are low when compared to those in the rest of the nation; however, the number of methamphetamine laboratories seized in the region is increasing slowly, and laboratories have been encountered in both urban and rural locations. Regionally, NCLSS data indicate that the number of methamphetamine laboratories seized rose from 3 in 2002, to 8 in 2004, and 18 in 2005, reaching 11 by September 2006. Most were seized in the Seacoast area of eastern New Hampshire. In 2005 the Maine General Assembly restricted the availability of over-the-counter medications containing the precursors ephedrine and pseudoephedrine, and in 2006 both the New Hampshire and Vermont legislatures passed similar laws, while legislators in Connecticut, Massachusetts, and Rhode Island have proposed similar restrictions.

Methamphetamine transported primarily by mail

Mexican and Caucasian DTOs and OMGs are the primary transporters of methamphetamine available in the region. Methamphetamine shipments destined for the NER typically originate in California and southwestern states as well as Colorado and Oregon. These traffickers typically use the U.S. mail system to smuggle methamphetamine into the region and recently have begun structuring shipments sent through the mail to minimize the risk of seizure. Law enforcement officials suspect that traffickers are "shotgunning" multiple small loads into the NER so that even if one package is seized, most of the drug will reach its destination. Caucasian independent distributors and small criminal groups are the dominant wholesale and retail distributors of the drug in the region.

Methamphetamine, possibly precursors, being smuggled from Canada

Canada has emerged as a source for methamphetamine trafficked by Asian DTOs and OMGs, and possibly for ephedrine and pseudoephedrine encountered in the region. Canada-based Asian polydrug traffickers transport methamphetamine from areas in eastern Canada to the NER for distribution.

New York/New Jersey OCDETF Region

Methamphetamine threat rising; Mexican DTOs smuggling ice methamphetamine into region

The methamphetamine threat in the New York/New Jersey (NY/NJ) Region is low but increasing, especially in some areas with large Hispanic populations. Availability is rising, driven by an influx of higher purity ice methamphetamine being transported into the area by Mexican organizations based in the Southwest and Mexico. Reporting from law enforcement and public health agencies throughout the city of New York indicates that the abuse of ice methamphetamine is increasing, particularly within the gay male community and nightclub scene of New York City. Law enforcement and treatment personnel are monitoring this situation closely because these populations have long been on the cutting edge of drug trends that later spread to the general population. Ice methamphetamine abuse also is increasing among the Asian community, particularly in the southern section of Queens. These abusers appear to be supplied by Asian traffickers who ship ice methamphetamine from the West Coast.

Local production low and falling

Methamphetamine production poses a low threat in the NY/NJ Region, with most activity concentrated in rural areas, particularly Upstate New York. The number of clandestine methamphetamine laboratories seized in the region is low and stable, according to law enforcement officials in the region, in part as a result of an increase in ice methamphetamine being transported from the Southwest Border, rendering local production less necessary. Additionally, legislation enacted in New York and New Jersey has been instrumental in combating local methamphetamine production. New Jersey enacted legislation that restricts the sale of ephedrine and pseudoephedrine products, and New York introduced legislation to either schedule or place point-of-sale restrictions on these precursors. Most laboratories in the region are small-scale operations run by young Caucasian males, who produce the drug for their own use and for sale to close associates. These clandestine laboratory operators predominantly produce user-level amounts, although there have been several cases in southern New York State and in the Watertown area where larger, multiounce quantities were manufactured.

Mexican DTOs dominate methamphetamine trade

The vast majority of the methamphetamine consumed in the region is transported from Mexico and the western United States by Mexican DTOs, using well-established transportation and distribution networks that, since the mid-1990s, have gradually extended into the NY/NJ Region. Local Mexican wholesale distributors transport multipound quantities of methamphetamine into the region from Mexico and from transshipment locations in Southwest Border states, California and, increasingly, Atlanta. Most methamphetamine is transported overland by private and commercial vehicles. DTOs also use parcel delivery services and couriers on buses, trains, and commercial aircraft to transport the drug. Mexican DTOs also are the principal wholesale distributors of methamphetamine in the region. Moreover, these Mexican DTOs, along with Hispanic street gangs, control much of the midlevel and retail distribution in the region's cities and towns. Caucasian independent dealers and OMGs are the predominant retail dealers in rural areas of the region, where most methamphetamine is distributed and consumed.

Pacific OCDETF Region

Region has most pervasive methamphetamine threat

Methamphetamine is increasingly available in the Pacific Region, particularly ice methamphetamine, which has become the predominant form of the drug available in most areas of the region. According to NDTS 2006 data, 92.2 percent of law enforcement agencies in the Pacific Region report that methamphetamine is the greatest drug threat in their jurisdictions, a higher percentage than for any other region in the country (see Appendix A, Map 2). Throughout most of the Pacific Region, the rate of methamphetamine abuse is very high; for instance, in Hawaii, methamphetamine abuse rates are extremely high, indicating that methamphetamine is significantly more abused than marijuana.

TEDS data for Hawaii show that in 2004 (the last year for which such data are available), primary methamphetamine admissions (2,381 or 41%) accounted for twice as many admissions to publicly funded treatment facilities in Hawaii as marijuana admissions (1,209 or 20.8%). Conversely, nationwide in 2004 primary treatment admissions for methamphetamine accounted for 8 percent of all drug treatment admissions, while marijuana accounted for 16 percent of all admissions to publicly funded treatment facilities. Furthermore, Community Epidemiology Work Group (CEWG) findings indicate that, in Hawaii, methamphetamine accounted for 58 percent of drug treatment admissions in the state during 2005. Additionally, CEWG data for the state (available only through June 2005) reveal a 25 percent increase in medical examiner reports of positive decedent toxicology for methamphetamine, a 20 percent increase in occupancy of treatment spaces for methamphetamine treatment, and a 20 percent increase in methamphetamine-related cases reported by the Honolulu Police Department during that time.

Lower methamphetamine purity levels in some areas

Methamphetamine availability is high throughout most of the Pacific Region; however, law enforcement reporting from the region indicates a decrease in the purity of the drug in some areas. Law enforcement officials in California, Hawaii, and Nevada have reported lower purity methamphetamine, particularly at the midlevel and retail level. For instance, law enforcement in Las Vegas report that local distributors are limiting the amount of methamphetamine that mid- and retail-level buyers can purchase because of decreased supplies of ice methamphetamine. The lower purity observed and reported by law enforcement may be a result of decreased availability that has forced mid- and retail-level distributors to cut the drug to stretch supplies.

Chemical controls decrease production, but chemical diversion continues

Methamphetamine production has decreased significantly in the Pacific Region, largely a result of successful law enforcement operations and regulatory efforts to control precursor chemicals. Most states in the Pacific Region have enacted legislation to regulate the sale of ephedrine or pseudoephedrine, and several states have scheduled the substances to further restrict their use. Most states report decreased production levels since enacting these controls. Nonetheless, precursor chemical diversion has persisted in the region, with wholesale quantities being smuggled in from Canada and Mexico to operators of major and large-scale laboratories. Many of the Mexican DTOs operating large-scale laboratories in the region have moved production operations to either Mexico or very remote rural areas, particularly in the Central Valley region of California, in an attempt to decrease the risk of detection from sustained, intense law enforcement pressure.

Mexican groups produce large quantities of methamphetamine, primarily in California

Methamphetamine continues to be produced in large-scale laboratories located primarily in the Central Valley of California for distribution throughout the region and the country. Mexican DTOs and criminal groups that continue to produce methamphetamine in the region operate both superlabs and major laboratories (those capable of producing between 2 and 9 pounds of methamphetamine per production cycle). According to NCLSS, 6 superlabs were seized in the Pacific Region through September 2006, compared with 29 in 2005 and 48 in 2004. Although superlab seizures are relatively few and decreasing, 5 of the 6 laboratories seized in 2006 were relatively large, capable of producing more than 20 pounds of methamphetamine per production cycle. Additionally, 4 major laboratories were seized in the region through September 2006. While major laboratories do not have the production capability of superlabs, they can produce significantly more methamphetamine than small-scale laboratories.

Methamphetamine is distributed by Mexican traffickers from the Pacific Region to drug markets throughout the country

Methamphetamine produced in the Pacific Region and methamphetamine smuggled from Mexico are distributed to drug markets in the region and in other regions of the United States. Mexican DTOs and criminal groups operating large-scale methamphetamine laboratories in the region distribute significant quantities of the drug that they produce to drug markets throughout the country. Mexican DTOs and criminal groups also dominate distribution of methamphetamine that is smuggled from Mexico, distributing the drug in the Pacific Region as well as to markets throughout the country. As demand for methamphetamine spreads into new drug markets and as precursor controls curb local production, methamphetamine distribution from the Pacific Region by these groups most likely will increase.

Southeast OCDETF Region

Ice distribution and abuse up dramatically

Methamphetamine poses a significant threat to the Southeast Region. The distribution and abuse of ice methamphetamine have increased dramatically in the Southeast over the past several years, primarily as a result of two factors. First, Mexican DTOs have fostered an increase in ice availability throughout the region by using transportation and distribution networks established for cocaine and marijuana to smuggle and sell massive quantities of ice and by aggressively marketing the drug. Second, abusers have been increasingly drawn to the drug's long-lasting high, declining price, and smokable form.

Abuse spreading beyond traditional users

Interviews of law enforcement and public health agencies throughout the Southeast Region indicate that methamphetamine abuse is expanding among users and in locations that historically have not been associated with the drug. Previously, almost all methamphetamine abused in the Southeast was used by lower-income Caucasians in rural areas, and they almost exclusively abused powder methamphetamine. Now, a growing number of methamphetamine abusers in the Southeast are middle- and upper-income Caucasians, African Americans, and Hispanics who live in cities and suburban areas and abuse ice. A substantial portion of these users are teenagers and young adults involved in the club scene, a venue where many new ice abusers are introduced to the drug.

Local methamphetamine production is declining as more ice is transported into the region and precursor restrictions take hold

Overall production of methamphetamine within the Southeast is declining. Seizure data and reports from law enforcement officials throughout the region indicate a reduction in the number of laboratories in the Southeast. In fact, NCLSS data show that the number of methamphetamine laboratories seized in the region decreased from 2,241 in 2004 to 1,327 in 2005 and 521 through September 2006. The influx of Mexico-produced ice has rendered local production less necessary, and restrictions in every Southeast state limiting access to products containing ephedrine and pseudoephedrine have made production of methamphetamine more difficult.

Mexican DTOs primary suppliers:

Mexican DTOs supply most of the ice available in the Southeast. These DTOs produce the vast majority of the drug in laboratories in Mexico and transport it to markets throughout the region, often via distribution hubs, including Atlanta. The Mexican DTOs that distribute ice frequently are polydrug organizations, and they traffic ice using many of the same relatively secure methods and networks used to transport the other drugs that they distribute. Mexican DTOs supply African American, Caucasian, other Hispanic, and Asian distribution groups as well as OMGs, who sell midlevel or retail quantities of ice in the region. Mexican DTOs do not typically sell ice at the street level.

Aggressive marketing expanding ice availability

Mexican DTOs are aggressively marketing ice in the Southeast. Law enforcement officials report that Mexican DTOs frequently front pound quantities or more of the drug to local distributors in order to build a customer base for the drug without having to pay for supplies up front. Mexican DTOs' willingness to take the risk of fronting ice—sometimes to distributors they do not even know—suggests that they have ready access to a supply and are making a concerted effort to further expand the market for this drug. Mexican DTOs are quite likely attracted to the ice market not only because of the profitability of selling ice, but also because they have strong connections to producers, which allow them to operate independently of Colombian and other suppliers (as in the cocaine trade) and to adjust production to meet demand.

Southwest OCDETF Region

Increasing quantities of methamphetamine smuggled into the Southwest Region from Mexico

The amount of methamphetamine smuggled across the Southwest Border has increased considerably in recent years, resulting in increased transshipment and abuse of the drug throughout the Southwest. EPIC data show that the total amount of methamphetamine seized along the Southwest Border increased from 1,935 kilograms in 2004 to 2,481 kilograms in 2005. Data for 2006 are incomplete; however, through July 2006 officials report seizing approximately 602 kilograms of methamphetamine along the Southwest Border. The increase in methamphetamine seizures at or between ports of entry (POEs) on the Southwest Border most likely reflects increased methamphetamine production in Mexico since 2002. Production capability of Mexico-based methamphetamine laboratories is largely an intelligence gap; methamphetamine production in Mexico is dependent greatly upon the acquisition of ephedrine, particularly from China, by laboratory operators in Mexico. The amount of ephedrine available for methamphetamine production is unknown, and Mexican DTOs are not the only consumers of this precursor. The International Narcotics Control Strategy Report further indicates that Mexican DTOs must compete for ephedrine shipments with criminal groups in Southeast Asia, particularly Burma, that produce billions of methamphetamine tablets annually and also are increasing production.

Declining domestic methamphetamine production offset by increased production in Mexico

Methamphetamine production in both large-scale and small-scale laboratories has decreased significantly in the Southwest Region. However, methamphetamine continues to be produced in superlabs in southern California and in small-scale laboratories located throughout the Southwest Region. Many Mexican DTOs operating large-scale laboratories in southern California have transferred production operations to Mexico, where they can more easily obtain precursor chemicals, while small-scale domestic producers have begun to purchase rather than produce the drug. The methamphetamine threat will very likely remain high if producers in Mexico continue to produce enough methamphetamine to offset additional decreases in domestic production and increased demand for the drug in the United States.

Precursor control legislation has contributed to decreased methamphetamine production in the Southwest Region

Methamphetamine laboratory seizures have declined significantly over the past several years, primarily as a result of regulatory efforts to control precursor chemical diversion, the influx of powder and ice methamphetamine from Mexico, and law enforcement efforts. In fact, NCLSS data show that the number of methamphetamine laboratory seizures in the Southwest Region decreased from 1,415 in 2003, to 955 in 2004, to 391 in 2005, and 173 through September 2006. Most states in the Southwest Region currently schedule ephedrine or pseudoephedrine and/or have point-of-sale restrictions, including restrictions on quantity, packaging, and/or display. Local municipalities also have passed laws regulating precursor chemicals in parts of the region, including Cottonwood and Tucson, Arizona, and Albuquerque, New Mexico. Local precursor laws often are put in place where statewide regulations are not implemented or to complement state legislation. These laws primarily impact small-scale laboratories because operators of these laboratories typically obtain precursor chemicals from retail outlets. Increasing transportation and distribution of Mexico-produced methamphetamine in the region have offset the drop in local production, thereby sustaining availability of the drug.

The Southwest Region is the primary entry point for ice methamphetamine supplied to most consumer markets in the United States

Methamphetamine smuggled from Mexico is distributed in market areas in the Southwest Region as well as throughout the United States. Ice methamphetamine is becoming the predominant form of the drug seized in and transshipped from the region and may pose an even more severe threat as a result of increased demand, purity, and profit potential. Methamphetamine produced and smuggled into the Southwest Region from Mexico is distributed primarily from Dallas/Fort Worth, Houston, Los Angeles, Phoenix, and San Diego to markets throughout the United States.

West Central OCDETF Region

Methamphetamine production has decreased significantly in the region; however, local production continues to pose a significant threat to the public and environment:

NCLSS data reveal that seizures of methamphetamine laboratories decreased significantly in the West Central Region from 3,082 in 2004 to 1,705 in 2005 to 560 through September 2006 as a result of a combination of factors, including increasing availability of Mexico-produced ice methamphetamine, aggressive law enforcement efforts, public awareness campaigns, and precursor chemical control legislation. Although methamphetamine production levels have decreased significantly, 64.7 percent of NDTS 2006 respondents in the West Central Region report that the level of methamphetamine production is moderate to high in their jurisdictions. According to NCLSS data, laboratory cleanup costs in 2005 totaled $3,989,37 1[2] for federal, state, and local law enforcement agencies in the West Central Region, down from $4,575,803 in 2004.

Mexican DTOs are the primary transporters and wholesale distributors of methamphetamine in the region

Mexican DTOs and local independent dealers use sophisticated networks to transport large quantities of methamphetamine from Mexico and the Pacific and Southwest Regions to market areas in the West Central Region, typically by private and commercial vehicles and, to a lesser extent, parcel delivery services and couriers aboard buses, trains, and commercial aircraft. Mexican and Caucasian criminal groups, Caucasian and Native American local independent dealers, street gangs, and OMGs distribute midlevel and retail-level quantities of methamphetamine.

Methamphetamine abuse continues to increase in the region

Increasing demand for methamphetamine in the region has been fueled in part by the increasing availability of ice methamphetamine supplied by Mexican traffickers. TEDS data indicate that the number of individuals seeking treatment for methamphetamine abuse at public treatment facilities in the West Central Region increased nearly 68 percent from 18,444 in 2000 to 30,936 in 2004. CEWG reporting shows that in 2005 and through midyear 2006, methamphetamine abuse indicators in Denver (the only West Central state represented in CEWG) were higher than those for cocaine and heroin.

Increasing availability and abuse of methamphetamine associated with increasing violence and property crime

Law enforcement reporting indicates that much of the crime throughout the West Central Region has a methamphetamine nexus. Abusers and distributors throughout the region increasingly commit crimes such as burglary, automobile theft, currency counterfeiting, home invasion, and forgery. The majority of law enforcement agencies in the West Central Region that responded to the NDTS 2006 indicate that methamphetamine contributes greatly to crime in their areas; 71.3 percent report that methamphetamine is the drug that most contributes to violent crime, and 74.4 percent report that methamphetamine is the drug that most contributes to property crime.

Appendix A. Maps

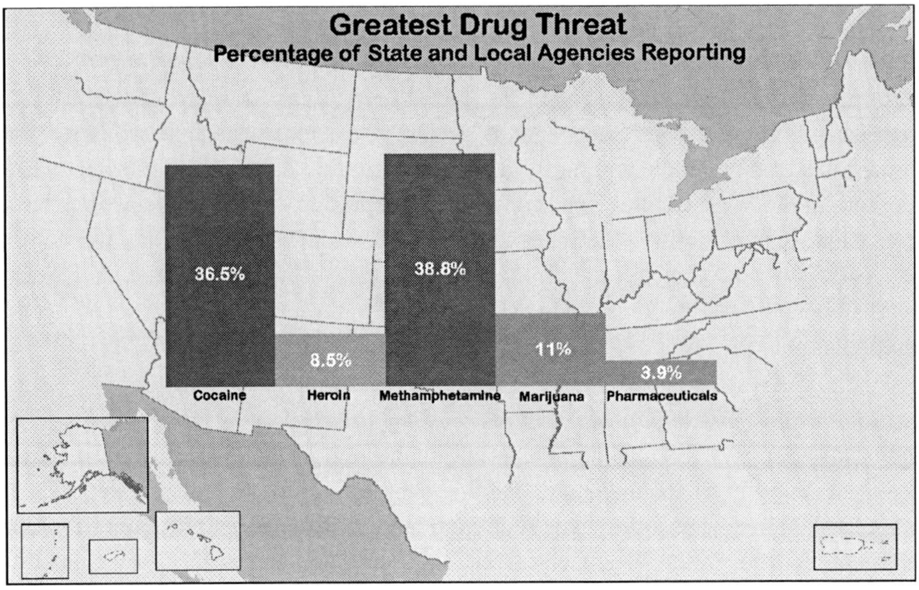

Map 1. National Drug Threat Survey 2006 greatest drug threat as reported by state and local agencies.

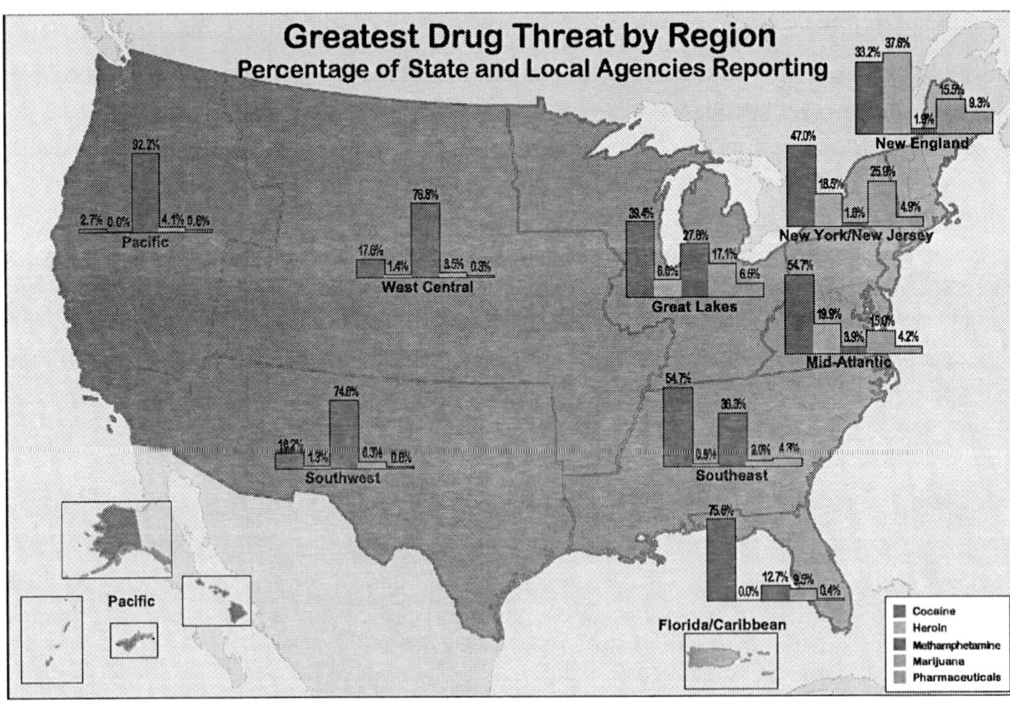

Map 2. National Drug Threat Survey 2006 greatest drug threat by OCDETF region.

APPENDIX B. TABLES

Table 1. Trends in Percentage of Past Year Methamphetamine Use, 2002–2005

	2002	2003	2004	2005
Individuals (12 and older)	0.7	0.6	0.6	0.5
Adolescents (12-17)	0.9	0.7	0.6	0.7
Adults (18-25)	1.7	1.6	1.6	1.5
Adults (26 and older)	0.4	0.4	0.4	0.3

Source: National Survey on Drug Use and Health.

Table 2. Adolescent Trends in Percentage of Past Year Methamphetamine Use, 2000–2005

	2000	2001	2002	2003	2004	2005
8th Grade	2.5	2.8	2.2	2.5	1.5	1.8
10th Grade	4.0	3.7	3.9	3.3	3.0	2.9
12th Grade	4.3	3.9	3.6	3.2	3.4	2.5

Source: Monitoring the Future.

Table 3. Federal Methamphetamine Seizures, in Kilograms, 2000–2006.

Drug	2000	2001	2002	2003	2004	2005	2006*
Methamphetamine	3,471.0	3,971.0	2,478.0	3,856.0	3,127.0	4,767.0	601.9

Source: Federal-Wide Drug Seizure System.
*Data for 2006 are incomplete.

Table 4. Methamphetamine-Related Arrests, United States, 2001–2006

Drug	2001	2002	2003	2004	2005	2006*
Methamphetamine	7,363	6,231	6,055	5,893	6,090	1,504

Source: Drug Enforcement Administration.
*Data for 2006 are incomplete.

Table 5. Average Purity of Methamphetamine Samples Tested by Percentage, 2002–2005

	2002	2003	2004	2005
Kilogram	43	66	78	80
Ounce	37	54	58	68
Gram	49	59	61	69

Source: Drug Enforcement Administration.

Sources

In addition to the sources listed below, numerous state and local law enforcement agencies throughout the United States provided valuable input to this chapter through their participation in the National Drug Threat Survey.

Executive Office of the President
- Office of National Drug Control Policy
  - High Intensity Drug Trafficking Areas
    - Appalachia Atlanta
    - Central Florida
    - Central Valley California
    - Chicago
    - Gulf Coast
    - Hawaii
    - Houston
    - Lake County Los Angeles Michigan
    - Midwest
    - Milwaukee
    - Nevada
    - New England
    - New York/New Jersey
    - Northern California
    - North Florida North Texas Northwest
    - Ohio
    - Oregon
    - Philadelphia/Camden
    - Puerto Rico/U.S. Virgin Islands
    - Rocky Mountain
    - South Florida Southwest Border
    - Washington/Baltimore

National Center on Addiction and Substance Abuse Columbia University
Partnership Attitude Tracking Study
Royal Canadian Mounted Police
United Nations International Narcotics Control Board

U.S. Department of Agriculture
- U.S. Forest Service
  - National Forest System

U.S. Department of Defense
- Defense Intelligence Agency
- Joint Interagency Task Force/West
- Joint Task Force
- Naval Criminal Investigative Service

U.S. Air Force

U.S. Department of Health and Human Services
- Centers for Disease Control and Prevention
- National Institutes of Health
  - National Institute on Drug Abuse
    - Community Epidemiology Work Group
    - Monitoring the Future
- Substance Abuse and Mental Health Services Administration
  - Drug Abuse Warning Network
  - National Survey on Drug Use and Health
  - Treatment Episode Data Set

U.S. Department of Homeland Security
- U.S. Customs and Border Protection
  - Border Patrol Intelligence Center
- U.S. Immigration and Customs Enforcement
- U.S. Coast Guard
  - Maritime Intelligence Center

U.S. Department of Justice
- Bureau of Justice Assistance
  - Western States Information Network
- Criminal Division
  - Organized Crime Drug Enforcement Task Force
- Drug Enforcement Administration
  - Atlanta Field Division
  - Boston Field Division
  - Caribbean Field Division
  - Chicago Field Division
  - Cocaine Signature Program
  - Dallas Field Division
  - Denver Field Division
  - Detroit Field Division
  - Domestic Cannabis Eradication/Suppression Program
  - Domestic Monitor Program
  - El Paso Field Division
  - El Paso Intelligence Center
  - National Clandestine Laboratory Seizure System
  - Federal-Wide Drug Seizure System
  - Houston Field Division
  - Los Angeles Field Division
  - Miami Field Division
  - National Forensic Laboratory Information System
  - Newark Field Division
  - New Orleans Field Division

New York Field Division
Office of Diversion Control
Philadelphia Field Division
Phoenix Field Division
San Diego Field Division
San Francisco Field Division
Seattle Field Division
Special Operations Division
St. Louis Field Division
System to Retrieve Information From Drug Evidence
Washington, D.C., Field Division

U.S. Department of State
International Narcotics Control Strategy Report
U.S. Government Accountability Office
U.S. Sentencing Commission

End Notes

[1] Treatment Episode Data Set (TEDS) 2004 data are the most current and comprehensive data available. However, other drug consequence data such as Drug Abuse Warning Network (DAWN) Live and local drug treatment data reported by the Community Epidemiology Work Group (CEWG) are current through middle to late 2005 and indicate a similar trend continuing in 2005.

[2] This figure includes the total cleanup cost for the entire state of Illinois.

In: Methamphetamine: Background, Controls and Issues ISBN: 978-1-60692-548-5
Editor: Andrea S. Sandoval

Chapter 4

PRESIDENTIAL DETERMINATION ON THE MAJOR METHAMPHETAMINE PRECURSOR CHEMICAL EXPORTING AND IMPORTING COUNTRIES

United States Department of State

MEMORANDUM FOR THE SECRETARY OF STATE

Subject: Presidential Determination under Section 490(b)(1)(A) of the Foreign Assistance Act Relating to the Largest Exporting and Importing Countries of Certain Precursor Chemicals

Pursuant to Section 490(b)(1)(A) of the Foreign Assistance Act, I hereby determine that the top five exporting and importing countries of pseudoephedrine and ephedrine in 2005 (Belgium, China, Germany, India, Indonesia, Mexico, Singapore, South Africa, South Korea, Switzerland, Taiwan, and the United Kingdom) have cooperated fully with the United States or have taken adequate steps on their own to achieve full compliance with the goals and objectives established by the United Nations Convention Against Illicit Traffic in Narcotic Drugs and Psychotropic Substances.

You are directed to publish this determination in the *Federal Register,* and are authorized and directed to transmit to Congress the report under Section 722 of the Combat Methamphetamine Epidemic Act.

Justification for Presidential Determination on the Major Methamphetamine Precursor Chemical Exporting and Importing Countries

Section 489(a)(8)(A)(I) and (II) of the Foreign Assistance Act of 1961 (FAA) has been amended by Section 722 of the Combat Methamphetamine Epidemic Act of 2005 (CMEA) (Title VII, P.L. 109-177) to require that the annual International Narcotics Control Strategy

Report (INSCR) include the identification of the five countries exporting the largest amount of pseudoephedrine, ephedrine, and phenylpropanolamine (including salts, optical isomers or salts of optical isomers, and also including any products or substances containing such chemicals) during calendar year 2006. Section 722 also requires the identification of the five countries importing the largest amounts of the chemicals noted above during calendar year 2006, with the highest rate of diversion of such chemicals for the illicit production of methamphetamine (either in that country or in another country). The statute requires that the identification be based on a comparison of legitimate demand for the chemicals as compared to the actual or estimated amount imported into the country.

Section 490(b) of the FAA has been amended by the CMEA and requires the President to certify that the top five exporting and importing countries have fully cooperated with the United States to prevent these substances from being used to produce methamphetamine or have taken adequate steps on their own to achieve full compliance with the 1988 United Nations Convention against Illicit Traffic in Narcotic Drugs and Psychotropic Substances. Absent a Presidential Determination, fifty percent of the foreign assistance allocated in FY 2007 for the designated countries must be withheld.

In complying with the Section 722 requirements, the Departments of State and Justice have determined that phenylpropanolomine is not a methamphetamine precursor chemical, although it can be used as an amphetamine precursor chemical. In 2000, the Food and Drug Administration issued warnings concerning significant health risks associated with phenylpropanolomine, and as a result, manufacturers voluntarily removed the chemical compound from its over-the-counter medicines. The largest U.S. producer ceased production, and today the chemicals are imported only for limited use by veterinarians. The Global Trade Atlas, the source relied upon in this chapter to determine the top five exporters and importers of ephedrine and pseudoephedrine, does not include data on the export or import of phenylpropanolomine, and no other source of reliable data has been identified. Therefore, it has not been included in this determination. Data on exports and imports of products containing pseudoephedrine and ephedrine are commercial and proprietary and are not available. Data on legitimate demand for these substances are not available at this time. Therefore, this listing of the top five importers does not necessarily demonstrate that these countries have the highest levels of diversion. A U.S. resolution adopted by the March 2006 United Nations Commission on Narcotic Drugs requested countries to provide voluntarily estimates of legitimate demand to the United Nations International Narcotics Control Board, and the estimates should be available for the 2008 determination.

The top five exporters and importers of pseudoephedrine and ephedrine have been identified using 2005 data from the commercially available Global Trade Atlas, which are the latest data available. The top five exporters of pseudoephedrine were Germany, India, China, Switzerland, and Taiwan. The top five exporters of ephedrine in 2005 were India, Germany, Singapore, China, and the United Kingdom. The top five importers of pseudoephedrine in 2005 were the United Kingdom, Mexico, South Africa, Switzerland, and Belgium. The top five importers of ephedrine in 2005 were Singapore, South Korea, Indonesia, South Africa, and the United Kingdom. For purposes of this determination, the United States has been excluded from these lists. Nevertheless, the United States was the largest importer of pseudoephedrine and ephedrine in 2005.

Data on 2005 exports and imports of pseudoephedrine and ephedrine and statements of explanation for these determinations are attached.

The rapidly changing and complex nature of the methamphetamine trafficking threat requires that U.S. government agencies cooperate closely with these countries, as well as work closely with other countries, so as to prevent harm to the health and well-being of people everywhere. Over the next year we will continue to address the threat of methamphetamine precursor chemical diversion and methamphetamine trafficking around the globe.

Certification Determinations Pursuant to the Combat Methamphetamine Epidemic Act

Top five exporters and importers of pseudoephedrine and ephedrine - 2005

Exporters (KGs)

Pseudoephedrine	**2005**
Germany	390,000
India	270,600
China	107,914
Switzerland	41,084
Taiwan	31,546
Sub-Total	**841,144**
United States	28,895
All Others	19,088
Total	**889,127**
Ephedrine	**2005**
India	217,106
Germany	51,000
Singapore	16,350
China	8,955
United Kingdom	4,000
Sub-Total	**297,411**
United States	5,542
All Others	6,083
Total	**309,036**

Importers (KGs)

Pseudoephedrine	**2005**
United Kingdom	203,000
Mexico	124,552*
South Africa	91,400

(Continued)

Pseudoephedrine	**2005**
Switzerland	67,800
Belgium	52,000
Sub-Total	**538,752**
United States	319,998
All Others	365,419
Total	**1,224,169**
Ephedrine	**2005**
Singapore	19,875
South Korea	17,550
Indonesia	16,177
South Africa	14,374
United Kingdom	14,000
Sub-Total	81,976
United States	178,657
All Others	57,274
Totals	**317,907**

Source: Global Trade Atlas (GTA), Global Trade Information Services, Inc. (www.gtis.com)

* The GTA reports Mexico's 2005 pseudoephedrine imports as 3,115,552 kilograms, of which 3,009,000 were imported from Germany. A cross-reference to Germany's reported exports to Mexico indicate that Germany exported only 18,000 kilograms to Mexico. Therefore, we have revised Mexican imports downward by 2,991,000 kilograms. The Government of Mexico has confirmed this revised data.

Statements of Explanation

Belgium

Belgium was the fifth largest non-U.S. importer of pseudoephedrine in 2005. The domestic pharmaceutical industry is the primary user, although as a trading nation, some may be resold. There is no evidence of widespread diversion to domestic methamphetamine manufacture.

The Belgians responded fully to U.S. requests for cooperation in chemical control and are generally very good at sharing information on precursor chemical matters. Belgium participates with the United States and other nations in cooperative multilateral chemical control initiatives such as Project Prism, targeting precursor chemicals used in the manufacture of synthetic drugs, including pseudoephedrine and ephedrine. During the past year, DEA's office in Brussels has cooperated with Belgian authorities on a number of investigations involving methamphetamine precursors that could have potentially impacted the U.S. drug supply.

Belgium is a party to the 1988 United Nations Convention against Illicit Traffic in Narcotic Drugs and Psychotropic Substance and is implementing its chemical control provisions.

China

China is one of the three largest manufacturers of pseudoephedrine and ephedrine; in 2005, it was the third largest exporter of pseudoephedrine and the fourth largest exporter of ephedrine. There are reports of domestic diversion that is smuggled into Burma for methamphetamine production. There are also reports of exports to Mexico that have been diverted to methamphetamine production. Exports of pharmaceutical preparations containing pseudoephedrine, which are not controlled by international conventions, have also been diverted to methamphetamine manufacture.

China fully cooperates with U.S. and Mexican initiatives to stem this diversion. In Hong Kong, Chinese authorities have agreed not to export pseudoephedrine and ephedrine and, significantly, pharmaceutical preparations containing them, to Mexico, Panama, and the United States until they receive positive responses from these countries to their pre-export notifications. They also require a positive response to pre-export notifications for all exports of bulk pseudoephedrine and ephedrine before authorizing shipments. China fully supported the negotiated text of the U.S.-drafted resolution targeting synthetic drug chemicals, including methamphetamine chemicals, at the March 2006 UN Commission on Narcotic Drugs. China is actively involved in law enforcement initiatives being developed pursuant to the International Narcotics Control Board's Projects Prism and Cohesion to strengthen chemical diversion control throughout the world, and serves as the Asia regional representative on the Project Prism Task Force.

Bilateral U.S./Chinese chemical control cooperation is excellent. DEA has Diversion Investigator positions in its Beijing and Hong Kong offices. During the past year, the DEA offices in Beijing and Hong Kong participated with Chinese authorities on a number of investigations involving methamphetamine precursors with the potential to impact the U.S. drug supply. In general, Chinese authorities are very good at sharing information on precursor chemical matters, as well as taking an aggressive stance against the potential diversion of large quantities of ephedra, a plant that can be used as a methamphetamine precursor.

China is a party to the 1988 United Nations Convention against Illicit Traffic in Narcotic Drugs and Psychotropic Substances and has chemical control laws and regulations meeting its chemical control provisions. Although committed to achieving the goals of the Convention, the size of its chemical industry is not matched by a law enforcement structure adequate to effectively monitor all its chemical production and international trade.

Germany

Germany is another of the three largest manufacturers of pseudoephedrine and ephedrine for its large licit pharmaceutical industry, and for export. In 2005, it was the largest exporter of pseudoephedrine and the third largest exporter of ephedrine.

Germany is one of the United States's closest chemical control partners, cooperating both bilaterally and multilaterally, to promote transnational chemical control initiatives. Germany was a strong supporter of the U.S. resolution targeting synthetic drug chemicals at the March 2006 Commission on Narcotic Drugs. A senior DEA Diversion Investigator from DEA's Frankfurt office is assigned to Germany's police/customs Joint Precursor Unit in Weisbaden. Germany strongly supported the international initiatives, Operation Purple and Operation Topaz, the global efforts to control the diversion of potassium permanganate and acetic anhydride, respectively. These projects are now part of the International Narcotics Control

Board's Project Cohesion. We also work together effectively in promoting Project Prism, targeting synthetic drug chemicals, and Germany is a leader in law enforcement initiatives under Project Prism.

Germany is a party to the 1988 United Nations Convention against Illicit Traffic in Narcotic Drugs and Psychotropic Substances and implements its chemicals control provisions. Its strong chemical control program is one of the most effective in meeting Convention requirements.

India

India is the third of the three largest producers of pseudoephedrine and ephedrine, both for the domestic pharmaceutical industry and for export. In 2005, it was the second largest exporter of pseudoephedrine and the largest non-U.S. exporter of ephedrine. There are reports of domestic diversion of these chemicals that are smuggled into neighboring Burma for methamphetamine manufacture.

India is a party to the 1988 United Nations Convention against Illicit Traffic in Narcotic Drugs and Psychotropic Substances, and it has the required controls on pseudoephedrine and ephedrine, although not on all 23 chemicals in the Convention. India has a system of letters of no objection for the export of pseudoephedrine and ephedrine and will not authorize exports until the receiving government approves the import.

U.S. and Indian authorities cooperate closely on letters of no objection and in other areas of chemical control. DEA has a Diversion Investigator assigned to its New Delhi office. The DEA New Delhi office cooperated with Indian authorities in the past year on a number of investigations involving methamphetamine precursors which could have potentially impacted the U.S. drug supply. Indian authorities are extremely good at sharing information on precursor control issues and frequently, in consultation with the International Narcotics Control Board and involved parties, do not allow suspect consignments of precursors to be shipped, if there are concerns regarding their legitimacy.

India fully supported the U.S.-drafted resolution targeting the diversion of synthetic drug precursors at the March 2006 UN Commission on Narcotic Drugs. It is also actively involved in law enforcement initiatives developed by the International Narcotics Control Board's Projects Prism and Cohesion to halt diversion throughout the world of precursor chemicals to illicit chemical trafficking and drug manufacturing organizations.

Indonesia

Indonesia was the third largest non-U.S. importer of ephedrine in 2005 for use by the domestic pharmaceutical industry. However, there are local methamphetamine laboratories capable of producing multi-hundred pound quantities of methamphetamine, indicating chemical diversion and/or the smuggling of precursors into the country. The methamphetamine is sold in local and regional markets. There is no firm evidence that methamphetamine manufactured in Indonesia, or chemicals transiting Indonesia, have reached the United States or Mexico.

U.S.-Indonesian chemical control cooperation is excellent, although not extensive, given the limited chemical diversion threat Indonesia poses to the United States and Mexico. DEA's office in Singapore is the primary point for counternarcotics cooperation and works well with Indonesian authorities. When requested, the Indonesians have cooperated fully with us in chemical control investigations. For example, in November 2005, the Indonesians seized a large clandestine methamphetamine laboratory in Cikande, Indonesia. Forensic scientists from DEA provided assistance in processing the precursor chemicals found in the laboratory. At present, Indonesians authorities working with DEA and other U. S. authorities, are also conducting a review of Indonesia's chemical control system and its chemical industry.

In 2005, DEA provided training in chemical diversion control to Indonesian officials, as well as several industry representatives. DEA will provide clandestine laboratory training in 2007. Indonesia is a party to the 1988 United Nations Convention against Illicit Traffic in Narcotic Drugs and Psychotropic Substances. Indonesia participates in Project Prism.

Mexico

In 2005, Mexico was the second largest non-U.S. pseudoephedrine importer. Pseudoephedrine imports serve an important pharmaceutical industry, but there is diversion to major methamphetamine laboratories. There is also false labeling of imports and probable smuggling of precursor chemicals.

The Government of Mexico (GOM) has reacted strongly to the diversion of precursors and the methamphetamine manufacture, implementing strict precursor chemical import quotas and internal chemical distribution controls. Within the last several years, Mexico has begun imposing import quotas tied to estimated legitimate national needs. A study conducted by the GOM estimated that there was an excess of imports of pseudoephedrine products of approximately 60 to 100 metric tons in 2004. The GOM reported that its efforts to control methamphetamine precursor chemicals reduced imports in 2005 by approximately 40 percent and, while a final number has yet to be determined, pseudoephedrine and ephedrine import permits are likely to be reduced to 70 metric tons in 2006. Mexican officials confirm that the 70-ton limit includes combination products containing pseudoephedrine and ephedrine.

Chemical control is one of the closest areas of U.S.-Mexican law enforcement cooperation. We are assisting the GOM as it tightens its chemical controls and Mexico is assisting the United States in preventing illicit sales of precursor chemicals or their smuggling into the United States. In addition, U.S.-Mexican cooperation in targeting methamphetamine trafficking and manufacturing organizations is at an all-time high.

Mexico is a party to the 1988 United Nations Convention against Illicit Traffic in Narcotic Drugs and Psychotropic Substances and has laws and regulations meeting its chemical control requirements. Mexico participates in Project Prism.

Singapore

Singapore was the largest non-U.S. importer of ephedrine in 2005 and the third-largest exporter. The quantities not re-exported are used primarily by the domestic pharmaceutical industry. In 2006, there was no known production of illicit narcotics or precursor chemicals in Singapore.

The country is a party to the 1988 United Nations Convention against Illicit Traffic in Narcotic Drugs and Psychotropic Substances and controls precursor chemicals, including pseudoephedrine and ephedrine, in accordance with its provisions. It will not authorize imports until it has issued a No Objection letter in response to the exporting country's pre-export notification. Pre-export notifications are issued on all exports. All transshipment cases are treated as an import followed by an export; therefore, the same procedures apply. The government conducts rigorous site visits on companies dealing with controlled chemicals to ensure awareness of the requirements and compliance with them.

Singapore participates in Project Prism and is actively involved in law enforcement initiatives developed under the project to halt worldwide diversion of precursors to illicit chemical trafficking and drug manufacturing organizations. DEA has an office in Singapore that works closely with Singapore authorities on joint investigations and precursor control issues.

South Africa

In 2005, South Africa was the third largest non-U.S. importer of pseudoephedrine and the fourth largest non-U.S importer of ephedrine. The imports are for use by the domestic pharmaceutical industry, which markets both locally and regionally. There is some methamphetamine manufactured in the country for the local market. Cape Town, where the increase in demand for treatment of methamphetamine abuse has been dramatic, is the center of consumption. With few exceptions, there is little evidence that pseudoephedrine and ephedrine imported into South Africa, or methamphetamine manufactured there, reaches the United States or Mexico.

South Africa is a party to the 1988 United Nations Convention against Illicit Traffic in Narcotic Drugs and Psychotropic Substances and has import and export controls on the 23 chemicals listed in its tables. The authorities work closely with industry in implementing the controls, and the system is considered the best in Southern Africa.

DEA has an office in Pretoria responsible for all counternarcotics matters, including chemical control. Cooperation with the South African Police and prosecutorial authorities is excellent. In the past year, DEA's Pretoria office participated with South African authorities on a number of investigations involving methamphetamine precursors with a potential to impact the U.S. drug market.

South Africa participates in Project Prism and is a member of the Project Prism Task Force, serving as the focal point for Africa. It is actively involved in chemical control operations developed under Project Prism procedures.

South Korea

In 2005, South Korea was the second largest non-U.S. importer of ephedrine. It is used by the domestic pharmaceutical industry and there have been no exports of ephedrine, pseudoephedrine, or products containing them since 2003. No clandestine laboratories have been found in South Korea since 2004.

South Korea is a party to the 1988 United Nations Convention against Illicit Traffic in Narcotic Drugs and Psychotropic Substances and complies with its chemical control provisions. The DEA Office in Seoul cooperates closely with South Korean authorities on all counternarcotics issues. This cooperation includes joint investigations regarding diversion of precursors. DEA has also worked with South Korean authorities and other regional partners on investigations targeting precursors being diverted from other parts of Southeast Asia.

In 2006, DEA held two one-week training seminars on Chemical and Precursor Diversion, co-hosted by the Korean Customs Service and the Korean Food and Drug Administration. South Korea participates in Project Prism, the voluntary multilateral operation tracking synthetic drug chemicals.

Switzerland

Switzerland is the fourth largest importer and exporter of pseudoephedrine. The imports are for both the large domestic pharmaceutical industry and for re-export. There is no evidence that pseudoephedrine is being diverted to methamphetamine manufacture.

In 2005, Switzerland ratified the 1988 United Nations Convention against Illicit Traffic in Narcotic Drugs and Psychotropic Substance and is bound by its chemical control provisions. Even before ratification it had strong controls on its international chemical commerce. This allowed it to play an active and constructive role in the U.S.-chaired G-8 Chemical Action Task Force that in the early 1990's developed procedures to assist countries as they implemented the Convention's chemical provisions. Swiss regulatory authorities are very vigilant on chemical control issues, including verifying the legitimacy of end-users.

Switzerland has become a participant in Project Prism and is actively involved in operations conducted under its auspices. The DEA office in Switzerland interacts with both regulatory and law enforcement officials on chemical control issues. Cooperation on chemical investigations is very good.

Taiwan

According to official Taiwan data and the Global Trade Atlas, Taiwan was the fifth largest exporter of pseudoephedrine. However, the data are misleading because a criminal investigation has revealed that during the period 2003-2005, a Taiwan company that had reported exports included in its trade data had actually diverted the chemical to local drug manufacturer for local consumption. Nevertheless, the data show that exports by the sixth-largest exporter were sufficiently small that Taiwan would remain the fifth largest exporter despite the falsely reported exports. The source of the pseudoephedrine exports is limited local production and imports.

DEA cooperates with Taiwan authorities on the full range of counternarcotics issues, and has excellent working relationships with all law enforcement and regulatory agencies involved in precursor control. U.S. and Taiwan authorities have cooperated and continue to cooperate in joint precursor investigations. In 2006, DEA provided in-service training, including chemical control training, to over one hundred Taiwan law enforcement officers.

Taiwan is not a member of the United Nations and, therefore, cannot be a party to the 1988 United Nations Convention against Illicit Traffic in Narcotic Drugs and Psychotropic Substances. Nevertheless, Taiwan authorities have amended and passed legislation consistent with the goals and objectives of the Convention. This includes forwarding pre- export notifications to the United States regarding precursor shipments. Taiwan cannot participate in Project Prism because it is a UN-run project. In 2006, the Executive Yuan Anti-Drug Council identified international counternarcotics cooperation and chemical controls as one of the four major areas of its anti-drug policy.

United Kingdom

In 2005, the United Kingdom was the largest non-U.S. importer of pseudoephedrine, the fifth largest importer of ephedrine, and the fifth largest non-U.S. exporter of ephedrine. Most of the imports are for a large pharmaceutical industry. Methamphetamine is growing in notoriety and use, and several small methamphetamine laboratories have been seized. Recognizing the dangers of this substance, in January 2007, methamphetamine was reclassified by British authorities as a Class A drug, bringing it in line with other drugs such as heroin and cocaine. Prior to the reclassification, methamphetamine was a Class B drug.

The United Kingdom is a party to the 1988 United Nations Convention against Illicit Traffic in Narcotic Drugs and Psychotropic Substances and effectively enforces laws and regulations in accordance with its chemical control provisions.

The United Kingdom is a close partner with the United States in chemical control, both bilaterally and multilaterally. British law enforcement agencies are regularly involved in a wide range of precursor chemical investigations, some of which have led to law enforcement success in the United States as well.

The British have been very active with the United States and others in the design and implementation of Project Prism, and support and participate in chemical initiatives developed under its auspices.

In: Methamphetamine: Background, Controls and Issues
Editor: Andrea S. Sandoval
ISBN: 978-1-60692-548-5

Chapter 5

PUSHING BACK AGAINST METH: A PROGRESS REPORT ON THE FIGHT AGAINST METHAMPHETAMINE IN THE U.S.

Office of National Drug Control Policy

SUMMARY OF FINDINGS

This chapter highlights good news for America: a nationwide drop in methamphetamine laboratory incidents. This is a pattern observed, to varying degrees, in nearly every State. In 2004, there were approximately 17,750 methamphetamine laboratory incident seizures by law enforcement in the United States. In 2005, this number was 12,500 – a decline of more than 30%. Although 2006 numbers are not yet final, early 2006 data suggests that the decline is continuing at about the same pace.

The primary reason for this positive trend is the enactment of various State laws, starting with Oklahoma in April 2004, which implemented restrictions on transactions involving products containing certain chemicals (primarily, ephedrine and pseudoephedrine) that can be used to make methamphetamine. By early 2006, more than 40 States had implemented some type of new restriction on retail transactions involving these products. Then, on September 30, 2006, the Combat Methamphetamine Epidemic Act of 2005 (CMEA) went fully into effect. The law set a nationwide baseline standard for how to legally sell these products, which include some popular over-the-counter cold medications.

Although the CMEA is effective nationwide, the State laws, which vary widely in content, are concurrently in effect. The most notable provisions of the Federal law are also addressed by many of the State laws: where products containing these chemicals can be sold, how and where the products must be stored, what amount may be purchased or sold in a single transaction or in a month, and whether purchasers must show identification and sign a logbook. If the State law is less strict than the Federal CMEA on a certain issue, then compliance with the State provision is insufficient, and the Federal law, as a practical matter, is controlling. Conversely, if the State law is stricter on a certain issue than the Federal CMEA, then the State law, as a practical matter, is the controlling standard on that point. (In both cases, of course, retailers and others subject to the laws must show compliance with both.) Unsurprisingly, some States are a hybrid of the two situations, with the State law more lenient in some respects and stricter in others.

This chapter attempts to describe the various restrictions in all 50 States and compare them to the Federal CMEA standard implemented in September 2006.[1] It is not intended as a legal guide, and should not be used by retailers or others to gauge their own compliance. This chapter attempts to measure the impact of the various State laws in light of the declines in methamphetamine production in the State, and it also notes changes in positive drug tests for amphetamine in the workplace. In some States, enactment of the law was followed by a swift and sudden decline in methamphetamine laboratory incidents – sometimes, by as much as 75% or more. In some other States, however, the decline was less dramatic. This chapter may be helpful to State policymakers interested in understanding the effect of various types of restrictions on the sale of these chemicals, or in considering further restrictions at the State level.

A Note About Methodology

In reviewing the number of methamphetamine laboratory incidents, this chapter relies on the Drug Enforcement Administration's Clandestine Laboratory Seizure System (CLSS). State and local law enforcement agencies report their methamphetamine laboratory incident seizures to CLSS, and these typically become reliable six months after the month measured, meaning that for most States, data is only available through April 2006. However, some States centrally track their own data, and where available, these numbers – which may be as recent as October 2006 – were used.

The implementation dates of the various State laws range from April 2004 (Oklahoma) to November 2006 (South Carolina). States for which three or fewer months of data are available were generally listed as "data not yet available."

This chapter intentionally omits discussion of special exemptions to State laws. For example, some State laws apply to all products containing pseudoephedrine except those in liquid or gelatin capsule form; other State laws exempt certain pediatric products. Instead of listing each of these exemptions, interested parties are urged to carefully review the actual State law or consult an attorney.

This chapter is a State-by-State analysis of national-level data. The quality of State-level information is contingent upon the data provided by each State.

The report sought to utilize the most reliable and recent information available regarding State laws, methamphetamine laboratory incident seizures and positive workplace tests for amphetamines. The Administration welcomes input or information from State officials in possession of more timely information concerning State laws, methamphetamine laboratory incident seizures or other relevant data. Contact information is available at www.methresources.gov/ContactUs.aspx.

UNITED STATES: THE COMBAT METHAMPHETAMINE EPIDEMIC ACT OF 2005

Summary

The Combat Methamphetamine Epidemic Act of 2005 (CMEA) went into effect in two stages. First, on April 8th , 2006, purchase limits, mail order restrictions and blister-pack requirements went into effect. Since April 8th , there has been a nationwide sales limit of 3.6 grams of products containing pseudoephedrine or ephedrine within a 24-hour period, and a 30-day purchase limit of 9 grams. Additionally, all non-liquid forms of the product are required to be in blister packs or similar packaging.

On September 30th , the rest of CMEA, including the product placement and identification/logbook requirements, went into effect. These provisions require that all single-entity and multi-active products containing any of those three chemicals – called "listed chemicals" in the bill – be kept behind a store counter or in a locked cabinet. The CMEA does not restrict the sale of products containing listed chemicals to pharmacies, and does not classify these chemicals as Schedule V controlled substances. The CMEA requires purchasers of products containing listed chemicals to provide photo identification, and to sign a logbook with information about the purchase.

FEDERAL STANDARD: THE UNITED STATES COMBAT METHAMPHETAMINE ACT

Effective Dates:	4/8/2006 9/30/2006
Sales locations limited to pharmacies?	No
Behind the counter/locked cabinet?	Yes
All listed chemicals*?	Yes
Daily sales limit:	3.6 g
30-day purchase limit:	9
Identification/logbook requirement?	Yes

* "Listed chemicals" means any product containing ephedrine (EPH), pseudoephedrine (PSE), or phenylpropanolamine (PPA).

State	Amph Positives,	2000 (Jan-(Jan-May) Quest Amph Positives, 2001	Quest Amph Positives, 2002 (Jan-May)	Quest Amph Positives, 2003 (Jan-May)	Quest Amph Positives, 2004 (Jan-May)	Quest Amph Positives, 2005 (Jan-May)	Quest Amph Positives, 2006 (Jan-May)	% Change 2005-2006
National	0.25%	0.29%	0.32%	0.35%	0.41%	0.48%	0.42%	-12.40%

Nationwide Data Round-up

Nationally, monthly methamphetamine laboratory incidents have been decreasing since reaching a high of 2,049 in March 2004. In 2004 there were about 17,750 methamphetamine laboratory incidents, compared to approximately 12,500 incidents in 2005 – a drop of more than 30%. In the first four months of 2006 – the most recent period of time for which this data is available – there were 3,160 methamphetamine laboratory incidents reported, compared to 6,472 and 7,208 in the same time period in 2005 and 2004, respectively. This represents a 51.1% decline from 2005 and 56.1% decline from 2004, although late data entries will probably increase final tallies of laboratory incidents by a small number. It is important to note that the CMEA became fully effective on September 30th, 2006, and therefore the nationwide decline in methamphetamine laboratory incidents is due to the various State laws on which the CMEA is based, not the CMEA itself. Additionally, workplace drug testing results showed a 12.4% decrease in positive tests for amphetamine, measuring the first five months in 2006, compared to the same period one year earlier.

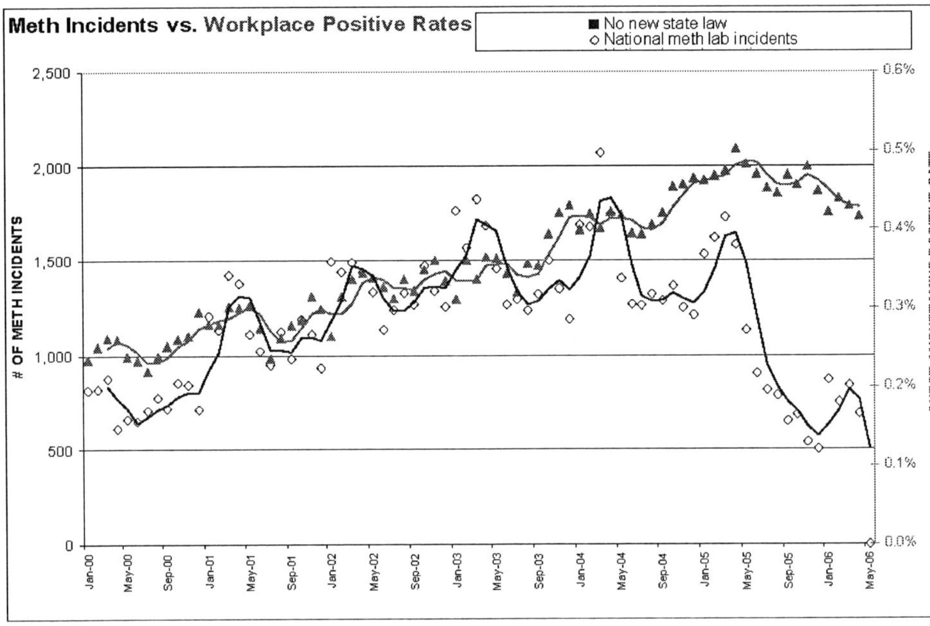

ALABAMA

62% decline in meth lab incidentspositive amphetamine workplace tests: +3.6%

Federal Standard: The United States Combat Methamphetamine Act		**Alabama State Law: Less strict than Federal standard**	
Effective Dates:	4/8/2006	Effective Date:	July 1, 2005
	9/30/2006	Meth lab reduction:	62%
Sales locations limited to pharmacies?	**No**	**Sales locations limited to pharmacies?**	**No**
Behind the counter/locked cabinet?	**Yes**	**Behind the counter/locked cabinet?**	**Yes**
All listed chemicals?	**Yes**	*All listed chemicals?*	*PSE, EPH*
Daily sales limits:	**3.6 g**	*Transaction limit:*	*2 pkg/6 g*
30-day purchase limit:	**9 g**	*30-day purchase limit:*	--
Identification/logbook requirement?	**Yes**	**Identification/logbook requirement?**	**Yes**

"Listed chemicals" means any product containing ephedrine (EPH), pseudoephedrine (PSE), or phenylpropanolamine (PPA). Items in bold indicate the controlling standard in the state. Items in *italics* indicate that the provision is trumped by a stricter standard.

Summary

Alabama's methamphetamine precursor law took effect on July 1st, 2005, except for the registration requirement, which was effective on October 1, 2005.

Alabama's law covers all products containing pseudoephedrine or ephedrine, and has purchase limits that are less strict than the CMEA. In a single sale, 2 packages or 6 grams can be sold – less strict than the CMEA. Although Alabama has a 6 gram purchase limit per month, this is only activated with the "intent to manufacture methamphetamine," and is thus not a universal limit. Products in which the sole ingredient is pseudoephedrine or ephedrine can only be sold in blister packs.

Alabama does not limit sales of products containing methamphetamine precursor chemicals like pseudoephedrine to pharmacies, and does not classify products containing those chemicals as Schedule V drugs under the State scheduling scheme. Like the CMEA, Alabama has an identification and logbook requirement. Sole ingredient products must be kept behind the store counter or in a locked container; multi-active products can be kept under video surveillance (although the CMEA is stricter on this point).

State	Quest Amph Positives, 2000 (Jan-May)	Quest Amph Positives, 2001 (Jan-May)	Quest Amph Positives, 2002 (Jan-May)	Quest Amph Positives, 2003 (Jan-May)	Quest Amph Positives, 2004 (Jan-May)	Quest Amph Positives, 2005 (Jan-May)	Quest Amph Positives, 2006 (Jan-May)	% Change 2005-2006
AL	0.33%	0.34%	0.38%	0.41%	0.52%	0.50%	0.51%	3.63%

Note: On October 1, 2009, no product containing ephedrine or pseudoephedrine may be sold, unless the product is made with "lock technology" to prevent conversion into methamphetamine.

Alabama Data Round-up

In Alabama, methamphetamine laboratory incidents declined just over 62% in the period from July 1st, 2005, to April 30, 2006 (98 incidents), compared to the year before (260 incidents). Workplace drug testing results showed a 3.63% increase in positive tests for amphetamine, measuring the first five months in 2006, compared to the same period one year earlier.

ALASKA

Meth lab incident data not available positive amphetamine workplace tests: -46.9%

Federal Standard: The United States Combat Methamphetamine Act		**Alaska State Law: Slightly stricter than Federal standard.**	
Effective Dates:	4/8/2006	*Effective Date:*	June 6, 2006
	9/30/2006	Meth lab reduction:	unavailable
Sales locations limited to pharmacies?	No	**Sales locations limited to pharmacies?**	**No**
Behind the counter/locked cabinet?	**Yes**	**Behind the counter/locked cabinet?**	**Yes**
All listed chemicals?	**Yes**	**All listed chemicals?**	**Yes**
Daily sales limits:	**3.6 g**	**Daily sales limits:**	**3.6 g**
30-day purchase limit:	*9 g*	**30-day purchase limit:**	**6 g**
Identification/logbook requirement?	Yes	**Identification/logbook requirement?**	**Yes**

"Listed chemicals" means any product containing ephedrine (EPH), pseudoephedrine (PSE), or phenylpropanolamine (PPA). Items in bold indicate the controlling standard in the state. Items in italics indicate that the provision is trumped by a stricter standard.

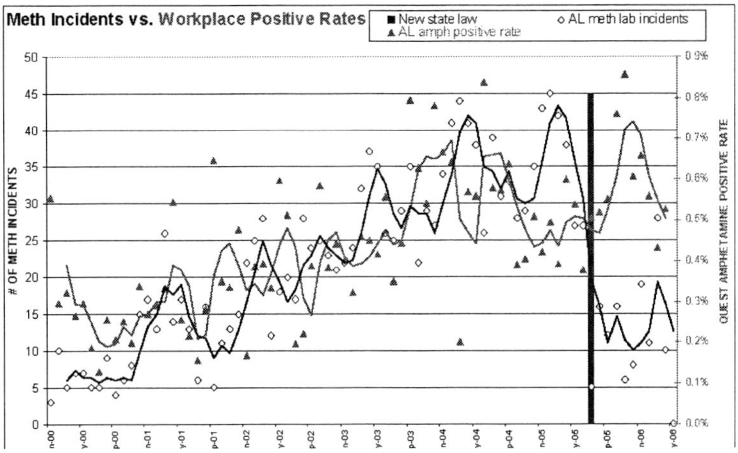

Summary

Alaska's precursor laws took effect on June 6th, 2006. Alaska's legislation basically incorporated the CMEA by reference, and without significant difference between the two, the Federal CMEA is the controlling standard in Alaska. One area in which Alaska's law is stricter is the 6 gram monthly purchase limit on pseudoephedrine.

Alaska does not limit sales of products containing methamphetamine precursor chemicals like pseudoephedrine to pharmacies, and does not classify products containing those chemicals as Schedule V drugs under the State scheduling scheme.

State	Quest Amph Positives, 2000 (Jan-May)	Quest Amph Positives, 2001 (Jan-May)	Quest Amph Positives, 2002 (Jan-May)	Quest Amph Positives, 2003 (Jan-May)	Quest Amph Positives, 2004 (Jan-May)	Quest Amph Positives, 2005 (Jan-May)	Quest Amph Positives, 2006 (Jan-May)	% Change 2005-2006
AK	0.18%	0.07%	0.25%	0.19%	0.33%	0.47%	0.25%	-46.93%

Alaska Data Round-up

Alaska's precursor legislation became effective in June 2006, and is too new to measure any change resulting from the new law. Over the last few years, 167 laboratory incidents were reported to the DEA. Workplace drug testing results showed a 46.9% decrease in positive tests for amphetamine, measuring the first five months in 2006, compared to the same period one year earlier.

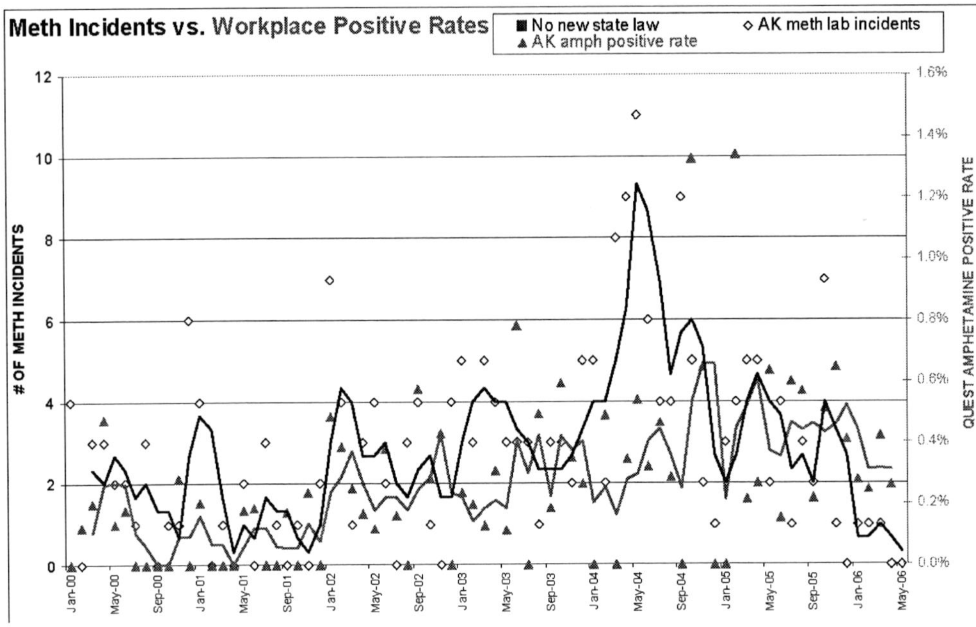

ARIZONA

70% decline in meth lab incidents positive amphetamine workplace tests: -3.5%

Federal Standard: The United States Combat Methamphetamine Act		Arizona State Law: Less strict than Federal standard	
Effective Dates:	4/8/2006 9/30/2006	*Effective Date:* October 31, 2005 Meth lab reduction: 70%	
Sales locations limited to pharmacies?	**No**	**Sales locations limited to pharmacies?**	**No**
Behind the counter/locked cabinet?	**Yes**	**Behind the counter/locked cabinet?**	**Yes**
All listed chemicals?	**Yes**	**All listed chemicals?**	**Yes**
Daily sales limits:	**3.6 g**	*Transaction limit:*	*3 pkg/9 g*
30-day purchase limit:	**9 g**	*30-day purchase limit:*	*n/a*
Identification/logbook requirement?	**Yes**	*Identification/logbook requirement?*	*No*

"Listed chemicals" means any product containing ephedrine (EPH), pseudoephedrine (PSE), or phenylpropanolamine (PPA). Items in bold indicate the controlling standard in the state. Items in *italics* indicate that the provision is trumped by a stricter standard.

Summary

Arizona's methamphetamine precursor law went into effect on October 31st; 2005. The Arizona law is less strict than the CMEA, meaning that the CMEA standard is controlling in Arizona in most respects.

Before the CMEA went into effect, under Arizona's law, all products containing pseudoephedrine, ephedrine or phenylpropanolamine were required to be kept behind a store counter or in a locked cabinet. There was a 9 gram limit on daily purchases and no limit on monthly purchases. There was no identification and logbook requirement in Arizona.

Arizona does not limit sales of products containing methamphetamine precursor chemicals like pseudoephedrine to pharmacies, and does not classify products containing those chemicals as Schedule V drugs under the State scheduling scheme.

State	Quest Amph Positives, 2000 (Jan-May)	Quest Amph Positives, 2001 (Jan-May)	Quest Amph Positives, 2002 (Jan-May)	Quest Amph Positives, 2003 (Jan-May)	Quest Amph Positives, 2004 (Jan-May)	Quest Amph Positives, 2005 (Jan-May)	Quest Amph Positives, 2006 (Jan-May)	% Change 2005-2006
AZ	0.60%	0.50%	0.64%	0.68%	0.64%	0.81%	0.78%	-3.53%

Arizona Data Roundup

In Arizona, methamphetamine laboratory incidents declined 70% after the State law was implemented, with 18 methamphetamine laboratory incidents reported to DEA for the period from October 31st, 2005, to April 30th , 2006, compared to 61 incidents the same period on year earlier. Workplace drug testing results showed a 3.5% decrease in positive tests for amphetamine, measuring the first five months in 2006, compared to the same period one year earlier.

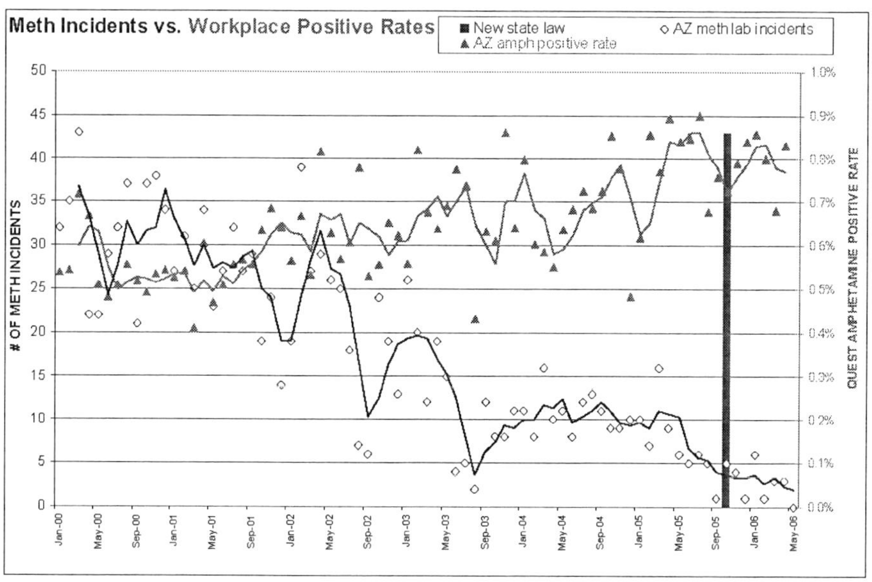

ARKANSAS

48% decline in meth lab incidents positive amphetamine workplace tests: -37.9%

Federal Standard: The United States Combat Methamphetamine Act		**Arkansas State Law: Stricter than the Federal standard**	
Effective Dates:	4/8/2006 9/30/2006	*Effective Date:* Meth lab reduction:	March 20, 2005 48%
Sales locations limited to pharmacies?	*No*	**Sales locations limited to pharmacies?**	**Yes**
Behind the counter/locked cabinet?	**Yes**	**Behind the counter/locked cabinet?**	**Yes**
All listed chemicals?	**Yes**	**All listed chemicals?**	**Yes**
Daily sales limits:	*3.6 g*	**Transaction limit:**	**3 g**
30-day purchase limit:	*9 g*	**30-day purchase limit:**	**5g EPH/9g PSE**
Identification/logbook requirement?	**Yes**	**Identification/logbook requirement?**	**Yes**

"Listed chemicals" means any product containing ephedrine (EPH), pseudoephedrine (PSE), or phenylpropanolamine (PPA). Items in bold indicate the controlling standard in the state. Items in *italics* indicate that the provision is trumped by a stricter standard.

Summary

Arkansas' methamphetamine precursor law went into effect March 20, 2005. Arkansas's legislation is stricter than the CMEA.

Products containing pseudoephedrine, ephedrine, or phenylpropanolamine are classified as Schedule V drugs under the State's scheduling scheme. Arkansas limits the sales of products containing pseudoephedrine to pharmacies, and single-entity and multi-active ingredient products must be kept behind the pharmacy counter. There is a 5 gram monthly purchase limit on ephedrine sales. There is also a 9 gram monthly purchase limit on pseudoephedrine, as in the CMEA. Arkansas has an identification and logbook requirement.

State	Quest Amph Positives, 2000 (Jan-May)	Quest Amph Positives, 2001 (Jan-May)	Quest Amph Positives, 2002 (Jan-May)	Quest Amph Positives, 2003 (Jan-May)	Quest Amph Positives, 2004 (Jan-May)	Quest Amph Positives, 2005 (Jan-May)	Quest Amph Positives, 2006 (Jan-May)	% Change 2005-2006
AR	0.48%	0.65%	0.65%	0.78%	0.92%	0.98%	0.61%	-37.92%

Arkansas Data Roundup

In Arkansas, methamphetamine laboratory incidents declined 48% after the law was implemented, with 364 incidents reported to DEA for the period from April 1, 2005 to March 31, 2006, compared to 706 incidents in the same period one year earlier. Workplace drug testing results showed a 37.9% decrease in positive tests for amphetamine, measuring the first five months in 2006, compared to the same period one year earlier.

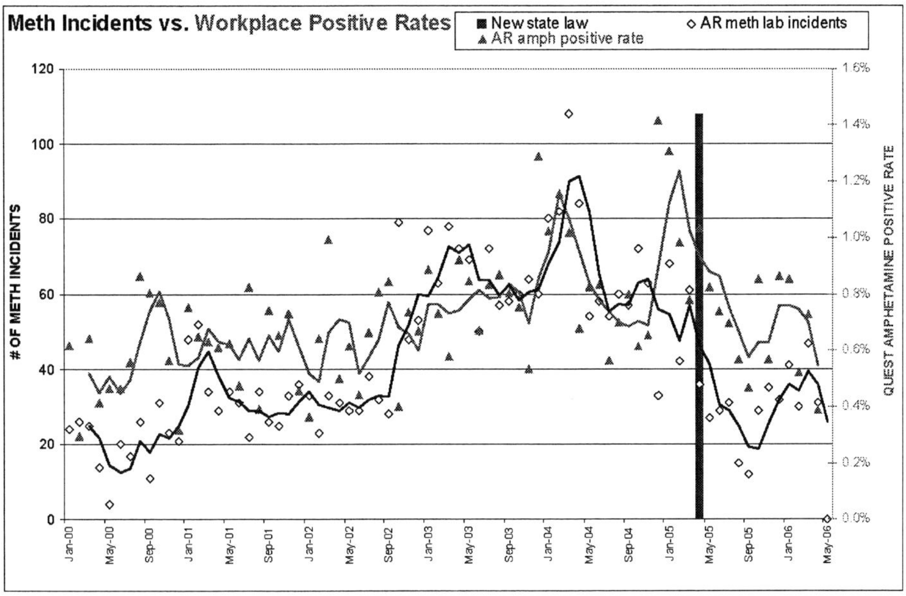

CALIFORNIA

44% decline in meth lab incidents positive amphetamine workplace tests: -25%

Federal Standard: The United States Combat Methamphetamine Act		**California State Law: Less strict than Federal standard**	
Effective Dates:	4/8/2006	*Effective Date:*	October 4, 2005
	9/30/2006	Meth lab reduction:	44%
Sales locations limited to pharmacies?	**No**	**Sales locations limited to pharmacies?**	**No**
Behind the counter/locked cabinet?	**Yes**	**Behind the counter/locked cabinet?**	**Yes**
All listed chemicals?	**Yes**	**All listed chemicals?**	**Yes**
Daily sales limits:	*3.6 g*	*Daily sales limits:*	*3 pkg/9 g*
30-day purchase limit:	*9 g*	*30-day purchase limit:*	--
Identification/logbook requirement?	Yes	**Identification/logbook requirement?**	**Yes**

"Listed chemicals"means any productcontaining ephedrine (EPH), pseudoephedrine (PSE), or phenylpropanolamine (PPA).Items in bold indicate the controlling standard in the state. Items in *italics* indicatethat the provision is trumped by a stricter standard.

Summary

California's methamphetamine precursor law went into effect October 4th 2005.The California Law is less strict than the CMEA, meaning that the CMEA standard is now the *de facto* California standard.

Prior to the effective dates of the CMEA, under California law, precursor chemicals were not required to be placed behind the counter or in a locked cabinet. The law placed a 3 package (9 gram) limit on daily purchases, with no limit on monthly purchases. California law contains an identification and logbook requirement and covers both single-ingredient and multi-active products containing listed chemicals.

California does not limit sales of products containing methamphetamine precursor chemicals like pseudoephedrine to pharmacies, and does not classify products containing those chemicals as Schedule V drugs under the State scheduling scheme.

State	Quest Amph Positives, 2000 (Jan-May)	Quest Amph Positives, 2001 (Jan-May)	Quest Amph Positives, 2002 (Jan-May)	Quest Amph Positives, 2003 (Jan-May)	Quest Amph Positives, 2004 (Jan-May)	Quest Amph Positives, 2005 (Jan-May)	Quest Amph Positives, 2006 (Jan-May)	% Change 2005-2006
CA	0.70%	0.71%	0.79%	0.81%	0.88%	0.89%	0.66%	-25.07%

California Data Roundup:

In California, methamphetamine laboratory incident seizures declined by 44% after the law went into effect, with 198 incidents reported to DEA for the period from October 4, 2005, to April 30, 2006, compared to 355 incidents in the same period one year earlier. Workplace drug testing results showed a 25% decrease in positive tests for amphetamine, measuring the first five months in 2006, compared to the same period one year earlier.

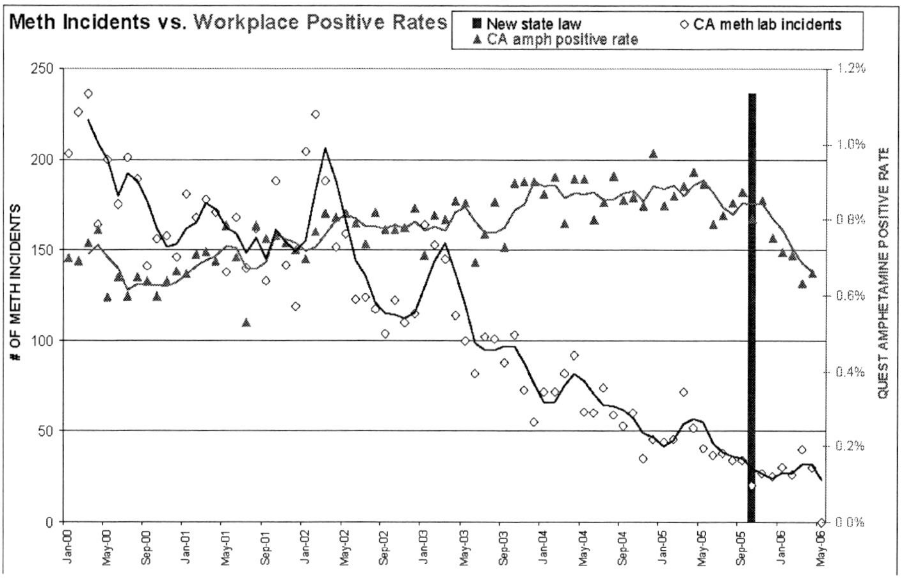

Colorado

50% decline in meth lab incidents positive amphetamine workplace tests: -29.3%

Federal Standard: The United States Combat Methamphetamine Act		**Colorado State Law: Less strict than Federal Standard**	
Effective Dates:	4/8/2006 9/30/2006	*Effective Date:* Meth lab reduction:	July 1, 2005 50%
Sales locations limited to pharmacies?	**No**	**Sales locations limited to pharmacies?**	**No**
Behind the counter/locked cabinet?	**Yes**	*Behind the counter/locked cabinet?*	*No*
All listed chemicals?	**Yes**	*All listed chemicals?*	*No*
Daily sales limits:	**3.6 g**	*Transaction limit:*	*3 pkg*
30-day purchase limit:	**9 g**	*30-day purchase limit:*	*None*
Identification/logbook requirement?	Yes	*Identification/logbook requirement?*	*No*

"Listed chemicals" means any productcontaining ephedrine (EPH), pseudoephedrine (PSE), or phenylpropanolamine (PPA).Items in bold indicatethe controlling standard in the state. Items in *italics* indicatethat the provision is trumped by a stricter standard.

Summary

Colorado's methamphetamine precursor law went into effect in two stages: on July 1st 2005, and again one year later, on July 1, 2006.The Colorado Law is less strict than the CMEA, making CMEA the *de facto* applicable standard in Colorado on most points.

After July 1st , 2005, retail sales were limited to three packages per sale. Since July 1st , 2006, there has been a 3.6 gram sales limit per person within a 24-hour period, virtually identical to CMEA's standard. The law's first iteration – the one that went into effect on July 1st , 2005 – did not require that methamphetamine precursors be placed behind the counter or in a locked cabinet. The July 1st , 2006 changes required products to be stored or displayed in an area of the store where the public is not allowed access, functionally the same as the CMEA standard.

Before July 1st , 2006, there was no identification or logbook requirement in Colorado (these requirements exist under both the existing State law and Federal CMEA). Colorado does not limit sales of products containing methamphetamine precursor chemicals like pseudoephedrine to pharmacies, and does not classify products containing those chemicals as Schedule V drugs under the State scheduling scheme.

State	Quest Amph Positives, 2000 (Ja n-Ma y)	Quest Amph Positives, 2001 (Jan-May)	Quest Amph Positives, 2002 (Jan-May)	Quest Amph Positives, 2003 (Jan-May)	Quest Amph Positives, 2004 (Jan-May)	Quest Amph Positives, 2005 (Jan-May)	Quest Amph Positives, 2006 (Ja n-Ma y)	% Change 2005-2006
CO	0.33%	0.26%	0.32%	0.31%	0.35%	0.52%	0.37%	-29.31%

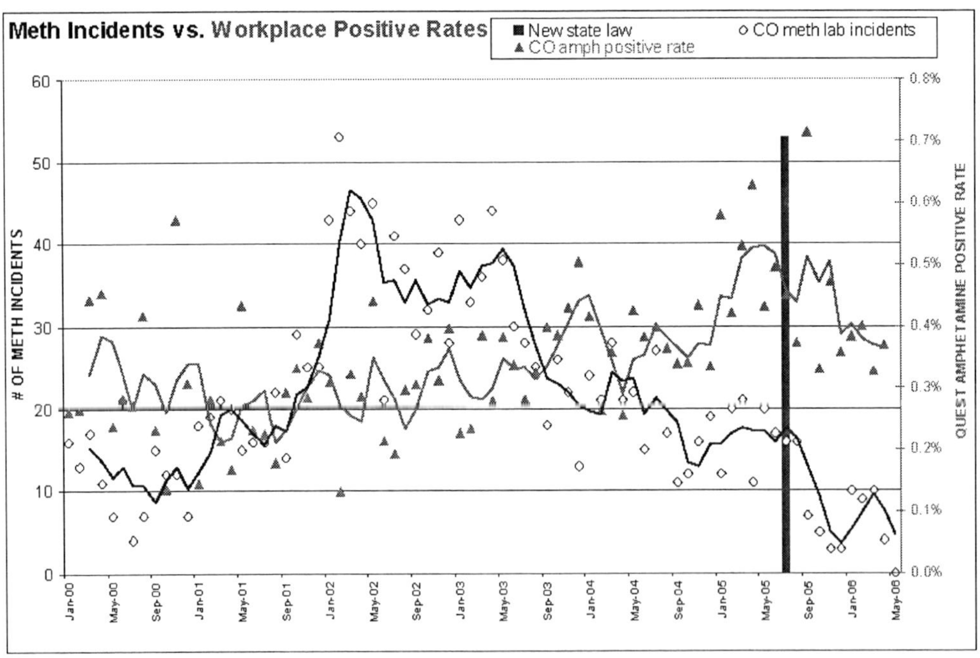

Colorado Data Roundup

The second stage of Colorado's methamphetamine precursor law went into effect in July 2006, so it is too soon to measure the impact of the law's second iteration. After the first iteration of the law went into effect on July 1st, 2005, methamphetamine laboratory incident seizures declined 50% in Colorado, with 83 incidents reported in the period from July 1st, 2005, to April 30th, 2006, compared to 166 incidents over the same period one year earlier. Workplace drug testing results showed a 29.3% decrease in positive tests for amphetamine, measuring the first five months in 2006, compared to the same period one year earlier.

CONNECTICUT

no state law/historically low lab numbers positive amphetamine workplace tests: +35.2%

Federal Standard: The United States Combat Methamphetamine Act		**Connecticut State Law: Less strict than Federal standard**	
Effective Dates:	4/8/2006 9/30/2006	*Effective Date:*	None
		Meth lab reduction:	n/a
Sales locations limited to pharmacies?	**No**	*Sales locations limited to pharmacies?*	*No*
Behind the counter/locked cabinet?	**Yes**	*Behind the counter/locked cabinet?*	*No*
All listed chemicals?	**Yes**	*All listed chemicals?*	*No*
Daily sales limits:	**3.6 g**	*Daily sales limits:*	*None*
30-day purchase limit:	**9 g**	*30-day purchase limit:*	*None*
Identification/logbook requirement?	Yes	*Identification/logbook requirement?*	*No*

"Listed chemicals" means any productcontaining ephedrine (EPH), pseudoephedrine (PSE), or phenylpropanolamine (PPA).Items in bold indicatethe controlling standard in the state. Items in *italics* indicatethat the provision is trumped by a stricter standard.

Summary

Connecticut, which has enjoyed low numbers of methamphetamine laboratory incidents, did not implement any methamphetamine precursor controls before the Combat Meth Act took effect September 30th 2006. In other words, the CMEA is the controlling standard in Connecticut. It also means that Connecticut does not limit sales of products containing methamphetamine precursors like pseudoephedrine to pharmacies, and does not classify these products as Schedule V drugs under the State's scheduling scheme.

Connecticut Data Roundup

Since January of 2000, Connecticut has only reported five methamphetamine laboratory incident seizures. Workplace drug testing results showed 35.2% increase in positive tests for amphetamine, measuring the first five months in 2006, compared to the same period one year earlier.

State	Quest Amph Positives, 2000 (Ja n-Ma y)	Quest Amph Positives, 2001 (Jan-May)	Quest Amph Positives, 2002 (Jan-May)	Quest Amph Positives, 2003 (Jan-May)	Quest Amph Positives, 2004 (Jan-May)	Quest Amph Positives, 2005 (Jan-May)	Quest Amph Positives, 2006 (Ja n-Ma y)	% Change 2005-2006
CT	0.10%	0.07%	0.14%	0.17%	0.20%	0.17%	0.23%	35.23%

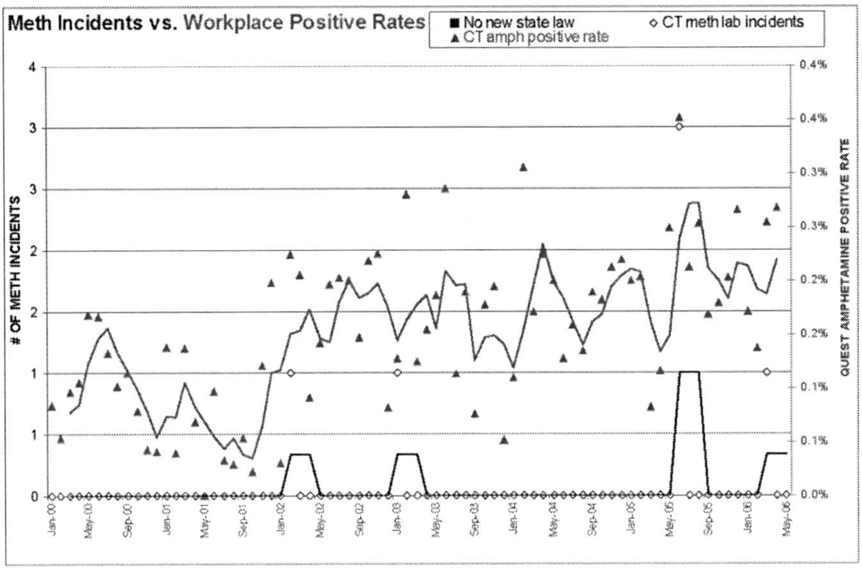

DELAWARE

n/a (see Data Round-up) positive amphetamine workplace tests: +7.5%

Federal Standard: The United States Combat Methamphetamine Act		**Delaware State Law: Similar to Federal standard**	
Effective Dates:	4/8/2006 9/30/2006	*Effective Date:* Meth lab reduction:	October 1, 2005 100%*
Sales locations limited to pharmacies?	**No**	**Sales locations limited to pharmacies?**	**No**
Behind the counter/locked cabinet?	**Yes**	**Behind the counter/locked cabinet?**	**Yes**
All listed chemicals?	**Yes**	*All listed chemicals?*	*EPH, PSE*
Daily sales limits:	**3.6 g**	*Daily sales limits:*	*None*
30-day purchase limit:	**9 g**	**30-day saleslimit:**	**9 g**
Identification/logbook requirement?	Yes	**Identification/logbook requirement?**	**Yes**

"Listed chemicals" means any productcontaining ephedrine (EPH), pseudoephedrine (PSE), or phenylpropanolamine (PPA).Items in bold indicatethe controlling standard in the state. Items in *italics* indicatethat the provision is trumped by a stricter standard.

Summary

Delaware's state methamphetamine law took effect on October 1st , 2005. Delaware's precursor restrictions are barely stricter than the CMEA, although most standards in Delaware are identical to the CMEA. Functionally, the CMEA standard applies in Delaware.

There is a 30-day sales limit of 9 grams in Delaware – the same as the CMEA. State law does not contain a daily sales limit, so the CMEA's 3.6 gram limit applies. State law contains an identification and logbook requirement.

State	Quest Amph Positives, 2000 (Ja n-Ma y)	Quest Amph Positives, 2001 (Jan-May)	Quest Amph Positives, 2002 (Jan-May)	Quest Amph Positives, 2003 (Jan-May)	Quest Amph Positives, 2004 (Jan-May)	Quest Amph Positives, 2005 (Jan-May)	Quest Amph Positives, 2006 (Ja n-Ma y)	% Change 2005-2006
DE	0.19%	0.29%	0.24%	0.35%	0.40%	0.42%	0.45%	7.47%

What makes Delaware barely stricter than the CMEA standard is the fact that although Delaware law does not expressly limit the sales of products containing these chemicals to pharmacies, the identification must be checked by a licensed pharmacist, sales clerk, or pharmacy technician. Products containing pseudoephedrine or ephedrine must be kept behind a checkout counter, pharmacy counter, or locked storage container. The State does not limit sales of products containing methamphetamine precursor chemicals like pseudoephedrine to pharmacies, and does not classify products containing those chemicals as Schedule V drugs under the State scheduling scheme.

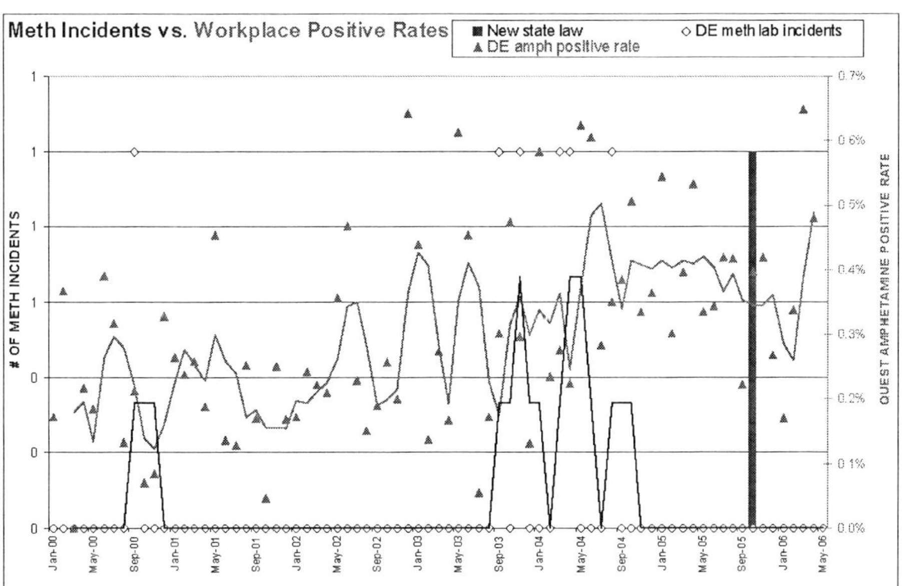

Delaware Data Roundup

In Delaware, only four methamphetamine laboratory incident seizures have been reported to DEA over the last few years. None of these have occurred since the State law was implemented on October 1st, 2005. Workplace drug testing results showed a 7.5% increase in positive tests for amphetamine, measuring the first five months in 2006, compared to the same period one year earlier.

FLORIDA

22% decline in meth lab incidents positive amphetamine workplace tests: -.06%

Federal Standard: The United States Combat Methamphetamine Act		Florida State Law: Less Strict than Federal Standard	
Effective Dates:	4/8/2006 9/30/2006	*Effective Date:* Meth lab reduction:	July 1, 2005 22%
Sales locations limited to pharmacies?	**No**	**Sales locations limited to pharmacies?**	**No**
Behind the counter/locked cabinet?	**Yes**	**Behind the counter/locked cabinet?**	**Yes**
All listed chemicals?	**Yes**	*All listed chemicals?*	*all single-entity*
Daily sales limits:	**3.6 g**	*Daily sales limits:*	*3 pkg/9 g*
30-day purchase limit:	**9 g**	*30-day purchase limit:*	--
Identification/logbook requirement?	**Yes**	*Identification/logbook requirement?*	*No*

"Listed chemicals" means any productcontaining ephedrine (EPH), pseudoephedrine (PSE), or phenylpropanolamine (PPA).Items in bold indicatethe controlling standard in the state. Items in *italics* indicatethat the provision is trumped by a stricter standard.

Summary

Florida's methamphetamine precursor law went into effect July 1st 2005. The Florida Law is less strict than the CMEA, meaning that the CMEA is the controlling standard in Florida.

Florida's law limits sales of products containing only ephedrine, pseudoephedrine, or phenylpropanolamine (meaning, single-ingredient but not multi-active products) to 9 grams or 3 packages. It also requires these products to be kept behind store counters. Florida law does not contain an identification or logbook requirement (although the Federal CMEA has now imposed this standard nationwide).

State	Quest Amph Positives, 2000 (Ja n-Ma y)	Quest Amph Positives, 2001 (Jan-May)	Quest Amph Positives, 2002 (Jan-May)	Quest Amph Positives, 2003 (Jan-May)	Quest Amph Positives, 2004 (Jan-May)	Quest Amph Positives, 2005 (Jan-May)	Quest Amph Positives, 2006 (Ja n-Ma y)	% Change 2005-2006
FL	0.12%	0.14%	0.15%	0.18%	0.18%	0.24%	0.24%	-0.61%

Florida does not limit sales of products containing methamphetamine precursor chemicals like pseudoephedrine to pharmacies, and does not classify products containing those chemicals as Schedule V drugs under the State scheduling scheme.

Florida Data Roundup:

In Florida, methamphetamine laboratory incident seizures declined by about 22% after the State law was made effective on July 1st , 2005, with 173 incidents reported to DEA for the period from July 1st , 2005, to April 30th, 2006, compared to 221 incidents over the same period one year earlier. Workplace drug testing results showed a 0.6% decrease in positive tests for amphetamine, measuring the first five months in 2006, compared to the same period one year earlier.

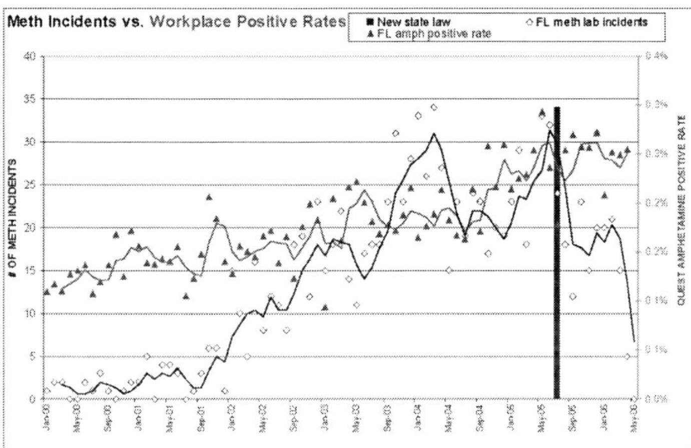

GEORGIA

43% decline in meth lab incidents positive amphetamine workplace tests: -25.5%

Federal Standard: The United States Combat Methamphetamine Act		**Georgia State Law: Less Strict than the Federal Standard**	
Effective Dates:	4/8/2006 9/30/2006	*Effective Date:*	July 1, 2005
		Meth lab reduction:	43%
Sales locations limited to pharmacies?	**No**	**Sales locations limited to pharmacies?**	**No**
Behind the counter/locked cabinet?	**Yes**	**Behind the counter/locked cabinet?**	**Yes**
All listed chemicals?	**Yes**	*All listed chemicals*	*single-entity PSE only*
Daily sales limits:	**3.6 g**	*Transaction limit:*	*3 pkg/9 g*
30-day purchase limit:	**9 g**	*30-day purchase limit:*	*None*
Identification/logbook requirement?	**Yes**	*Identification/logbook requirement?*	*No*

"Listed chemicals" means any productcontaining ephedrine (EPH), pseudoephedrine (PSE), or phenylpropanolamine (PPA).Items in bold indicatethe controlling standard in the state. Items in *italics* indicatethat the provision is trumped by a stricter standard.

Summary

Georgia's methamphetamine precursor law went into effect on July 1, 2005.The Georgia Law is less strict than the CMEA, making CMEA the applicable standard in Georgia.

Georgia's law applies only to products containing pseudoephedrine (not those containing ephedrine or phenylpropanolamine), and imposes a three package or nine gram limit – less strict than the CMEA. Like the CMEA, the state law requires that the products be placed behind the counter or in a locked cabinet.

There was no identification or logbook requirement in Georgia prior to the passage of the CMEA. Georgia does not limit sales of products containing methamphetamine precursor chemicals like pseudoephedrine to pharmacies, and does not classify products containing those chemicals as Schedule V drugs under the State scheduling scheme.

State	Quest Amph Positives, 2000 (Ja n-Ma y)	Quest Amph Positives, 2001 (Jan-May)	Quest Amph Positives, 2002 (Jan-May)	Quest Amph Positives, 2003 (Jan-May)	Quest Amph Positives, 2004 (Jan-May)	Quest Amph Positives, 2005 (Jan-May)	Quest Amph Positives, 2006 (Ja n-Ma y)	% Change 2005-2006
GA	0.19%	0.26%	0.43%	0.57%	0.64%	0.75%	0.56%	-25.54%

Georgia Data Roundup

In Georgia, methamphetamine laboratory incident seizures declined 43% after the State implemented its methamphetamine precursor control law, with 155 incidents reported to DEA for the period from July 1st, 2005, to April 30th , 2006, compared to 273 incidents reported in the same period one year earlier. Workplace drug testing results showed a 25.5% decrease in positive tests for amphetamine, measuring the first five months in 2006, compared to the same period one year earlier.

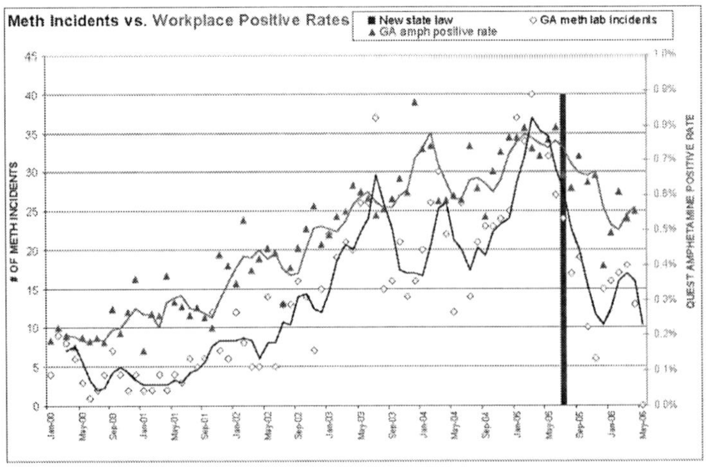

HAWAII

n/a (see Data Round-up) positive amphetamine workplace tests:-37.9%

Federal Standard: The United States Combat Methamphetamine Act		Hawaii State Law: Less Strict than the Federal Standard	
Effective Dates:	4/8/2006 9/30/2006	*Effective Date:*	July 5, 2005
		Meth lab reduction:	n/a
Sales locations limited to pharmacies?	**No**	**Sales locations limited to pharmacies?**	**No**
Behind the counter/locked cabinet?	**Yes**	*Behind the counter/locked cabinet?*	*No*
All listed chemicals?	**Yes**	*All listed chemicals?*	*PSE only*
Daily sales limits:	**3.6 g**	*Transaction limit:*	*3 pkg/9 g*
30-day purchase limit:	**9 g**	*30-day purchase limit:*	--
Identification/logbook requirement?	**Yes**	**Identification/logbook requirement?**	**Yes**

"Listed chemicals" means any productcontaining ephedrine (EPH), pseudoephedrine (PSE), or phenylpropanolamine (PPA).Items in bold indicatethe controlling standard in the state. Items in *italics* indicatethat the provision is trumped by a stricter standard.

Summary

Hawaii's methamphetamine precursor legislation went into effect in two stages: on July 5th, 2006 and October 1st , 2006. The law is less strict than the CMEA, meaning that the CMEA is the controlling standard in Hawaii.

On July 5th , 2006, Hawaii's law imposed a three package or nine gram sales limit. The law only applied to products containing pseudoephedrine, and required that these products be kept behind store counters, under video surveillance, or in the direct line of sight of a sales employee. The law that went into effect on October 1st was functionally the same as the CMEA (which also went into effect on October 1st), so Hawaii generally became a state in which the CMEA is the operating standard.

Hawaii does not limit sales of products containing methamphetamine precursor chemicals like pseudoephedrine to pharmacies, and does not classify products containing those chemicals as Schedule V drugs under the State scheduling scheme

State	Quest Amph Positives, 2000 (Ja n-Ma y)	Quest Amph Positives, 2001 (Jan-May)	Quest Amph Positives, 2002 (Jan-May)	Quest Amph Positives, 2003 (Jan-May)	Quest Amph Positives, 2004 (Jan-May)	Quest Amph Positives, 2005 (Jan-May)	Quest Amph Positives, 2006 (Ja n-Ma y)	% Change 2005-2006
HI	0.95%	1.47%	1.27%	1.36%	1.00%	1.15%	0.71%	-37.87%

Hawaii Data Roundup

Over the past four years, there have been 37 methamphetamine laboratory incident seizures reported in Hawaii. Although the State has faced a serious methamphetamine drug threat, law enforcement reports indicate that much of the methamphetamine consumed in the State comes from outside the State, as opposed to from methamphetamine laboratories located within the State. Since July 2005, there have only been two incidents reported to the DEA regarding laboratory seizures in Hawaii. Workplace drug testing results showed a 37.9% decrease in positive tests for amphetamine, measuring the first five months in 2006, compared to the same period one year earlier.

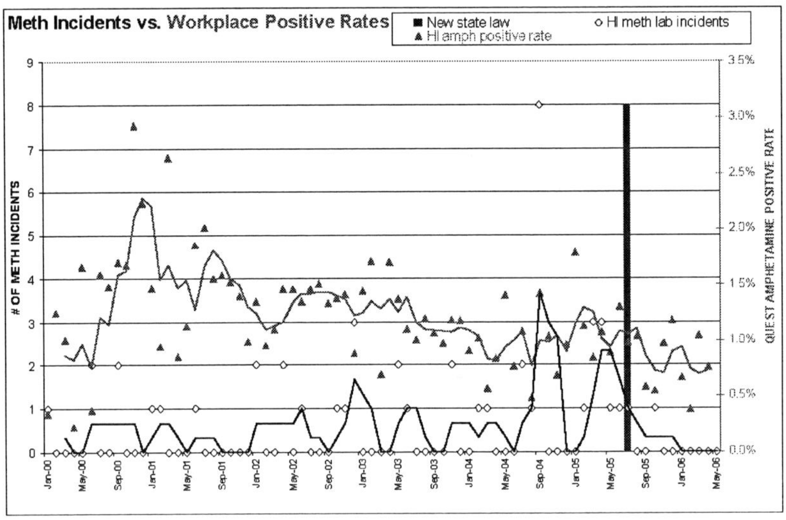

IDAHO

meth lab incident data not yet available positive amphetamine workplace tests: -34.8%

Federal Standard: The United States Combat Methamphetamine Act		Idaho State Law: Less Strict than the Federal Standard	
Effective Dates:	4/8/2006 9/30/2006	*Effective Date:*	March 3rd, 2006
		Meth lab reduction:	unavailable
Sales locations limited to pharmacies?	**No**	**Sales locations limited to pharmacies?**	**No**
Behind the counter/locked cabinet?	**Yes**	**Behind the counter/locked cabinet?**	**Yes**
All listed chemicals?	**Yes**	**All listed chemicals?**	**PSE**
Daily sales limits:	**3.6 g**	*Transactionlimit:*	*9 g*
30-day purchase limit:	**9 g**	**30-day purchase limit:**	**9 g**
Identification/logbook requirement?	**Yes**	*Identification/logbook requirement?*	*No*

"Listed chemicals" means any productcontaining ephedrine (EPH), pseudoephedrine (PSE), or phenylpropanolamine (PPA).Items in bold indicatethe controlling standard in the state. Items in *italics* indicatethat the provision is trumped by a stricter standard.

Summary

Idaho's methamphetamine precursor law went into effect on March 30th 2006.The Idaho Law is less strict than the CMEA, meaning that the nationwide CMEA standard is controlling in Idaho in most respects.

Under Idaho state law, products containing pseudoephedrine must be put in a locked display case or behind a counter, and the purchaser must show identification. Additionally, sales are limited to 9 grams per customer (this is both a daily and monthly limit). However, as noted, the CMEA's standard is stricter, and is controlling in Idaho.

Prior to the CMEA's enactment date, there was no ID and logbook requirement in Idaho. The State does not limit sales of products containing methamphetamine precursor chemicals like pseudoephedrine to pharmacies, and does not classify products containing those chemicals as Schedule V drugs under the State scheduling scheme.

State	Quest Amph Positives, 2000 (Ja n-Ma y)	Quest Amph Positives, 2001 (Jan-May)	Quest Amph Positives, 2002 (Jan-May)	Quest Amph Positives, 2003 (Jan-May)	Quest Amph Positives, 2004 (Jan-May)	Quest Amph Positives, 2005 (Jan-May)	Quest Amph Positives, 2006 (Ja n-Ma y)	% Change 2005-2006
ID	0.53%	0.47%	0.50%	0.58%	0.63%	0.62%	0.41%	-34.81%

Idaho Data Roundup

Idaho's methamphetamine precursor control law was effective on March 30th , 2006, and is therefore too new to measure any impact. However, methamphetamine laboratory incidents have generally been on a downward trend since an apparent peak in early 2003. Workplace drug testing results showed a 34.8% decrease in positive tests for amphetamine, measuring the first five months in 2006, compared to the same period one year earlier.

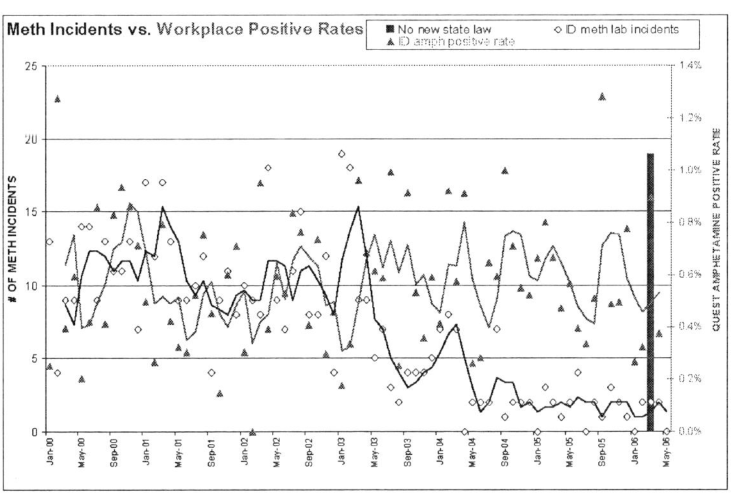

ILLINOIS

17% decline in meth lab incidents positive amphetamine workplace tests: +15.1%

Federal Standard: The United States Combat Methamphetamine Act		Illinois State Law: Stricter than the Federal Standard	
Effective Dates:	4/8/2006	*Effective Date:*	January 15, 2006
	9/30/2006	Meth lab reduction:	17%
Sales locations limited to pharmacies?	**No**	**Sales locations limited to pharmacies?**	*** see below**
Behind the counter/locked cabinet?	**Yes**	**Behind the counter/locked cabinet?**	**Yes**
All listed chemicals?	**Yes**	**All listed chemicals?**	**EPH, PSE**
Daily sales limits:	*3.6 g*	**Transaction limit:**	**2 pkg**
30-day purchase limit:	*9 g*	**30-day purchase limit:**	**7.5 g**
Identification/logbook requirement?	Yes	**Identification/logbook requirement?**	**Yes**

"Listed chemicals" means any productcontaining ephedrine (EPH), pseudoephedrine (PSE), or phenylpropanolamine (PPA).Items in bold indicatethe controlling standard in the state.Items in *italics* indicatethat the provision is trumped by a stricter standard.

Summary

Illinois' methamphetamine precursor legislation took effect January 15th , 2006. The law is stricter than the CMEA, although not wholly pharmacy-only.

Illinois law imposes a 7.5 gram limit on sales of products containing pseudoephedrine or ephedrine (compared to the federal CMEA standard, which is 9 grams). The daily limit is one convenience package (defined as containing 3.6 grams or less of pseudoephedrine or ephedrine, identical to the CMEA standard). All products containing pseudoephedrine or ephedrine are designated as Schedule V drugs, and this limits sales of these products to pharmacies or other authorized entities under the Illinois Controlled Substances Act, which includes some non-pharmacy retail establishments. Illinois state law, like the CMEA, contains an identification and logbook requirement.

State	Quest Amph Positives, 2000 (Ja n-Ma y)	Quest Amph Positives, 2001 (Jan-May)	Quest Amph Positives, 2002 (Jan-May)	Quest Amph Positives, 2003 (Jan-May)	Quest Amph Positives, 2004 (Jan-May)	Quest Amph Positives, 2005 (Jan-May)	Quest Amph Positives, 2006 (Ja n-Ma y)	% Change 2005-2006
IL	0.12%	0.15%	0.16%	0.18%	0.23%	0.22%	0.25%	15.17%

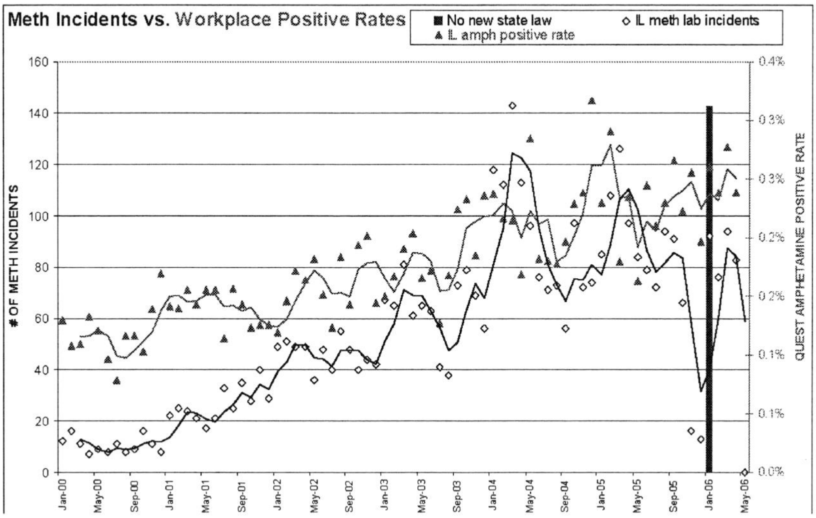

Illinois Data Roundup

In Illinois, methamphetamine laboratory incidents declined by 17% after the State's methamphetamine precursor control law went into effect on January 15, 2006, with 345 incidents reported to DEA for the period from January 15, 2006 to April 30th , 2006, compared to 416 incidents reported in the same period one year earlier. Workplace drug testing results showed a 15.1% increase in positive tests for amphetamine, measuring the first five months in 2006, compared to the same period one year earlier.

INDIANA

28% decline in meth lab incidents positive amphetamine workplace tests: -8.5%

Federal Standard: The United States Combat Methamphetamine Act		Indiana State Law: Similar to the Federal standard	
Effective Dates:	4/8/2006 9/30/2006	*Effective Date:*	July 1, 2005
		Meth lab reduction:	28%
Sales locations limited to pharmacies?	**No**	**Sales locations limited to pharmacies?**	**No**
Behind the counter/locked cabinet?	**Yes**	**Behind the counter/locked cabinet?**	**Yes**
All listed chemicals?	**Yes**	**All listed chemicals?**	**EPH, PSE**
Daily sales limits:	*3.6 g*	**Transaction limit:**	**3 g**
30-day purchase limit:	9 g	*7-day purchase limit:*	*3 g*
Identification/logbook requirement?	Yes	**Identification/logbook requirement?**	**Yes**

"Listed chemicals" means any productcontaining ephedrine (EPH), pseudoephedrine (PSE), or phenylpropanolamine (PPA).Items in bold indicatethe controlling standard in the state. Items in *italics* indicatethat the provision is trumped by a stricter standard.

Summary

Indiana's methamphetamine precursor law went into effect on July 1st , 2005. Indiana's law is similar to the CMEA, meaning that the CMEA standard is controlling in Indiana in most respects.

Indiana's law applies to products containing pseudoephedrine or ephedrine. There is a limit of three grams per purchase; there is also a limit of three grams purchase per week, which is apparently less strict than the CMEA's 9-gram limit per month. Like the CMEA, state law imposes an identification and logbook requirement.

Fundamentally, the CMEA is the functional standard in Indiana. The State does not limit sales of products containing methamphetamine precursor chemicals like pseudoephedrine to pharmacies, and does not classify products containing those chemicals as Schedule V drugs under the State scheduling scheme.

State	Quest Amph Positives, 2000 (Ja n-Ma y)	Quest Amph Positives, 2001 (Jan-May)	Quest Amph Positives, 2002 (Jan-May)	Quest Amph Positives, 2003 (Jan-May)	Quest Amph Positives, 2004 (Jan-May)	Quest Amph Positives, 2005 (Jan May)	Quest Amph Positives, 2006 (Ja n-Ma y)	% Change 2005-2006
IN	0.21%	0.30%	0.33%	0.40%	0.42%	0.44%	0.41%	-8.50%

Indiana Data Roundup

In Indiana, methamphetamine laboratory incident seizures declined by 28% after the State's methamphetamine precursor control law went into effect, with the State reporting 669 seizures from July 1st , 2005 to April 30th, 2006, compared to 934 over the same time period one year earlier. Workplace drug testing results showed a 8.5% decrease in positive tests for amphetamine, measuring the first five months in 2006, compared to the same period one year earlier.

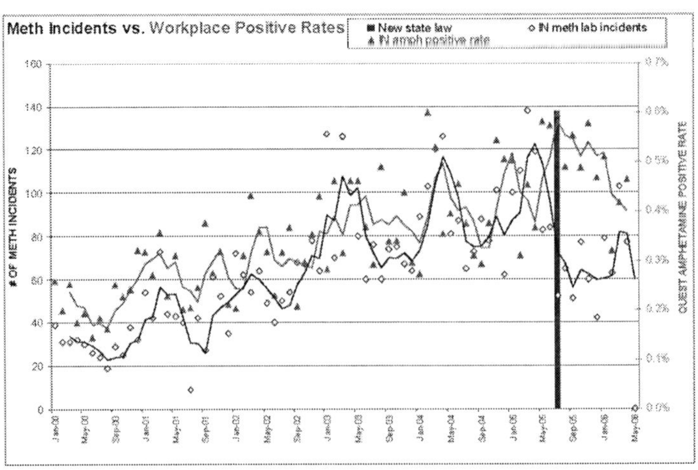

IOWA

70% decline in meth lab incidents positive amphetamine workplace tests: -31.1%

Federal Standard: The United States Combat Methamphetamine Act		Iowa State Law: Stricter than the Federal Standard	
Effective Dates:	4/8/2006 9/30/2006	*Effective Date:* Meth lab reduction:	July 1, 2005 74%
Sales locations limited to pharmacies?	*No*	Sales locations limited to pharmacies?	Yes
Behind the counter/locked cabinet?	**Yes**	Behind the counter/locked cabinet?	Yes
All listed chemicals?	**Yes**	All listed chemicals?	Yes
Daily sales limits:	*3.6 g*	Daily sales limits:	1 pkg/360 mg
30-day purchase limit:	*9 g*	30-day purchase limit:	7.5 g
Identification/logbook requirement?	Yes	Identification/logbook requirement?	Yes

"Listed chemicals" means any productcontaining ephedrine (EPH), pseudoephedrine (PSE), or phenylpropanolamine (PPA).Items in bold indicatethe controlling standard in the state. Items in *italics* indicatethat the provision is trumped by a stricter standard.

Summary

Iowa's methamphetamine precursor law went into effect on May 21st , 2005. Iowa's law is one of the strictest in the nation, and is stricter than the CMEA.

Iowa's law classifies products containing pseudoephedrine, ephedrine or phenylpropanolamine as Schedule V drugs, and limits sales of these products to pharmacies. (Products containing less than 120 milligrams of pseudoephedrine are exempt.) There is a 7.5 gram monthly limit on these products and a daily limit of one package within 24 hours. Iowa law contains an identification and logbook requirement.

Sta te	Quest Amph Positives, 2000 (Jan-May)	Quest Amph Positives, 2001 (Jan-May)	Quest Amph Positives, 2002 (Jan-May)	Quest Amph Positives, 2003 (Jan-May)	Quest Amph Positives, 2004 (Jan-May)	Quest Amph Positives, 2005 (Jan-May)	Quest Amph Positives, 2006 (Jan-May)	% Change 2005-2006
IA	0.27%	0.80%	0.73%	0.63%	0.59%	0.61%	0.42%	-31.10%

Iowa Data Roundup

In Iowa, methamphetamine laboratory incident seizures declined by 70% after the State's methamphetamine precursor control law went into effect, with the State reporting 350 seizures from May 21st, 2005 to April 30th, 2006, compared to 1154 over the same time period one year earlier. Workplace drug testing results showed a 31.1% decrease in positive tests for amphetamine, measuring the first five months in 2006, compared to the same period one year earlier.

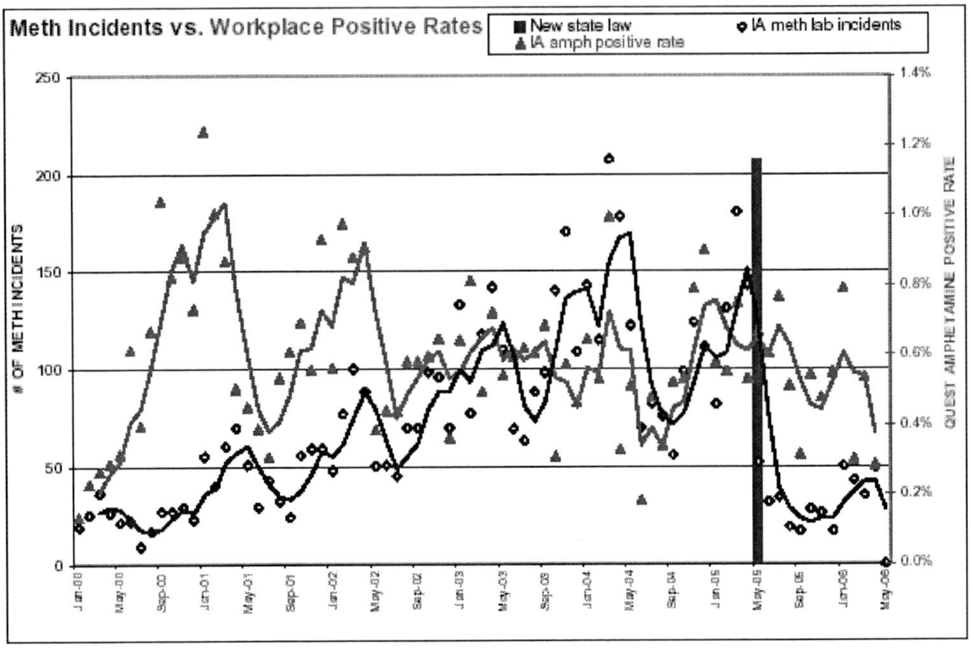

Kansas

54% decline in meth lab incidents positive amphetamine workplace tests: -15.1%

Federal Standard: The United States Combat Methamphetamine Act		**Kansas State Law: Stricter than the Federal Standard**	
Effective Dates:	4/8/2006 9/30/2006	Effective Date:	June 1, 2005
		Meth lab reduction:	54%
Sales locations limited to pharmacies?	*No*	**Sales locations limited to pharmacies?**	**Yes**
Behind the counter/locked cabinet?	**Yes**	**Behind the counter/locked cabinet?**	**Yes**
All listed chemicals?	**Yes**	**All listed chemicals?**	**EPH, PSE**
Daily sales limits:	*3.6 g*	**Daily sales limits:**	*** see below**
30-day purchase limit:	*9 g*	**30-day purchase limit:**	*** see below**
Identification/logbook requirement?	Yes	**Identification/logbook requirement?**	**Yes**

"Listed chemicals" means any productcontaining ephedrine (EPH), pseudoephedrine (PSE), or phenylpropanolamine (PPA).Items in bold indicatethe controlling standard in the state. Items in *italics* indicatethat the provision is trumped by a stricter standard.

Summary

Kansas's methamphetamine precursor law went fully into effect on June 1st, 2005 (some provisions became effective on April 28, 2005). Kansas law is one of the strictest in the nation, and is stricter than the CMEA.

Kansas's law classifies products containing pseudoephedrine or ephedrine – except those in liquid or gelatin capsule form – as Schedule V drugs. These products may only be sold at pharmacies, and must be stored behind pharmacy counters. Like the CMEA, Kansas law contains an identification and logbook requirement. In Kansas, no more than 24 dosage units may be sold to the same purchaser in a 48 hour period, and no more than four packages may be sold per customer per seven days.

State	Quest Amph Positives, 2000 (Ja n-Ma y)	Quest Amph Positives, 2001 (Jan-May)	Quest Amph Positives, 2002 (Jan-May)	Quest Amph Positives, 2003 (Jan-May)	Quest Amph Positives, 2004 (Jan-May)	Quest Amph Positives, 2005 (Jan-May)	Quest Amph Positives, 2006 (Ja n-Ma y)	% Change 2005-2006
KS	0.31%	0.42%	0.39%	0.46%	0.41%	0.78%	0.66%	-15.16%

Kansas Data Roundup

In Kansas, methamphetamine laboratory incident seizures declined by 54% after the State's methamphetamine precursor control law went into effect, with the State reporting 215 seizures from June 1st , 2005 to April 30th, 2006, compared to 470 over the same time period one year earlier. Workplace drug testing results showed a 15.1% decrease in positive tests for amphetamine, measuring the first five months in 2006, compared to the same period one year earlier.

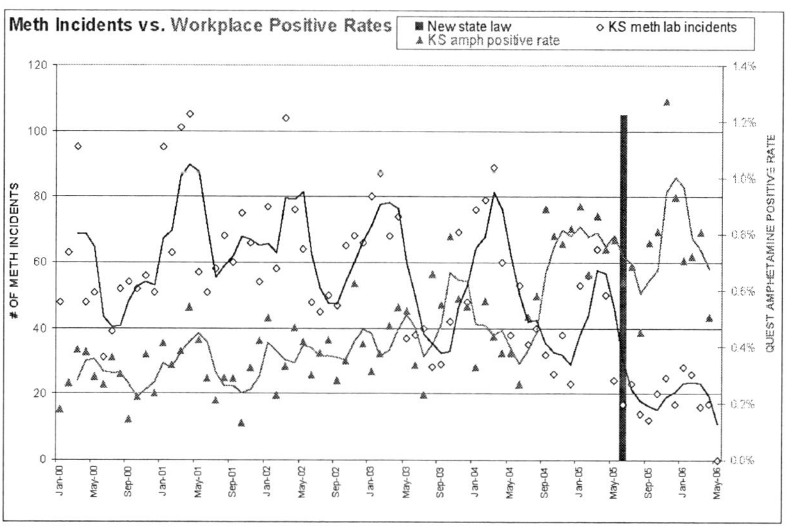

KENTUCKY

43% decline in meth lab incidents positive amphetamine workplace tests: -22.3%

Federal Standard: The United States Combat Methamphetamine Act		**Kentucky State Law: Stricter than the Federal Standard**	
Effective Dates:	4/8/2006 9/30/2006	*Effective Date:* Meth lab reduction:	June 20, 2005 43%
Sales locations limited to pharmacies?	**No**	**Sales locations limited to pharmacies?**	**Yes**
Behind the counter/locked cabinet?	**Yes**	**Behind the counter/locked cabinet?**	**Yes**
All listed chemicals?	**Yes**	**All listed chemicals?**	**Yes**
Daily sales limits:	**3.6 g**	**Transaction limit:**	**3 g**
30-day purchase limit:	**9 g**	**30-day purchase limit:**	**9 g**
Identification/logbook requirement?	**Yes**	**Identification/logbook requirement?**	**Yes**

"Listed chemicals" means any productcontaining ephedrine (EPH), pseudoephedrine (PSE), or phenylpropanolamine (PPA).Items in bold indicatethe controlling standard in the state. Items in *italics* indicatethat the provision is trumped by a stricter standard.

Summary

Kentucky's methamphetamine precursor law went into effect June 20th, 2005. Kentucky's law is stricter than the CMEA, and basically imposes a pharmacy-only standard.

Kentucky's law applies to all products containing pseudoephedrine, ephedrine, or phenylpropanolamine. There are sales limits of 3 grams per transaction and 9 grams per month, similar to the CMEA. Kentucky limits sales of these products to stores where the products can be sold by a pharmacist, pharmacist technician or intern, and requires that the products be kept behind a pharmacy counter or in a locked case. Like the Federal CMEA, Kentucky state law contains an identification and logbook requirement

State	**Quest Amph Positives, 2000 (Jan-May)**	**Quest Amph Positives, 2001 (Jan-May)**	**Quest Amph Positives, 2002 (Jan-May)**	**Quest Amph Positives, 2003 (Jan-May)**	**Quest Amph Positives, 2004 (Jan-May)**	**Quest Amph Positives, 2005 (Jan-May)**	**Quest Amph Positives, 2006 (Jan-May)**	**% Change 2005-2006**
KY	0.21%	0.20%	0.28%	0.31%	0.37%	0.36%	0.28%	-22.35%

Kentucky Data Roundup

In Kentucky, methamphetamine laboratory incident seizures declined by 43% after the State's methamphetamine precursor control law went into effect, with the State reporting 304 seizures from June 20th, 2005 to April 30th, 2006, compared to 535 over the same time period one year earlier. Workplace drug testing results showed a 22.3% decrease in positive tests for amphetamine, measuring the first five months in 2006, compared to the same period one year earlier.

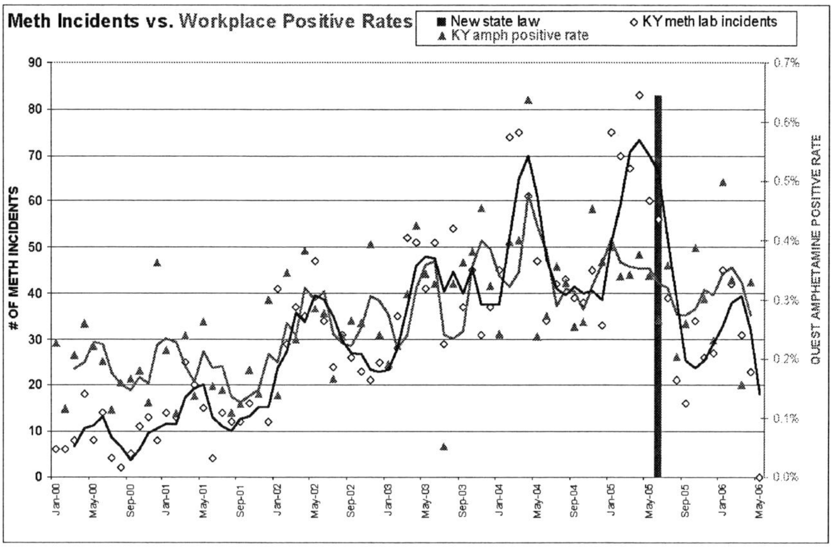

Louisiana

85%* decline in meth lab incidents positive amphetamine workplace tests: +0.5%

Federal Standard: The United States Combat Methamphetamine Act		Louisiana State Law: Less strict than the Federal Standard	
Effective Dates:	4/8/2006 9/30/2006	*Effective Date:*	August 15, 2005
		Meth lab reduction:	88%
Sales locations limited to pharmacies?	**No**	**Sales locations limited to pharmacies?**	**No**
Behind the counter/locked cabinet?	**Yes**	**Behind the counter/locked cabinet?**	**Yes**
All listed chemicals?	**Yes**	All listed chemicals?	Yes
Daily sales limits:	**3.6 g**	*Daily sales limits:*	*3 pkg/9 g*
30-day purchase limit:	**9 g**	**30-day purchase limit:**	**9 g**
Identification/logbook requirement?	**Yes**	**Identification/logbook requirement?**	**Yes**

"Listed chemicals" means any productcontaining ephedrine (EPH), pseudoephedrine (PSE), or phenylpropanolamine (PPA).Items in bold indicatethe controlling standard in the state. Items in *italics* indicatethat the provision is trumped by a stricter standard.

Summary

Louisiana's methamphetamine precursor law went into effect on August 15th, 2005. Louisiana's law is less strict than the CMEA, meaning that the federal CMEA standard is controlling in the State.

Louisiana's law applies to all products containing pseudoephedrine or ephedrine. There is a somewhat complicated system under state law involving differing sales limits for pharmacies and non-pharmacies, but these were largely rendered irrelevant by the Federal CMEA sales limits, which are stricter. Like the federal CMEA, there is an identification and logbook requirement.

Louisiana does not limit sales of products containing methamphetamine precursor chemicals like pseudoephedrine to pharmacies, and does not classify products containing those chemicals as Schedule V drugs under the State scheduling scheme.

State	Quest Amph Positives, 2000 (Ja n-Ma y)	Quest Amph Positives, 2001 (Jan-May)	Quest Amph Positives, 2002 (Jan-May)	Quest Amph Positives, 2003 (Jan-May)	Quest Amph Positives, 2004 (Jan-May)	Quest Amph Positives, 2005 (Jan-May)	Quest Amph Positives, 2006 (Ja n-Ma y)	% Change 2005-2006
LA	0.16%	0.23%	0.24%	0.25%	0.46%	0.64%	0.65%	0.46%

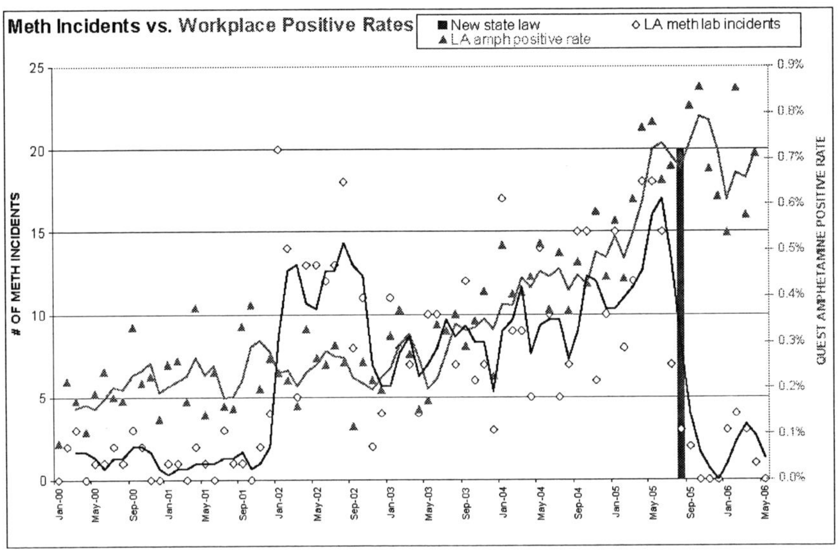

Louisiana Data Roundup

In Louisiana, methamphetamine laboratory incident seizures declined by 85% after the State's methamphetamine precursor control law went into effect, with the State reporting 16 seizures from July 15th, 2005 to April 30th , 2006, compared to 106 over the same time period one year earlier. Workplace drug testing results showed a .5% increase in positive tests for amphetamine, measuring the first five months in 2006, compared to the same period one year earlier.

*Note: Hurricane Katrina hit New Orleans in August of 2005, soon after the law went into effect. This most likely had a significant impact on the reduction in meth lab incidents and the number of workplace tests conducted.

MAINE

data not yet available positive amphetamine workplace tests: +39.4%

Federal Standard: The United States Combat Methamphetamine Act		Maine State Law: Stricter than the Federal Standard	
Effective Dates:	4/8/2006	*Effective Date:*	April 6, 2006
	9/30/2006	Meth lab reduction:	Not Available
Sales locations limited to pharmacies?	*No*	**Sales locations limited to pharmacies?**	**Yes**
Behind the counter/locked cabinet?	**Yes**	**Behind the counter/locked cabinet?**	**Yes**
All listed chemicals?	**Yes**	**All listed chemicals?**	**Yes**
Daily sales limits:	*3.6 g*	**Transaction limit:**	**3 pkg/3 g**
30-day purchase limit:	**9 g**	**30-day purchase limit:**	**9 g**
Identification/logbook requirement?	**Yes**	**Identification/logbook requirement?**	**Yes**

"Listed chemicals" means any productcontaining ephedrine (EPH), pseudoephedrine (PSE), or phenylpropanolamine (PPA).Items in bold indicatethe controlling standard in the state. Items in *italics* indicatethat the provision is trumped by a stricter standard.

Summary

Maine's methamphetamine precursor law went into effect on April 6th , 2006. Maine's law is stricter than the CMEA in several respects.

Maine's law applies to all products containing ephedrine, pseudoephedrine or in solid form, or those in liquid form designated as precursors by state regulation. The state law limits sales to pharmacies, but unlike Oklahoma, does not require that the products be kept behind a counter. Rather, most products may be kept in a locked location or an area not accessible by the public. The law requires dispensation only by a licensed pharmacist or an employee under the supervision of a pharmacist. The state law's monthly limit is the same as the federal CMEA's limit – 9 grams.

Maine's state law does not classify products containing pseudoephedrine or ephedrine as Schedule V drugs.

State	Quest Amph Positives, 2000 (Ja n-Ma y)	Quest Amph Positives, 2001 (Jan-May)	Quest Amph Positives, 2002 (Jan-May)	Quest Amph Positives, 2003 (Jan-May)	Quest Amph Positives, 2004 (Jan-May)	Quest Amph Positives, 2005 (Jan-May)	Quest Amph Positives, 2006 (Ja n-Ma y)	% Change 2005-2006
ME	0.05%	0.00%	0.04%	0.20%	0.13%	0.22%	0.31%	39.41%

Maine Data Roundup

Maine's methamphetamine precursor control law went into effect on April 6th, 2006, and is therefore too new to measure any impact. However, there have only been 16 methamphetamine laboratory incident seizures reported to the DEA since January 2000 from Maine. Workplace drug testing results showed a 39.4% increase in positive tests for amphetamine, measuring the first five months in 2006, compared to the same period one year earlier.

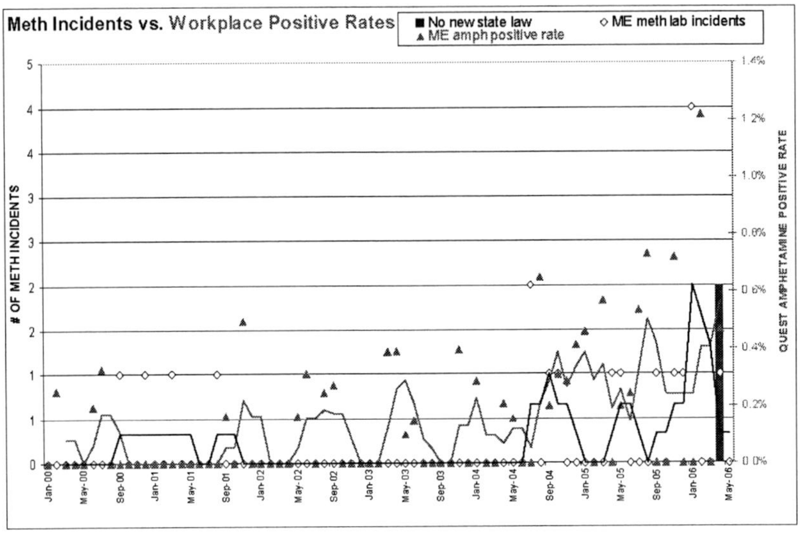

MARYLAND

no state law/historically low lab numbers positive amphetamine workplace tests: +33.9%

Federal Standard: The United States Combat Methamphetamine Act		**Maryland State Law: No state law, only CMEA applies**	
Effective Dates:	4/8/2006	*Effective Date:*	None
	9/30/2006	Meth lab reduction:	n/a
Sales locations limited to pharmacies?	**No**	*Sales locations limited to pharmacies?*	*No*
Behind the counter/locked cabinet?	**Yes**	*Behind the counter/locked cabinet?*	*No*
All listed chemicals?	**Yes**	*All listed chemicals?*	*No*
Daily sales limits:	**3.6 g**	*Daily sales limits:*	*None*
30-day purchase limit:	**9 g**	*30-day purchase limit:*	*None*
Identification/logbook requirement?	**Yes**	*Identification/logbook requirement?*	*No*

"Listed chemicals" means any productcontaining ephedrine (EPH), pseudoephedrine (PSE), or phenylpropanolamine (PPA).Items in bold indicatethe controlling standard in the state. Items in *italics* indicatethat the provision is trumped by a stricter standard.

Summary

Maryland, which has enjoyed low numbers of methamphetamine laboratory incidents, did not implement any methamphetamine precursor controls before the Combat Meth Act took effect September 30th 2006. In other words, the CMEA is the controlling standard in Maryland. It also means that Maryland does not limit sales of products containing methamphetamine precursors like pseudoephedrine to pharmacies, and does not classify these products as Schedule V drugs under the State's scheduling scheme.

State	Quest Amph Positives, 2000 (Ja n-Ma y)	Quest Amph Positives, 2001 (Jan-May)	Quest Amph Positives, 2002 (Jan-May)	Quest Amph Positives, 2003 (Jan-May)	Quest Amph Positives, 2004 (Jan-May)	Quest Amph Positives, 2005 (Jan-May)	Quest Amph Positives, 2006 (Ja n-Ma y)	% Change 2005-2006
MD	0.09%	0.12%	0.18%	0.17%	0.22	0.20%	0.26%	33.96%

Maryland Data Roundup

Maryland did not implement a methamphetamine precursor control law at the State level. However, since January of 2000, Maryland has only reported less than ten methamphetamine lab incidents. Workplace drug testing results showed a 33.9% increase in positive tests for amphetamine, measuring the first five months in 2006, compared to the same period one year earlier.

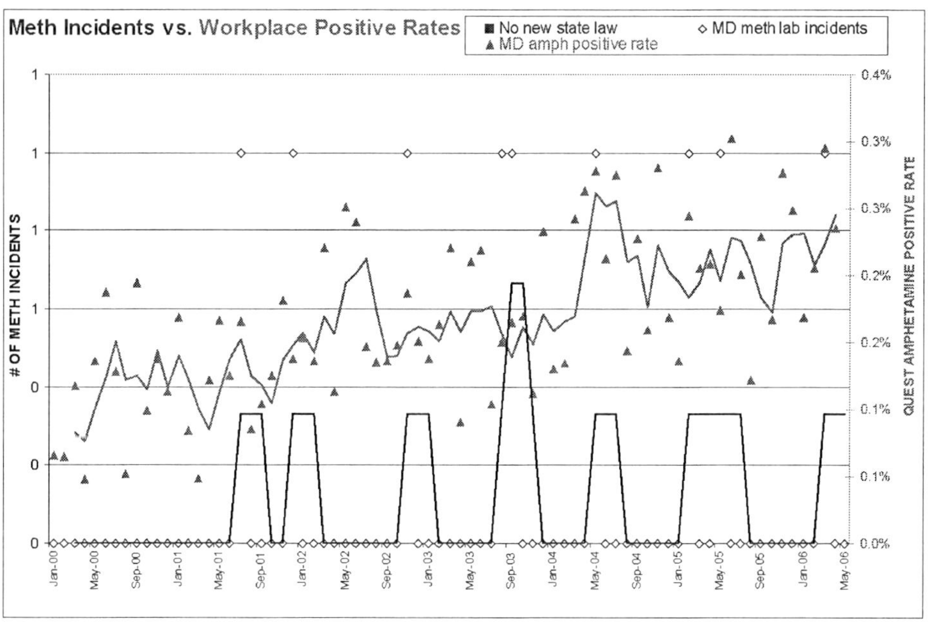

MASSACHUSETTS

no state law/historically low lab numbers positive amphetamine workplace tests: -16.2%

Federal Standard: The United States Combat Methamphetamine Act		**Massachusetts State Law: No State law, only CMEA applies**	
Effective Dates:	4/8/2006 9/30/2006	*Effective Date:* Meth lab reduction:	None n/a
Sales locations limited to pharmacies?	**No**	*Sales locations limited to pharmacies?*	*No*
Behind the counter/locked cabinet?	**Yes**	*Behind the counter/locked cabinet?*	*No*
All listed chemicals?	**Yes**	*All listed chemicals?*	*No*
Daily sales limits:	**3.6 g**	*Daily sales limits:*	*None*
30-day purchase limit:	**9 g**	*30-day purchase limit:*	*None*
Identification/logbook requirement?	**Yes**	*Identification/logbook requirement?*	*No*

"Listed chemicals" means any productcontaining ephedrine (EPH), pseudoephedrine (PSE), or phenylpropanolamine (PPA).Items in bold indicatethe controlling standard in the state. Items in *italics* indicatethat the provision is trumped by a stricter standard.

Summary

Massachusetts, which has enjoyed low numbers of methamphetamine laboratory incidents, did not implement any methamphetamine precursor controls before the Combat Meth Act took effect September 30th 2006. In other words, the CMEA is the controlling standard in Massachusetts. It also means that the State does not limit sales of products containing methamphetamine precursors like pseudoephedrine to pharmacies, and does not classify these products as Schedule V drugs under the State's scheduling scheme.

State	Quest Amph Positives, 2000 (Ja n-Ma y)	Quest Amph Positives, 2001 (Jan-May)	Quest Amph Positives, 2002 (Jan-May)	Quest Amph Positives, 2003 (Jan-May)	Quest Amph Positives, 2004 (Jan-May)	Quest Amph Positives, 2005 (Jan-May)	Quest Amph Positives, 2006 (Ja n-Ma y)	% Change 2005-2006
MA	0.16%	0.18%	0.12%	0.16%	0.24%	0.33%	0.27%	-16.26%

Massachusctts Data Roundup

Massachusetts did not implement a methamphetamine precursor control law at the State level. However, since January of 2000, the State has only reported less than ten methamphetamine lab incidents. Workplace drug testing results showed a 16.2% decrease in positive tests for amphetamine, measuring the first five months in 2006, compared to the same period one year earlier.

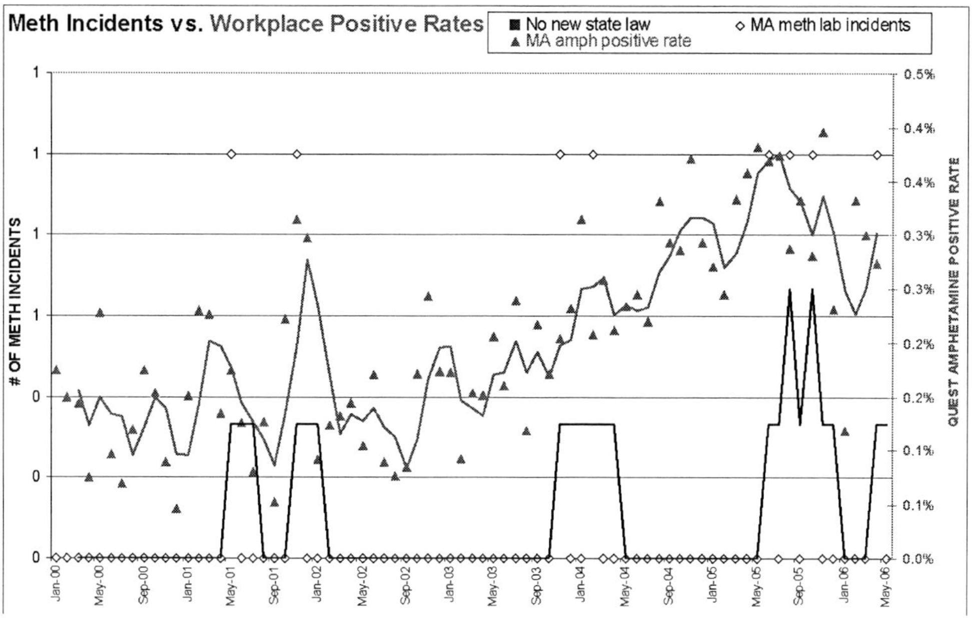

MICHIGAN

16% decline in meth lab incidents positive amphetamine workplace tests: +73.3%

Federal Standard: The United States Combat Methamphetamine Act		Michigan State Law: Similar to the Federal Standards	
Effective Dates:	4/8/2006	Effective Date:	July 20, 2005
	9/30/2006	Meth lab reduction:	16%
Sales locations limited to pharmacies?	**No**	**Sales locations limited to pharmacies?**	**No**
Behind the counter/locked cabinet?	**Yes**	**Behind the counter/locked cabinet?**	**Yes**
All listed chemicals?	**Yes**	*All listed chemicals?*	*EPH, PSE*
Daily sales limits:	*3.6 g*	**Daily sales limits:**	**2 pkg**
30-day purchase limit:	**9 g**	*30-day purchase limit:*	*None*
Identification/logbook requirement?	**Yes**	**Identification/logbook requirement?**	**Yes**

"Listed chemicals" means any productcontaining ephedrine (EPH), pseudoephedrine (PSE), or phenylpropanolamine (PPA).Items in bold indicatethe controlling standard in the state. Items in *italics* indicatethat the provision is trumped by a stricter standard.

Summary:

Michigan's methamphetamine precursor law went into effect in two stages: December 15th, 2005, and July 17th , 2006. Michigan state law is approximately as strict as the CMEA, meaning that for most purposes, the CMEA is the controlling standard in Michigan.

Most of the State provisions went into effect on December 15th, 2005. The law limited single sales of products containing pseudoephedrine or ephedrine to two packages or 48 capsules, which in most cases will probably be more restrictive than the Federal CMEA standard. Although the State law does not limit sales of the products to pharmacies, the law provides retailers with a somewhat complex list of options, including keeping the products behind the counter, in a locked cabinet, under video surveillance, or within 20 feet of the counter with certain other requirements. Some of these requirements are less strict than the Federal CMEA and are thus obviated by the Federal law. Like the Federal CMEA, Michigan's law contains an identification and logbook requirement.

Michigan does not classify products containing those chemicals as Schedule V drugs under the State scheduling scheme.

State	Quest Amph Positives, 2000 (Ja n-Ma y)	Quest Amph Positives, 2001 (Jan-May)	Quest Amph Positives, 2002 (Jan-May)	Quest Amph Positives, 2003 (Jan-May)	Quest Amph Positives, 2004 (Jan-May)	Quest Amph Positives, 2005 (Jan-May)	Quest Amph Positives, 2006 (Ja n-Ma y)	% Change 2005-2006
MI	0.08%	0.09%	0.18%	0.19%	0.19%	0.29%	0.51%	73.26%

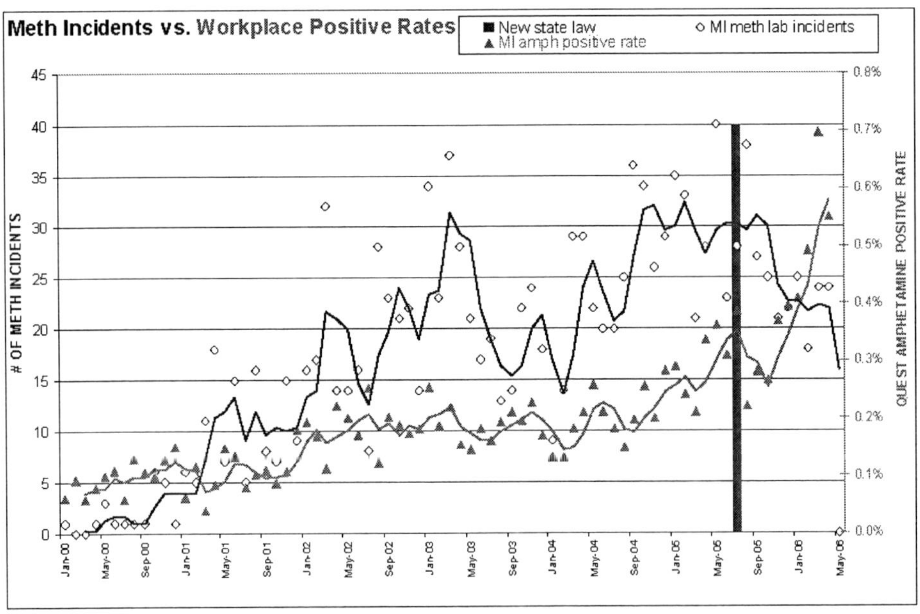

Michigan Data Roundup

In Michigan, methamphetamine laboratory incident seizures declined by 16% after the State's methamphetamine precursor control law went into effect, with the State reporting 224 seizures from July 20th, 2005 to April 30th , 2006, compared to 267 over the same time period one year earlier. Workplace drug testing results showed a 73.3% increase in positive tests for amphetamine, measuring the first five months in 2006, compared to the same period one year earlier.

Minnesota

70% decline in meth lab incidents positive amphetamine workplace tests: -4.9%

Federal Standard: The United States Combat Methamphetamine Act		**Michigan State Law: Similar to the Federal Standards**	
Effective Dates:	4/8/2006	Effective Date:	July 20, 2005
	9/30/2006	Meth lab reduction:	70 %
Sales locations limited to pharmacies?	**No**	**Sales locations limited to pharmacies?**	**No**
Behind the counter/locked cabinet?	**Yes**	**Behind the counter/locked cabinet?**	**Yes**
All listed chemicals?	**Yes**	*All listed chemicals?*	*EPH, PSE*
Daily sales limits:	*3.6 g*	**Daily sales limits:**	**2 pkg**
30-day purchase limit:	**9 g**	*30-day purchase limit:*	*None*
Identification/logbook requirement?	**Yes**	**Identification/logbook requirement?**	**Yes**
"Listed chemicals" means any productcontaining ephedrine (EPH), pseudoephedrine (PSE), or phenylpropanolamine (PPA).Items in bold indicatethe controlling standard in the state. Items in *italics* indicatethat the provision is trumped by a stricter standard.			

Summary

Minnesota's methamphetamine precursor law went into effect June 3rd, 2005. Minnesota's law is stricter than the CMEA.

Most products containing pseudoephedrine or ephedrine can only be sold at a pharmacy, and must be kept behind the pharmacy counter. There is a 2 package or 6 gram limit on daily purchases, which is less strict than the CMEA, but there is a 6 gram monthly purchase limit, which is stricter than the CMEA. State law also contains an identification and logbook requirement.

State	**Quest Amph Positives, 2000 (Ja n-Ma y)**	**Quest Amph Positives, 2001 (Jan-May)**	**Quest Amph Positives, 2002 (Jan-May)**	**Quest Amph Positives, 2003 (Jan-May)**	**Quest Amph Positives, 2004 (Jan-May)**	**Quest Amph Positives, 2005 (Jan-May)**	**Quest Amph Positives, 2006 (Ja n-Ma y)**	**% Change 2005-2006**
MN	0.25%	0.42%	0.40%	0.38%	0.48%	0.59%	0.56%	-4.90%

Minnesota Data Roundup

In Minnesota, methamphetamine laboratory incident seizures declined by 70% after the State's methamphetamine precursor control law went into effect, with the State reporting 42 seizures from June 3rd , 2005 to April 30th , 2006, compared to 138 over the same time period one year earlier. Workplace drug testing results showed a 4.9% decrease in positive tests for amphetamine, measuring the first five months in 2006, compared to the same period one year earlier.

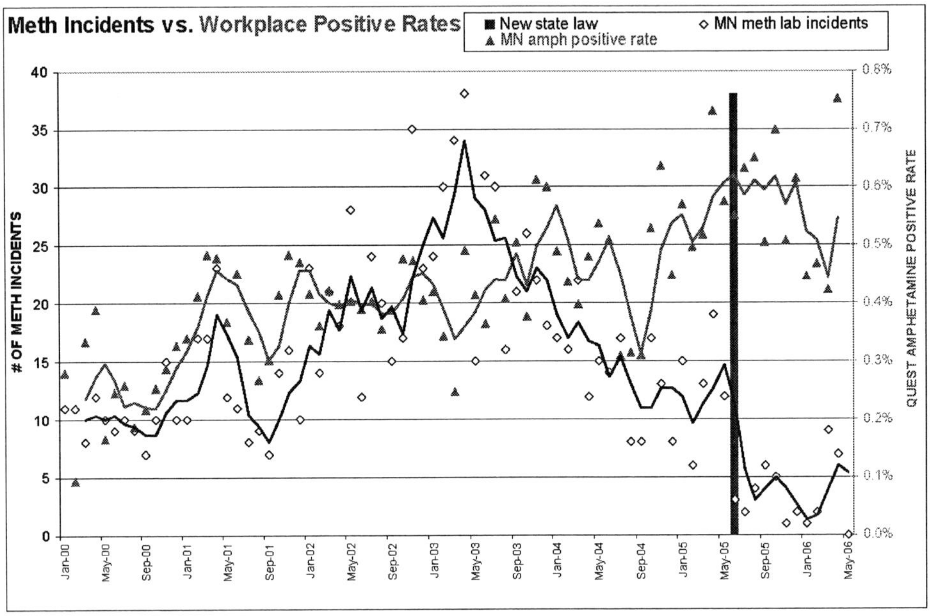

MISSISSIPPI

68%* decline in meth lab incidents positive amphetamine workplace tests: -51.4%

Federal Standard: The United States Combat Methamphetamine Act		Mississippi State Law. Less strict than the Federal Standard	
Effective Dates:	4/8/2006 9/30/2006	*Effective Date:* Meth lab reduction:	July 1, 2005 68%
Sales locations limited to pharmacies?	**No**	**Sales locations limited to pharmacies?**	**No**
Behind the counter/locked cabinet?	**Yes**	**Behind the counter/locked cabinet?**	**Yes**
All listed chemicals?	**Yes**	**All listed chemicals?**	**EPH, PSE**
Daily sales limits:	**3.6 g**	**Transaction limit:**	**2 pkg/6 g**
30-day purchase limit:	**9 g**	**30-day purchase limit:**	**9 g**
Identification/logbook requirement?	**Yes**	**Identification/logbook requirement?**	**Yes**

"Listed chemicals" means any productcontaining ephedrine (EPH), pseudoephedrine (PSE), or phenylpropanolamine (PPA).Items in bold indicatethe controlling standard in the state. Items in *italics* indicatethat the provision is trumped by a stricter standard.

Summary

Mississippi's methamphetamine precursor law went into effect July 1st , 2005. The Mississippi law is not quite as strict as the CMEA, so the CMEA is the controlling standard in Mississippi.

Mississippi's law places a 9 gram monthly limit on purchases of products containing pseudoephedrine or ephedrine. The daily purchase limit is 6 grams. The law requires that products containing only pseudoephedrine or ephedrine be placed behind the counter or in a locked cabinet. Multi-active products -- meaning, products containing one of those chemicals as well as other active ingredients – may also be placed under video surveillance or kept within 30 feet of the store's cashiers. There is an ID and logbook requirement in Mississippi.

Mississippi does not limit sales of products containing methamphetamine precursor chemicals like pseudoephedrine to pharmacies, and does not classify products containing those chemicals as Schedule V drugs under the State scheduling scheme.

State	Quest Amph Positives, 2000 (Ja n-Ma y)	Quest Amph Positives, 2001 (Jan-May)	Quest Amph Positives, 2002 (Jan-May)	Quest Amph Positives, 2003 (Jan-May)	Quest Amph Positives, 2004 (Jan-May)	Quest Amph Positives, 2005 (Jan-May)	Quest Amph Positives, 2006 (Ja n-Ma y)	% Change 2005-2006
MS	0.09%	0.24%	0.25%	0.45%	0.25%	0.55%	0.27%	-51 .40%

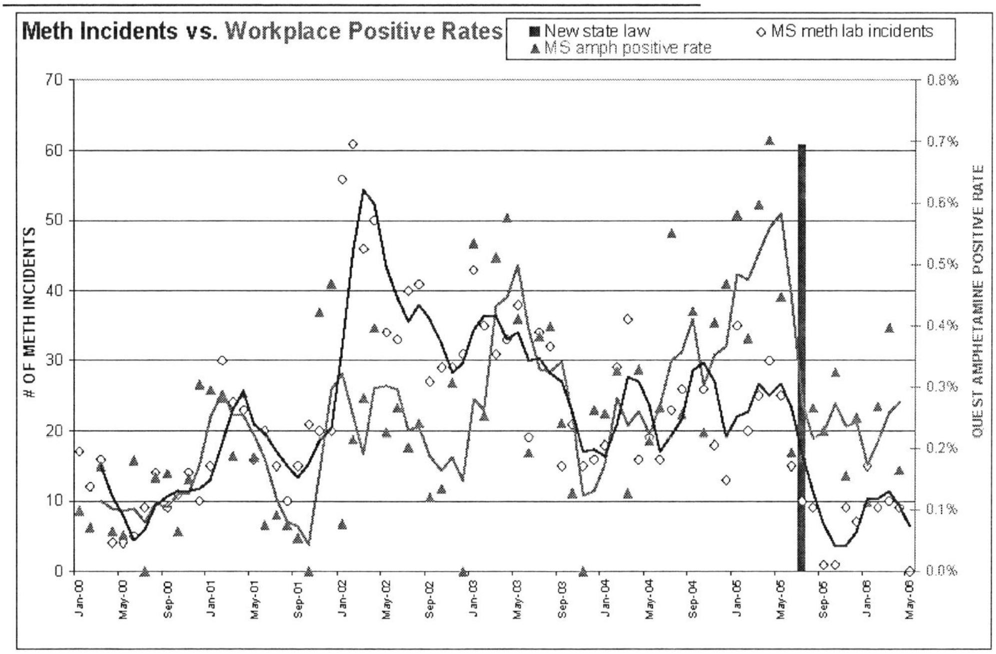

Mississippi Data Roundup

In Mississippi, methamphetamine laboratory incident seizures declined by 68% after the State's methamphetamine precursor control law went into effect, with the State reporting 80 seizures from July 1st , 2005 to April 30th, 2006, compared to 253 over the same time period one year earlier. Workplace drug testing results showed a 51.4% decrease in positive tests for amphetamine, measuring the first five months in 2006, compared to the same period one year earlier.

*Note: Hurricane Katrina hit Mississippi in August of 2005, soon after the law went into effect. This most likely was a significant factor in the reduction in meth lab incidents.

MISSOURI

45% decline in meth lab incidents positive amphetamine workplace tests: -27.1%

Federal Standard: The United States Combat Methamphetamine Act		**Missouri State Law: Stricter than the Federal Standard**	
Effective Dates:	4/8/2006 9/30/2006	*Effective Date:* Meth lab reduction:	July 15, 2005 45%
Sales locations limited to pharmacies?	*No*	**Sales locations limited to pharmacies?**	**Yes**
Behind the counter/locked cabinet?	**Yes**	**Behind the counter/locked cabinet?**	**Yes**
All listed chemicals?	**Yes**	**All listed chemicals? EPH, PSE**	
Daily sales limits:	**3.6 g**	**Daily sales limits:**	**n/a**
30-day purchase limit:	**9 g**	**30-day purchase limit:**	**9 g**
Identification/logbook requirement?	**Yes**	**Identification/logbook requirement?**	**Yes**

"Listed chemicals" means any productcontaining ephedrine (EPH), pseudoephedrine (PSE), or phenylpropanolamine (PPA).Items in bold indicatethe controlling standard in the state. Items in *italics* indicatethat the provision is trumped by a stricter standard.

Summary

Missouri's methamphetamine precursor law went into effect July 15th, 2005. The Missouri law is stricter than the CMEA in many important respects.

Missouri's law applies to both single-entity and multi-active products containing pseudoephedrine or ephedrine, and imposes a 9 gram monthly purchase limit – the same as the Federal CMEA's monthly purchase limit.

The State's scheduling scheme is somewhat complicated. Generally, single-entity ephedrine products are classified as Schedule IV. Single-entity pseudoephedrine products, and multi-active products containing either pseudoephedrine or ephedrine are classified as Schedule V products, and may only be sold by a registered pharmacist or pharmacy technician. These products must be kept behind the pharmacy counter, and purchasers must show identification and sign a logbook.

State	Quest Amph Positives, 2000 (Ja n-Ma y)	Quest Amph Positives, 2001 (Jan-May)	Quest Amph Positives, 2002 (Jan-May)	Quest Amph Positives, 2003 (Jan-May)	Quest Amph Positives, 2004 (Jan-May)	Quest Amph Positives, 2005 (Jan-May)	Quest Amph Positives, 2006 (Ja n-Ma y)	% Change 2005-2006
MO	0.38%	0.49%	0.43%	0.33%	0.51%	0.59%	0.43%	-27.10%

Missouri Data Roundup

In Missouri, methamphetamine laboratory incident seizures declined by 45% after the State's methamphetamine precursor control law went into effect, with the State reporting 1,325 seizures from July 15th, 2005 to April 30th , 2006, compared to 2,418 over the same time period one year earlier. Workplace drug testing results showed a 27.1% decrease in positive tests for amphetamine, measuring the first five months in 2006, compared to the same period one year earlier.

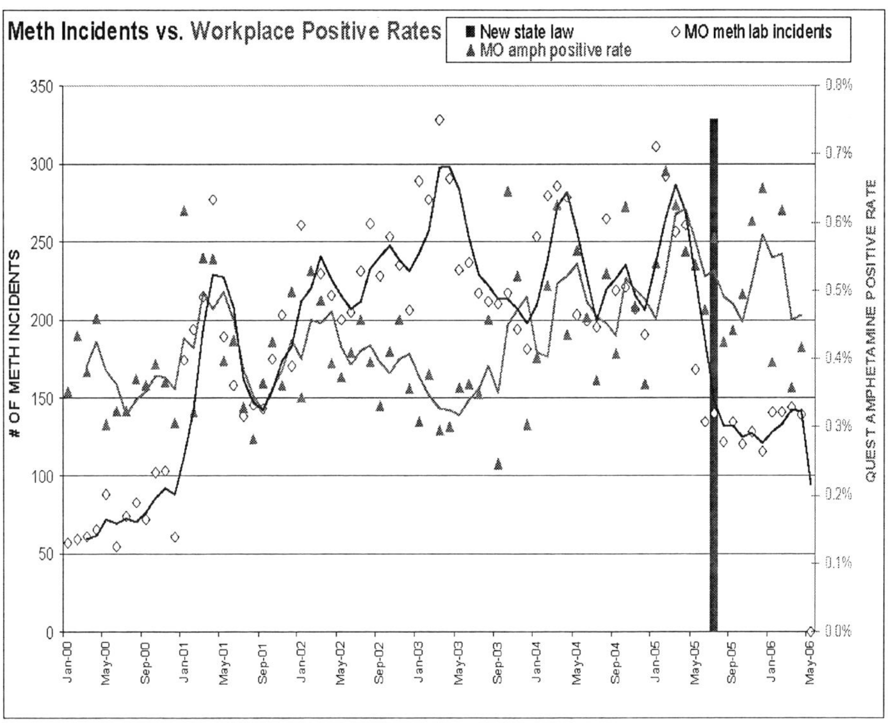

MONTANA

68% decline in meth lab incidents positive amphetamine workplace tests: -69.4%

Federal Standard: The United States Combat Methamphetamine Act		Montana State Law: Stricter than Federal Standard	
Effective Dates:	4/8/2006 9/30/2006	*Effective Date:*	July 1, 2005
		Meth lab reduction:	68%
Sales locations limited to pharmacies?	*No*	**Sales locations limited to pharmacies?**	**Mostly**
Behind the counter/locked cabinet?	**Yes**	**Behind the counter/locked cabinet?**	**Yes**
All listed chemicals?	**Yes**	*All listed chemicals?*	*EPH, PSE*
Daily sales limits:	**3.6 g**	*Daily sales limit:*	-
30-day purchase limit:	**9 g**	**30-day saleslimit:**	**9 g**
Identification/logbook requirement?	**Yes**	**Identification/logbook requirement?**	**Yes**

"Listed chemicals" means any productcontaining ephedrine (EPH), pseudoephedrine (PSE), or phenylpropanolamine (PPA).Items in bold indicatethe controlling standard in the state. Items in *italics* indicatethat the provision is trumped by a stricter standard.

Summary

Montana's methamphetamine precursor law went into effect July 1st 2005.The Montana law is stricter than the CMEA in several important respects.

Montana's law applies to single-entity and multi-active products containing pseudoephedrine or ephedrine (except for products in liquid or gelatin capsule form), and imposes a sales limit of nine grams in a 30-day period. The law limits sales of products containing pseudoephedrine or ephedrine to pharmacies, except in counties without a pharmacy; in these counties, the Montana Department of Justice may certify retail establishments to sell the products, subject to the same requirements on product placement, sales limits, and the like. In any case, the products must be kept behind pharmacy or store counters. There is an identification and logbook requirement in Montana.

State	Quest Amph Positives, 2000 (Ja n-Ma y)	Quest Amph Positives, 2001 (Jan-May)	Quest Amph Positives, 2002 (Jan-May)	Quest Amph Positives, 2003 (Jan-May)	Quest Amph Positives, 2004 (Jan-May)	Quest Amph Positives, 2005 (Jan-May)	Quest Amph Positives, 2006 (Ja n-Ma y)	% Change 2005-2006
MT	0.00%	0.39%	0.11%	0.41%	0.44%	0.90%	0.27%	-69.49%

Montana Data Roundup

In Montana, methamphetamine laboratory incident seizures declined by 68% after the State's methamphetamine precursor control law went into effect, with the State reporting 17 seizures from July 1st , 2005 to April 30th, 2006, compared to 53 over the same time period one year earlier. Workplace drug testing results showed a 69.4% decrease in positive tests for amphetamine, measuring the first five months in 2006, compared to the same period one year earlier.

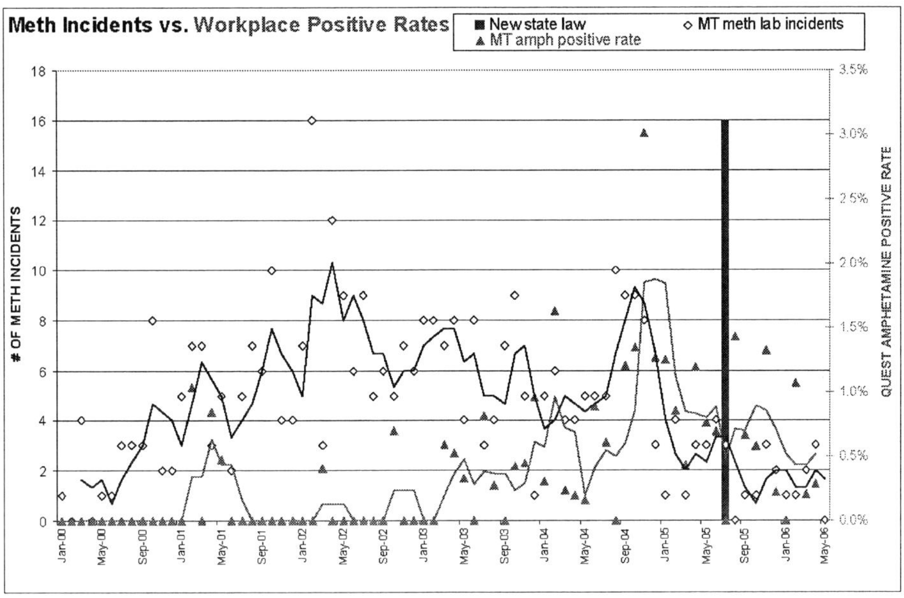

NEBRASKA

85% decline in meth lab incidents positive amphetamine workplace tests: -24.9%

Federal Standard: The United States Combat Methamphetamine Act		**Nebraska State Law: Stricter than Federal Standard**	
Effective Dates:	4/8/2006 9/30/2006	*Effective Date:*	September 1st, 2005
		Meth lab reduction:	85%
Sales locations limited to pharmacies?	**No**	**Sales locations limited to pharmacies?**	**No**
Behind the counter/locked cabinet?	**Yes**	**Behind the counter/locked cabinet?**	**Yes**
All listed chemicals?	**Yes**	**All listed chemicals?**	**EPH, PSE**
Daily sales limits:	*3.6 g*	**Daily sales limits:**	**1.44 g**
30-day purchase limit:	9 g	*30-day purchase limit:*	--
Identification/logbook requirement?	**Yes**	*Identification/logbook requirement?*	*ID only*

"Listed chemicals" means any productcontaining ephedrine (EPH), pseudoephedrine (PSE), or phenylpropanolamine (PPA).Items in bold indicatethe controlling standard in the state. Items in *italics* indicatethat the provision is trumped by a stricter standard.

Summary

Nebraska's methamphetamine precursor law went into effect September 1st , 2005.The Nebraska Law is stricter in some respects than the CMEA.

Nebraska's law applies to single-entity and multi-active products containing pseudoephedrine, and imposes a 24-hour purchase limit of 1.44 grams. State law requires that products containing the chemicals be kept behind a store counter or in a locked cabinet. The customer must show identification, but there is no logbook requirement under the State law (although the presence of this requirement under the Federal CMEA means that the logbook requirement does exist in Nebraska, as in the rest of the nation). The State does not limit sales of products containing methamphetamine precursor chemicals like pseudoephedrine to pharmacies, and does not classify products containing those chemicals as Schedule V drugs under the State scheduling scheme.

State	Quest Amph Positives, 2000 (Ja n-Ma y)	Quest Amph Positives, 2001 (Jan-May)	Quest Amph Positives, 2002 (Jan-May)	Quest Amph Positives, 2003 (Jan-May)	Quest Amph Positives, 2004 (Jan-May)	Quest Amph Positives, 2005 (Jan-May)	Quest Amph Positives, 2006 (Ja n-Ma y)	% Change 2005-2006
NE	0.30%	0.44%	0.41%	0.36%	0.38%	0.73%	0.55%	-24.86%

Nebraska Data Roundup

In Nebraska, methamphetamine laboratory incident seizures declined by 85% after the State's methamphetamine precursor control law went into effect, with the State reporting 35 seizures from September 1st, 2005 to April 30th , 2006, compared to 241 over the same time period one year earlier. Workplace drug testing results showed a 24.9% decrease in positive tests for amphetamine, measuring the first five months in 2006, compared to the same period one year earlier.

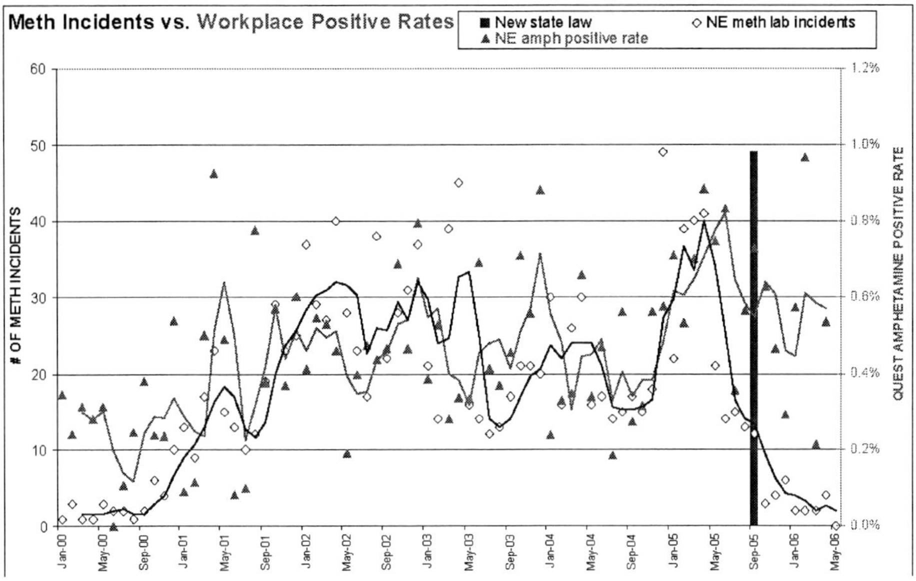

Nevada

no state law positive amphetamine workplace tests: -30.4%

Federal Standard: The United States Combat Methamphetamine Act		Nevada State Law: No state law, only CMEA applies	
Effective Dates:	4/8/2006 9/30/2006	*Effective Date:* Meth lab reduction:	None n/a
Sales locations limited to pharmacies?	**No**	*Sales locations limited to pharmacies?*	*No*
Behind the counter/locked cabinet?	**Yes**	*Behind the counter/locked cabinet?*	*No*
All listed chemicals?	**Yes**	*All listed chemicals?*	*No*
Daily sales limits:	**3.6 g**	*Daily sales limits:*	*None*
30-day purchase limit:	**9 g**	*30-day purchase limit:*	*None*
Identification/logbook requirement?	**Yes**	*Identification/logbook requirement?*	*No*
"Listed chemicals" means any productcontaining ephedrine (EPH), pseudoephedrine (PSE), or phenylpropanolamine (PPA).Items in bold indicatethe controlling standard in the state. Items in *italics* indicatethat the provision is trumped by a stricter standard.			

Summary

Nevada did not implement any methamphetamine precursor controls before the Combat Meth Act took effect September 30th 2006. In other words, the CMEA is the controlling standard in Nevada. It also means that the State does not limit sales of products containing methamphetamine precursors like pseudoephedrine to pharmacies, and does not classify these products as Schedule V drugs under the State's scheduling scheme.

State	Quest Amph Positives, 2000 (Ja n-Ma y)	Quest Amph Positives, 2001 (Jan-May)	Quest Amph Positives, 2002 (Jan-May)	Quest Amph Positives, 2003 (Jan-May)	Quest Amph Positives, 2004 (Jan-May)	Quest Amph Positives, 2005 (Jan-May)	Quest Amph Positives, 2006 (Ja n-Ma y)	% Change 2005-2006
NE	0.72%	0.97%	0.71%	0.75%	1.00%	0.99%	0.69%	-30.48%

Nevada Data Roundup

Nevada did not implement any methamphetamine precursor control legislation before the CMEA went into effect on September 30th , 2006. However, methamphetamine laboratory incidents look to be on a declining trend since peaking in 2003 and early 2004. Workplace drug testing results showed a 30.4% decrease in positive tests for amphetamine, measuring the first five months in 2006, compared to the same period one year earlier.

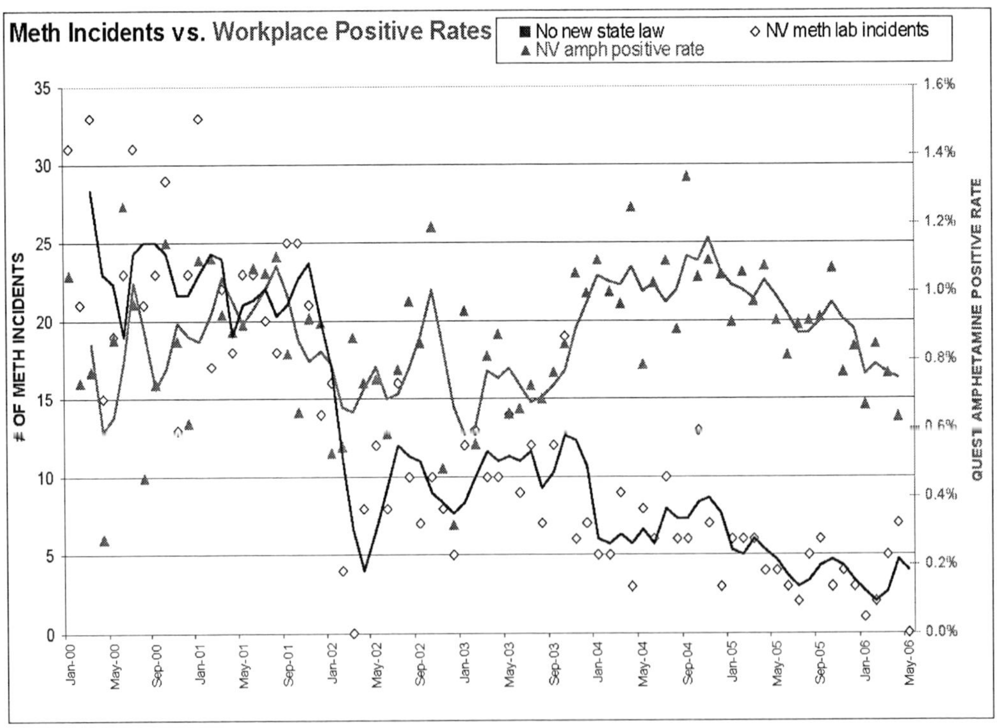

NEW HAMPSHIRE

no state law/historical low lab numbers positive amphetamine workplace tests: +25.3%

Federal Standard: The United States Combat Methamphetamine Act		New Hampshire State Law: No State Law, only CMEA applies	
Effective Dates:	4/8/2006	Effective Date:	None
	9/30/2006	Meth lab reduction:	n/a
Sales locations limited to pharmacies?	**No**	*Sales locations limited to pharmacies?*	*No*
Behind the counter/locked cabinet?	**Yes**	*Behind the counter/locked cabinet?*	*No*
All listed chemicals?	**Yes**	*All listed chemicals?*	*No*
Daily sales limits:	**3.6 g**	*Daily sales limits:*	*None*
30-day purchase limit:	**9 g**	*30-day purchase limit:*	*None*
Identification/logbook requirement?	**Yes**	*Identification/logbook requirement?*	*No*

"Listed chemicals" means any productcontaining ephedrine (EPH), pseudoephedrine (PSE), or phenylpropanolamine (PPA).Items in bold indicatethe controlling standard in the state. Items in *italics* indicatethat the provision is trumped by a stricter standard.

Summary

New Hampshire, which has enjoyed low numbers of methamphetamine laboratory incidents, did not implement any methamphetamine precursor controls before the Combat Meth Act took effect September 30th 2006. In other words, the CMEA is the controlling standard in New Hampshire. It also means that the State does not limit sales of products containing methamphetamine precursors like pseudoephedrine to pharmacies, and does not classify these products as Schedule V drugs under the State's scheduling scheme.

State	Quest Amph Positives, 2000 (Ja n-Ma y)	Quest Amph Positives, 2001 (Jan-May)	Quest Amph Positives, 2002 (Jan-May)	Quest Amph Positives, 2003 (Jan-May)	Quest Amph Positives, 2004 (Jan-May)	Quest Amph Positives, 2005 (Jan-May)	Quest Amph Positives, 2006 (Ja n-Ma y)	% Change 2005-2006
NH	0.14%	0.20%	0.18%	0.30%	0.34%	0.36%	0.45%	25.25%

New Hampshire Data Roundup

New Hampshire did not implement any state-level methamphetamine precursor control legislation prior to the CMEA's effective date of September 30th , 2006. In the last four years, the State has reported just eleven methamphetamine laboratory incident seizures to the DEA. Workplace drug testing results showed a 25.3% decrease in positive tests for amphetamine, measuring the first five months in 2006, compared to the same period one year earlier.

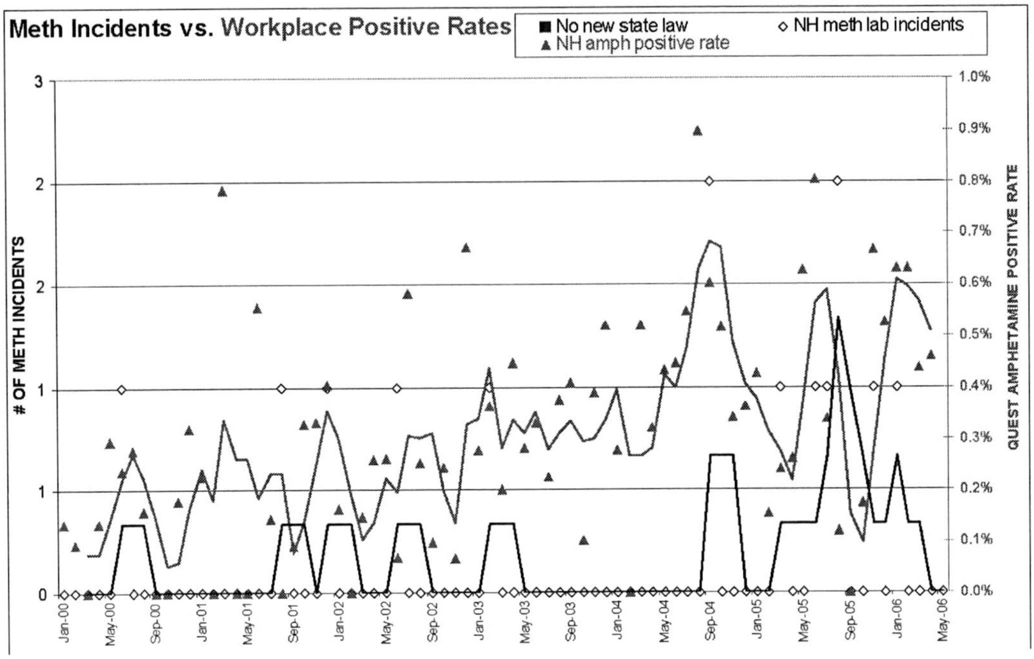

NEW JERSEY

data not yet available positive amphetamine workplace tests: -2.2%

Federal Standard: The United States Combat Methamphetamine Act		**New Jersey State Law: Less strict than Federal standards**	
Effective Dates:	4/8/2006	Effective Date:	November 24, 2005
	9/30/2006	Meth lab reduction:	n/a
Sales locations limited to pharmacies?	**No**	**Sales locations limited to pharmacies?**	**No**
Behind the counter/locked cabinet?	**Yes**	***Behind the counter/locked cabinet?***	***No***
All listed chemicals?	**Yes**	**All listed chemicals?**	**Yes**
Daily sales limits:	**3.6 g**	*Transaction limit:*	*3 pkg/9 g*
30-day purchase limit:	**9 g**	*30-day purchase limit:*	*None*
Identification/logbook requirement?	**Yes**	*Identification/logbook requirement?*	*No*

"Listed chemicals" means any productcontaining ephedrine (EPH), pseudoephedrine (PSE), or phenylpropanolamine (PPA).Items in bold indicatethe controlling standard in the state. Items in *italics* indicatethat the provision is trumped by a stricter standard.

Summary

New Jersey's methamphetamine precursor law went into effect November 23rd , 2005. The New Jersey law is less strict in most respects than the CMEA.

New Jersey's law simply imposes a single-transaction sales limit of three packages or nine grams of products containing pseudoephedrine, ephedrine, or (both single-entity and multi-active products). Although the State law does not require that the products be kept behind a store counter or in a locked cabinet, imposes no limit on monthly purchases, and contains no requirement as to purchasers showing identification or signing a logbook, these provisions are required nationwide under the Federal CMEA. New Jersey does not limit sales of products containing methamphetamine precursor chemicals like pseudoephedrine to pharmacies, and does not classify products containing those chemicals as Schedule V drugs under the State scheduling scheme.

State	Quest Amph Positives, 2000 (Ja n-Ma y)	Quest Amph Positives, 2001 (Jan-May)	Quest Amph Positives, 2002 (Jan-May)	Quest Amph Positives, 2003 (Jan-May)	Quest Amph Positives, 2004 (Jan-May)	Quest Amph Positives, 2005 (Jan-May)	Quest Amph Positives, 2006 (Ja n-Ma y)	% Change 2005-2006
NJ	0.09%	0.13%	0.15%	0.15%	0.14%	0.22%	0.21%	-2.18%

New Jersey Data Roundup

New Jersey has enjoyed relatively low numbers of methamphetamine laboratory incidents, reporting just five to the DEA in the past four years. As such, there is insufficient data to measure the impact of New Jersey's methamphetamine precursor control law. Workplace drug testing results showed a 2.2% decrease in positive tests for amphetamine, measuring the first five months in 2006, compared to the same period one year earlier.

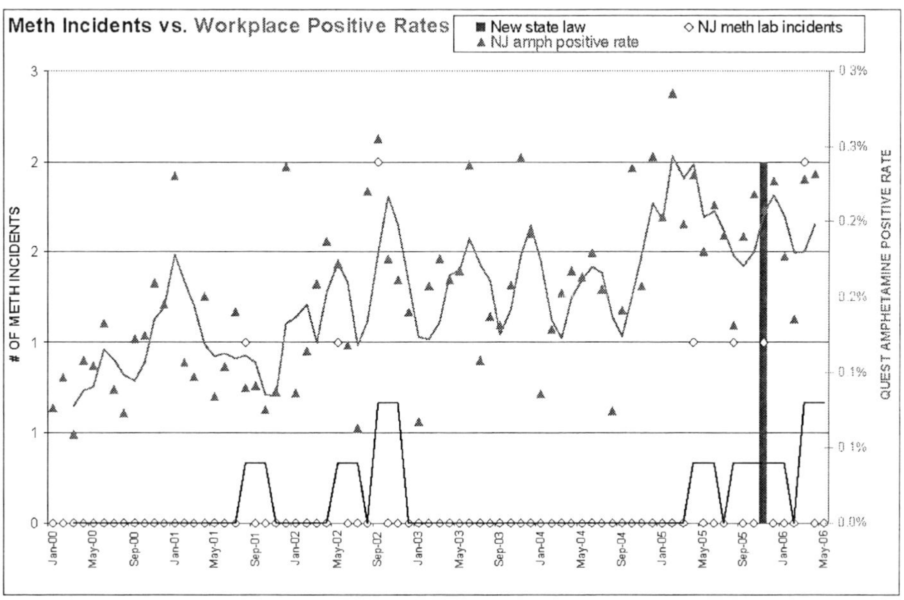

NEW MEXICO

51% decline in meth lab incidents positive amphetamine workplace tests: -60.5%

Federal Standard: The United States Combat Methamphetamine Act		New Jersey State Law: Less strict than Federal standards	
Effective Dates:	4/8/2006 9/30/2006	*Effective Date:*	July 1, 2006
		Meth lab reduction:	51%
Sales locations limited to pharmacies?	**No**	**Sales locations limited to pharmacies?**	**Yes**
Behind the counter/locked cabinet?	**Yes**	*Behind the counter/locked cabinet?*	**Yes**
All listed chemicals?	**Yes**	**All listed chemicals?**	**PSE**
Daily sales limits:	**3.6 g**	**Daily sales limits:**	***see below**
30-day purchase limit:	**9 g**	**30-day purchase limit:**	**9 g**
Identification/logbook requirement?	**Yes**	**Identification/logbook requirement?**	**Yes**

"Listed chemicals" means any productcontaining ephedrine (EPH), pseudoephedrine (PSE), or phenylpropanolamine (PPA).Items in bold indicatethe controlling standard in the state. Items in *italics* indicatethat the provision is trumped by a stricter standard.

Summary

New Mexico's methamphetamine precursor law went into effect in several stages: January 15th, 2005; September 30th , 2005, and July 1st 2006. Existing New Mexico law is stricter than the CMEA in several important respects.

As of July 1st , 2006, New Mexico's law classifies all products containing pseudoephedrine, except those in liquid form, as Schedule V drugs. The sales limits mirror Federal requirements, with a 3.6 gram daily limit and 9 gram monthly limit. Products containing pseudoephedrine may be sold only at pharmacies and by a licensed pharmacist, pharmacy intern, or pharmacy technician. The law requires that purchasers show identification and sign a logbook.

Prior to July 1st , 2006, the law was less restrictive, allowing sales at non-pharmacy retail stores, and imposing a somewhat complex system of requirements on product placement (for example, requiring products containing pseudoephedrine to be kept no more than 20 feet from a checkout counter or in a locked case accessible only by an employee, with different provisions for single-entity and multi-active pseudoephedrine products).

State	Quest Amph Positives, 2000 (Ja n-Ma y)	Quest Amph Positives, 2001 (Jan-May)	Quest Amph Positives, 2002 (Jan-May)	Quest Amph Positives, 2003 (Jan-May)	Quest Amph Positives, 2004 (Jan-May)	Quest Amph Positives, 2005 (Jan-May)	Quest Amph Positives, 2006 (Ja n-Ma y)	% Change 2005-2006
NM	0.42%	0.38%	0.51%	0.52%	0.76%	0.92%	0.36%	-60.47%

New Mexico Data Roundup

In New Mexico, methamphetamine laboratory incident seizures declined by 51% after the State's methamphetamine precursor control law (the first iteration) went into effect, with the State reporting 59 seizures from January 15th, 2005 to April 30th , 2006, compared to 120 over the same time period one year earlier. The most recent iteration was effective on July 1st, 2006, and is too recent to measure. Workplace drug testing results showed a 60.5% decrease in positive tests for amphetamine, measuring the first five months in 2006, compared to the same period one year earlier.

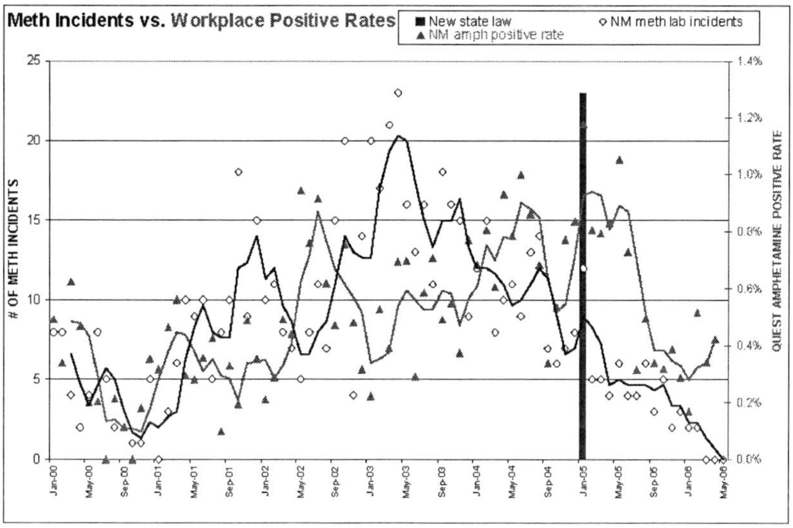

New York

no state law positive amphetamine workplace tests: +3.2%

Federal Standard: The United States Combat Methamphetamine Act		**New York State Law: No State Law, only CMEA applies**	
Effective Dates:	4/8/2006	*Effective Date:*	None
	9/30/2006	Meth lab reduction:	n/a
Sales locations limited to pharmacies?	**No**	*Sales locations limited to pharmacies?*	*No*
Behind the counter/locked cabinet?	**Yes**	*Behind the counter/locked cabinet?*	*No*
All listed chemicals?	**Yes**	*All listed chemicals?*	*No*
Daily sales limits:	**3.6 g**	*Daily sales limits:*	*None*
30-day purchase limit:	**9 g**	*30-day purchase limit:*	*None*
Identification/logbook requirement?	**Yes**	*Identification/logbook requirement?*	*No*

"Listed chemicals" means any productcontaining ephedrine (EPH), pseudoephedrine (PSE), or phenylpropanolamine (PPA).Items in bold indicatethe controlling standard in the state. Items in *italics* indicatethat the provision is trumped by a stricter standard.

Summary

New York did not implement any methamphetamine precursor controls before the Combat Meth Act took effect September 30th 2006. In other words, the CMEA is the controlling standard in New York. It also means that the State does not limit sales of products containing methamphetamine precursors like pseudoephedrine to pharmacies, and does not classify these products as Schedule V drugs under the State's scheduling scheme.

State	Quest Amph Positives, 2000 (Ja n-Ma y)	Quest Amph Positives, 2001 (Jan-May)	Quest Amph Positives, 2002 (Jan-May)	Quest Amph Positives, 2003 (Jan-May)	Quest Amph Positives, 2004 (Jan-May)	Quest Amph Positives, 2005 (Jan-May)	Quest Amph Positives, 2006 (Ja n-Ma y)	% Change 2005-2006
NY	0.06%	0.07%	0.07%	0.10%	0.11%	0.13%	0.13%	3.22%

New York Data Roundup

New York did not enact any significant methamphetamine precursor control legislation prior to the implementation of the Federal CMEA. Over the last four years, the State has reported 118 laboratory incident seizures to the DEA. Workplace drug testing results showed a 3.2% increase in positive tests for amphetamine, measuring the first five months in 2006, compared to the same period one year earlier.

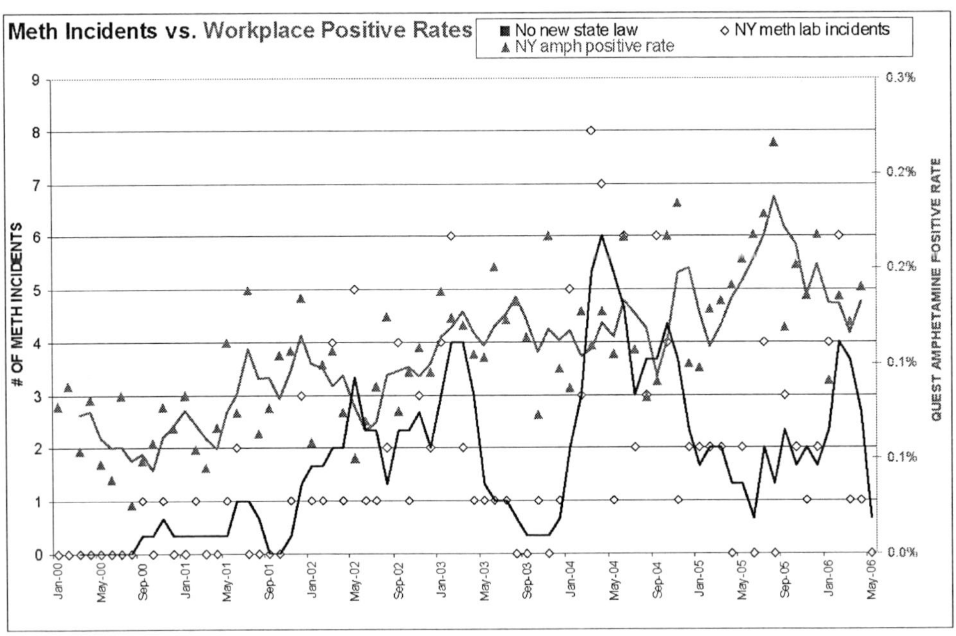

NORTH CAROLINA

27% decline in meth lab incidents positive amphetamine workplace tests: -11.1%

Federal Standard: The United States Combat Methamphetamine Act		North Carolina State Law: Stricter than the Federal Standards	
Effective Dates:	4/8/2006	*Effective Date:*	January 15, 2006
	9/30/2006	Meth lab reduction:	27%
Sales locations limited to pharmacies?	**No**	**Sales locations limited to pharmacies?**	**Yes**
Behind the counter/locked cabinet?	**Yes**	**Behind the counter/locked cabinet?**	**Yes**
All listed chemicals?	**Yes**	**All listed chemicals?**	**EPH, PSE**
Daily sales limits:	**3.6 g**	*Transaction limit:*	*2 pkg/6 g*
30-day purchase limit:	**9 g**	**30-day purchase limit:**	**3 pkg/9 g**
Identification/logbook requirement?	**Yes**	**Identification/logbook requirement?**	**Yes**
"Listed chemicals" means any productcontaining ephedrine (EPH), pseudoephedrine (PSE), or phenylpropanolamine (PPA).Items in bold indicatethe controlling standard in the state. Items in *italics* indicatethat the provision is trumped by a stricter standard.			

Summary

North Carolina's methamphetamine precursor law went into effect in two stages: January 15th, 2006, and August 3rd, 2006. The North Carolina law is stricter than the CMEA.

North Carolina's law imposes sales limits similar to those in the CMEA, of 3.6 grams per day, and 9 grams per month. (From January 15th until August 3rd , 2006, the purchase limits were 6 grams per day and 9 grams per month.) The current law applies to both single-entity and multi-active products containing pseudoephedrine or ephedrine. The law is somewhat unusual in that it references sales by retailers, but directly indicates that products containing pseudoephedrine may only be sold from, and kept behind, pharmacy counters. As a result, the law effectively imposes a pharmacy-only sales requirement on products containing pseudoephedrine, which is stricter than the Federal CMEA standard. These provisions were looser prior to August 3rd , 2006. There is an ID and logbook requirement in North Carolina.

State	Quest Amph Positives, 2000 (Ja n-Ma y)	Quest Amph Positives, 2001 (Jan-May)	Quest Amph Positives, 2002 (Jan-May)	Quest Amph Positives, 2003 (Jan-May)	Quest Amph Positives, 2004 (Jan-May)	Quest Amph Positives, 2005 (Jan-May)	Quest Amph Positives, 2006 (Ja n-Ma y)	% Change 2005-2006
NC	0.10%	0.21%	0.24%	0.25%	0.28%	0.38%	0.34%	-11.06%

North Carolina Data Roundup

In North Carolina, methamphetamine laboratory incident seizures declined by 27% after the State's methamphetamine precursor control law went into effect, with the State reporting 109 seizures from January 15th , 2006 to April 30th , 2006, compared to 150 over the same time period one year earlier. Workplace drug testing results showed a 11.1% decrease in positive tests for amphetamine, measuring the first five months in 2006, compared to the same period one year earlier

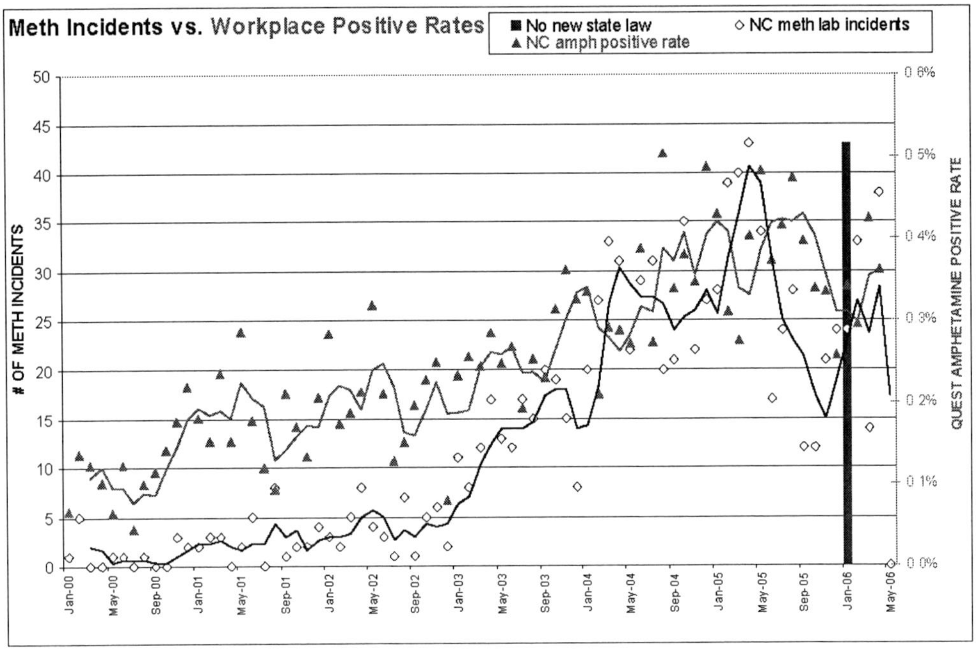

North Dakota

80% decline in meth lab incidents positive amphetamine workplace tests: -33.9%

Federal Standard: The United States Combat Methamphetamine Act		North Dakota State Law: Less strict than Federal Standards	
Effective Dates:	4/8/2006 9/30/2006	*Effective Date:* Meth lab reduction:	June 1, 2005 80%
Sales locations limited to pharmacies?	**No**	**Sales locations limited to pharmacies?**	**No**
Behind the counter/locked cabinet?	**Yes**	**Behind the counter/locked cabinet?**	**Yes**
All listed chemicals?	**Yes**	*All listed chemicals?*	*EPH, PSE*
Daily sales limits:	**3.6 g**	*Transactionlimit:*	*4 g*
30-day purchase limit:	**9 g**	*30-day purchase limit:*	--
Identification/logbook requirement?	**Yes**	**Identification/logbook requirement?**	**Yes**

"Listed chemicals" means any productcontaining ephedrine (EPH), pseudoephedrine (PSE), or phenylpropanolamine (PPA).Items in bold indicatethe controlling standard in the state. Items in

italics indicatethat the provision is trumped by a stricter standard.

Summary

North Dakota's methamphetamine precursor law went into effect June 1st 2005. The North Dakota law is less strict than the CMEA in several important respects.

North Dakota's law limits transactions of products containing pseudoephedrine or ephedrine to two packages, each of which may not contain more than two grams of the chemical. The State law imposes an identification and logbook requirement. The State law contains a somewhat different scheme for product placement than the CMEA, allowing either video surveillance of the products, or placement behind the counter. The CMEA appears to be slightly stricter on this point than North Dakota law, thereby controlling product placement in North Dakota. North Dakota does not limit sales of products containing methamphetamine precursor chemicals like pseudoephedrine to pharmacies, and does not classify products containing those chemicals as Schedule V drugs under the State scheduling scheme.

State	Quest Amph Positives, 2000 (Ja n-Ma y)	Quest Amph Positives, 2001 (Jan-May)	Quest Amph Positives, 2002 (Jan-May)	Quest Amph Positives, 2003 (Jan-May)	Quest Amph Positives, 2004 (Jan-May)	Quest Amph Positives, 2005 (Jan-May)	Quest Amph Positives, 2006 (Ja n-Ma y)	% Change 2005-2006
ND	0.12%	0.07%	0.08%	0.22%	0.26%	0.46%	0.30%	-33.93%

North Dakota Data Roundup

In North Dakota, methamphetamine laboratory incident seizures declined by 80% after the State's methamphetamine precursor control law went into effect, with the State reporting 49 seizures from June 1st , 2005, to April 30th , 2006, compared to 248 over the same time period one year earlier. Workplace drug testing results showed a 33.9% decrease in positive tests for amphetamine, measuring the first five months in 2006, compared to the same period one year earlier.

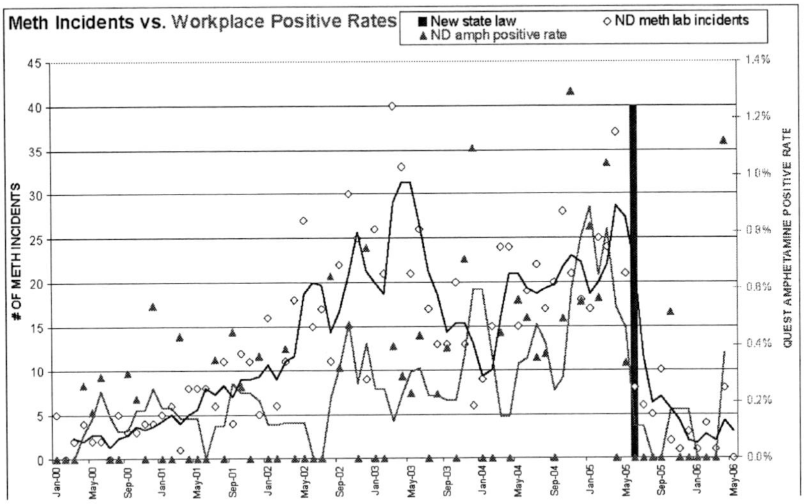

Ohio

data not yet available positive amphetamine workplace tests: +5.4%

Federal Standard: The United States Combat Methamphetamine Act		**Ohio State Law: Less strict than Federal Standards**	
Effective Dates:	4/8/2006 9/30/2006	*Effective Date:* Meth lab reduction:	February 9' 2006 unavailable
Sales locations limited to pharmacies?	**No**	**Sales locations limited to pharmacies?**	**No**
Behind the counter/locked cabinet?	**Yes**	**Behind the counter/locked cabinet?**	**Yes**
All listed chemicals?	**Yes**	*All listed chemicals?*	*single-entity PSE only*
Daily sales limits:	**3.6 g**	*Daily sales limits:*	*None*
30-day purchase limit:	**9 g**	**30-day purchase limit:**	**9 g**
Identification/logbook requirement?	**Yes**	**Identification/logbook requirement?**	**Yes**

"Listed chemicals" means any productcontaining ephedrine (EPH), pseudoephedrine (PSE), or phenylpropanolamine (PPA).Items in bold indicatethe controlling standard in the state. Items in *italics* indicatethat the provision is trumped by a stricter standard.

Summary

Ohio's methamphetamine precursor law went into effect May 17th , 2006.The Ohio Law is less strict than the CMEA in several important respects.

Ohio's law applies only to single-entity pseudoephedrine products. There is no daily sales/purchase limit under the State law, and there is a 9 gram monthly purchase limit, so the Federal CMEA's 3.6 daily purchase limit and 9 gram monthly purchase limit are the effective standard in Ohio. While it does not explicitly direct the products to be kept behind a store counter, it does require that the products be placed in such a manner that purchase is not possible without assistance from a store or pharmacy employee. The law contains an identification and logbook requirement. Ohio does not limit sales of products containing methamphetamine precursor chemicals like pseudoephedrine to pharmacies, and does not classify products containing those chemicals as Schedule V drugs under the State scheduling scheme.

State	Quest Amph Positives, 2000 (Ja n-Ma y)	Quest Amph Positives, 2001 (Jan-May)	Quest Amph Positives, 2002 (Jan-May)	Quest Amph Positives, 2003 (Jan-May)	Quest Amph Positives, 2004 (Jan-May)	Quest Amph Positives, 2005 (Jan-May)	Quest Amph Positives, 2006 (Ja n-Ma y)	% Change 2005-2006
OH	0.17%	0.15%	0.16%	0.21%	0.28%	0.34%	0.35%	5.43%

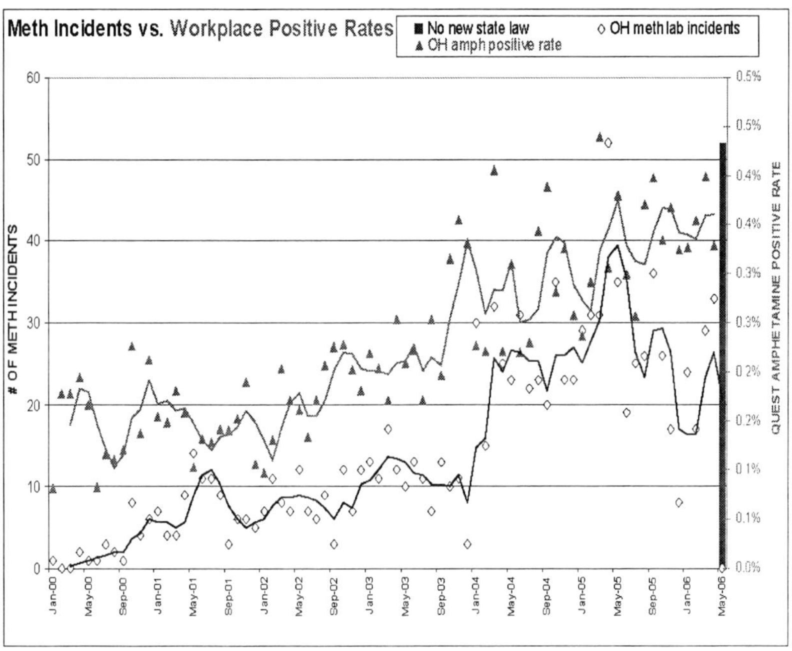

Ohio Data Roundup

Because Ohio's methamphetamine precursor control law went into effect in May 2006, the law is too recent to measure. Methamphetamine laboratory seizures in the State appear to have hit a peak in early 2005, generally declining since that time. Workplace drug testing results showed a 5.4% increase in positive tests for amphetamine, measuring the first five months in 2006, compared to the same period one year earlier.

OKLAHOMA

85% decline in meth lab incidents positive amphetamine workplace tests: -10.7%

Federal Standard: The United States Combat Methamphetamine Act		**Oklahoma State Law: Stricter than the Federal Standard**	
Effective Dates:	4/8/2006 9/30/2006	*Effective Date:* Meth lab reduction:	April 6, 2004 85%
Sales locations limited to pharmacies?	*No*	**Sales locations limited to pharmacies?**	**Yes**
Behind the counter/locked cabinet?	Yes	**Behind the counter/locked cabinet?**	**Yes**
All listed chemicals?	Yes	**All listed chemicals?**	**All PSE**
Daily sales limits:	*3.6 g*	**Daily sales limits:**	**--**
30-day purchase limit:	*9 g*	**30-day sales limit:**	**9 g**
Identification/logbook requirement?	**Yes**	**Identification/logbook requirement?**	**Yes**

"Listed chemicals" means any productcontaining ephedrine (EPH), pseudoephedrine (PSE), or phenylpropanolamine (PPA).Items in bold indicatethe controlling standard in the state. Items in italics indicatethat the provision is trumped by a stricter standard.

Summary

Oklahoma's methamphetamine precursor law went into effect April 6th , 2004, and was updated effective November 1, 2005. The Oklahoma Law is one of the strictest in the Nation, and is stricter than the CMEA. The law was also the first of its kind in the Nation, and served as the model for many States that subsequently implemented methamphetamine precursor control laws.

The Oklahoma law passed in April 20004 limited sales of sales of products containing pseudoephedrine (both single-entity and multi-active) to pharmacies, and requires that the products be placed behind the pharmacy counter. There is an identification and logbook requirement. The law places a 9 gram limit on monthly purchases. Oklahoma law also classifies products containing pseudoephedrine as Schedule V drugs.

The November 2005 updates to the law did not notably change the overall thrust of the law, addressing how information is collected and processed pursuant to the identification and logbook requirement

Oklahoma Data Roundup

In Oklahoma, methamphetamine laboratory incident seizures declined by 66% after the State's methamphetamine precursor control law first went into effect, with the State reporting 535 seizures from April 6, 2004, to October 30th , 2005, compared to 1572 over the same time period one year earlier. Then, after the second iteration of the law went into effect, methamphetamine laboratory incident seizures declined by 85% (compared to the period when no law was in effect), with 129 laboratory incident seizures reported from November 1st , 2005, to August 2006, compared to 862 in the same period before any State law was in effect. Workplace drug testing results showed a 10.7% decrease in positive tests for amphetamine, measuring the first five months in 2006, compared to the same period one year earlier.

State	Quest Amph Positives, 2000 (Ja n-Ma y)	Quest Amph Positives, 2001 (Jan-May)	Quest Amph Positives, 2002 (Jan-May)	Quest Amph Positives, 2003 (Jan-May)	Quest Amph Positives, 2004 (Jan-May)	Quest Amph Positives, 2005 (Jan-May)	Quest Amph Positives, 2006 (Ja n-Ma y)	% Change 2005-2006
OK	0.59%	0.75%	0.57%	0.62%	0.60%	0.85%	0.76%	-10.66%

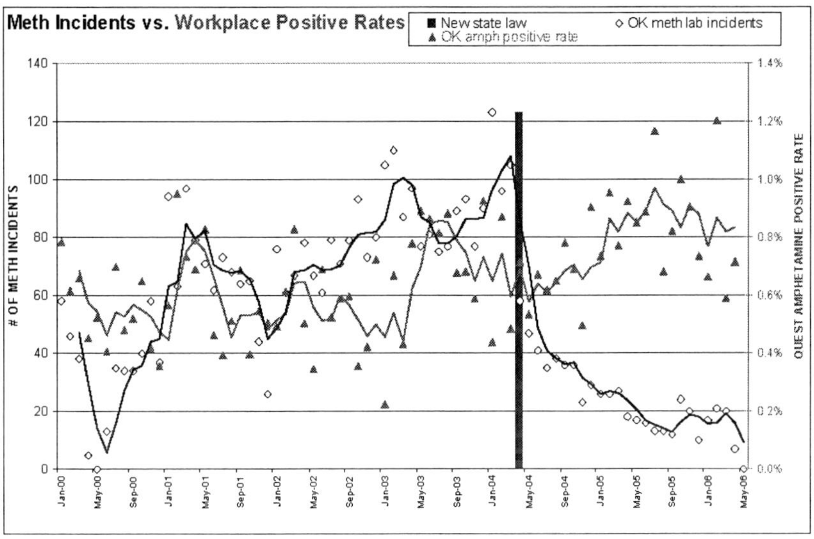

OREGON

87% decline in meth lab incidents positive amphetamine workplace tests: -29.1%

Federal Standard: The United States Combat Methamphetamine Act		Oregon State Law: Stricter than Federal Standard	
Effective Dates:	4/8/2006	*Effective Dates:*	11/15/04 * 4/14/05 * 7/1/06
	9/30/2006	Meth lab reduction:	41% 79% 87%
Sales locations limited to pharmacies?	*No*	**Sales locations limited to pharmacies?**	**Yes**
Behind the counter/locked cabinet?	*Yes*	**Behind the counter/locked cabinet?**	**n/a**
All listed chemicals?	*Yes*	**All listed chemicals?**	**Yes**
Daily sales limits:	*3.6 g*	**Transaction sales limit:**	**n/a**
30-day purchase limit:	*9 g*	**Purchase limit:**	**n/a**
Identification/logbook requirement?	*Yes*	**Identification/logbook requirement?**	**Yes**

"Listed chemicals" means any productcontaining ephedrine (EPH), pseudoephedrine (PSE), or phenylpropanolamine (PPA).Items in bold indicatethe controlling standard in the state. Items in *italics* indicatethat the provision is trumped by a stricter standard.

Summary

Oregon's methamphetamine precursor law is the strictest in the Nation. It went through three primary iterations. On November 15, 2004, the Oregon Board of Pharmacy implemented a rule requiring pseudoephedrine products, other than certain liquids and gel caps, be kept behind the counter and requiring photo identification. On May 14, 2005, a new rule went into effect requiring those pseudoephedrine products be kept behind the pharmacy counter and mandating photo identification and logbook entry for each sale. Finally, On July 1, 2006, a rule went into effect requiring a prescription for all products containing pseudoephedrine.

Oregon is the only state that completely prohibits the possession or use of any product containing pseudoephedrine without a prescription, classifying pseudoephedrine as a Schedule III drug under Oregon's controlled substance scheduling scheme. As such, products containing pseudoephedrine are, of course, only found behind pharmacy counters, as opposed to non-pharmacy retail outlets. Like other prescription drugs, identification is required, and as with all prescriptions, the transaction is recorded. Sales limits are not a relevant question, as the product is not sold over the counter.

State	Quest Amph Positives, 2000 (Ja n-Ma y)	Quest Amph Positives, 2001 (Jan-May)	Quest Amph Positives, 2002 (Jan-May)	Quest Amph Positives, 2003 (Jan-May)	Quest Amph Positives, 2004 (Jan-May)	Quest Amph Positives, 2005 (Jan-May)	Quest Amph Positives, 2006 (Ja n-Ma y)	% Change 2005-2006
OR	0.48%	0.39%	0.49%	0.72%	0.66%	0.64%	0.46%	-29.14%

Oregon Data Roundup

During the first iteration of methamphetamine precursor control (November 2004 to May 2005), Oregon recorded a total of 168 methamphetamine laboratory incidents, a drop of 41% from the same seven months a year prior (284 methamphetamine laboratory incidents from November 2003 to May 2004). During the second iteration, from June 2005 to June 2006 inclusive, there were 107 methamphetamine laboratory incidents. This was a 79% reduction, compared to the thirteen months prior to the first restriction (502 methamphetamine laboratory incidents). For the three months that the current iteration of the rule has been in place (July 2006 to August 2006), there were 13 methamphetamine laboratory incidents, an 87% reduction from the 100 laboratories seen during the same months before any restrictions were implemented. (There is also an 87% reduction using data for the most recent six months – April through September 2006, during which there were 30 metham phetam ine laboratories, compared to April through September 2004, during which there were 240.) Workplace drug testing results showed a 29.1% decrease in positive tests for amphetamine, measuring the first five months in 2006, compared to the same period one year earlier.

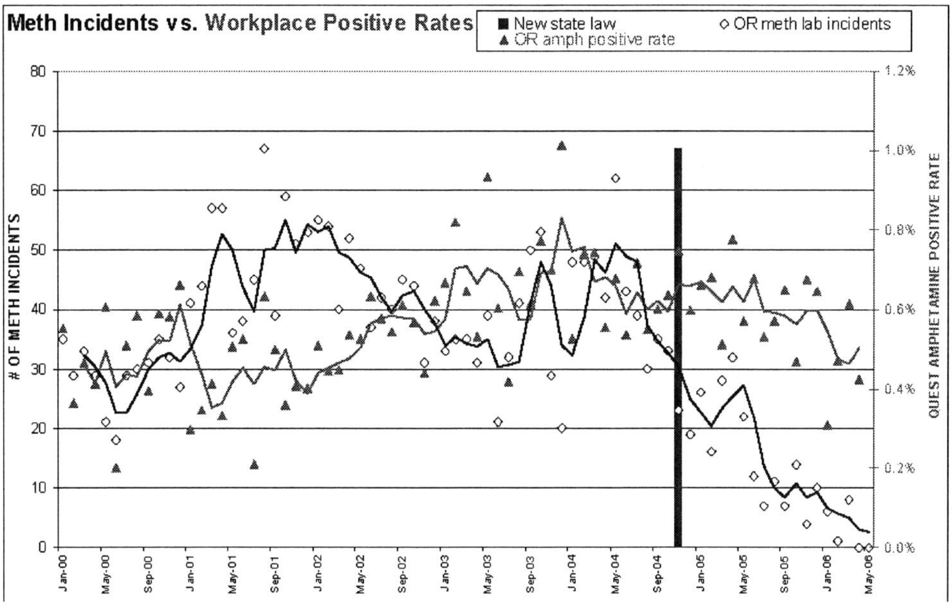

PENNSYLVANIA

no state law positive amphetamine workplace tests: +9.2%

Federal Standard: The United States Combat Methamphetamine Act		**Pennsylvania State Law: No state law, only CMEA applies**	
Effective Dates:	4/8/2006 9/30/2006	*Effective Date:* Meth lab reduction:	None n/a
Sales locations limited to pharmacies?	**No**	*Sales locations limited to pharmacies?*	*No*
Behind the counter/locked cabinet?	**Yes**	*Behind the counter/locked cabinet?*	*No*
All listed chemicals?	**Yes**	*All listed chemicals?*	*No*
Daily sales limits:	**3.6 g**	*Transaction limit:*	*No*
30-day purchase limit:	**9 g**	*30-day purchase limit:*	*None*
Identification/logbook requirement?	**Yes**	*Identification/logbook requirement?*	*No*

"Listed chemicals" means any productcontaining ephedrine (EPH), pseudoephedrine (PSE), or phenylpropanolamine (PPA).Items in bold indicatethe controlling standard in the state. Items in *italics* indicatethat the provision is trumped by a stricter standard.

Summary

Pennsylvania did not implement any methamphetamine precursor controls before the Combat Meth Act took effect September 30th 2006. In other words, the CMEA is the controlling standard in Pennsylvania. It also means that the State does not limit sales of products containing methamphetamine precursors like pseudoephedrine to pharmacies, and does not classify these products as Schedule V drugs under the State's scheduling scheme.

State	Quest Amph Positives, 2000 (Ja n-Ma y)	Quest Amph Positives, 2001 (Jan-May)	Quest Amph Positives, 2002 (Jan-May)	Quest Amph Positives, 2003 (Jan-May)	Quest Amph Positives, 2004 (Jan-May)	Quest Amph Positives, 2005 (Jan-May)	Quest Amph Positives, 2006 (Ja n-Ma y)	% Change 2005-2006
PA	0.13%	0.14%	0.17%	0.17%	0.20%	0.25%	0.27%	9.24%

Pennsylvania Data Roundup:

Pennsylvania did not implement any methamphetamine precursor controls before the Combat Meth Act took effect September 30th 2006. In 2004 and 2005, Pennsylvania recorded fewer than 190 methamphetamine laboratory incidents – often less than ten a month. Over the last four years, the State reported just over 300 methamphetamine laboratory incident seizures to the DEA. Workplace drug testing results showed a 9.2% increase in positive tests for amphetamine, measuring the first five months in 2006, compared to the same period one year earlier.

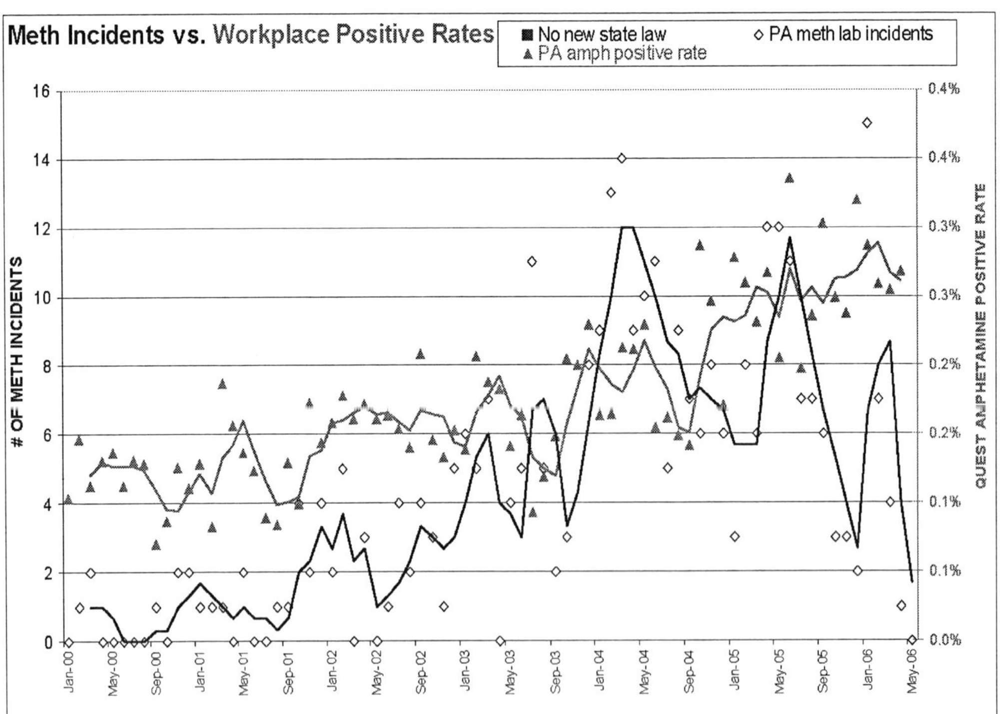

RHODE ISLAND

no state law positive amphetamine workplace tests: -24%

Federal Standard: The United States Combat Methamphetamine Act		Rhode Island State Law: No state law, only CMEA applies	
Effective Dates:	4/8/2006	*Effective Date:*	None
	9/30/2006	Meth lab reduction:	n/a
Sales locations limited to pharmacies?	**No**	*Sales locations limited to pharmacies?*	*No*
Behind the counter/locked cabinet?	**Yes**	*Behind the counter/locked cabinet?*	*No*
All listed chemicals?	**Yes**	*All listed chemicals?*	*No*
Daily sales limits:	**3.6 g**	*Daily sales limits:*	*None*
30-day purchase limit:	**9 g**	*30-day purchase limit:*	*None*
Identification/logbook requirement?	**Yes**	*Identification/logbook requirement?*	*No*

"Listed chemicals" means any productcontaining ephedrine (EPH), pseudoephedrine (PSE), or phenylpropanolamine (PPA).Items in bold indicatethe controlling standard in the state. Items in *italics* indicatethat the provision is trumped by a stricter standard.

Summary

Rhode Island, which has enjoyed low numbers of methamphetamine laboratory incidents, did not implement any methamphetamine precursor controls before the Combat Meth Act took effect September 30th 2006. In other words, the CMEA is the controlling standard in Rhode Island. It also means that the State does not limit sales of products containing methamphetamine precursors like pseudoephedrine to pharmacies, and does not classify these products as Schedule V drugs under the State's scheduling scheme.

State	Quest Amph Positives, 2000 (Ja n-Ma y)	Quest Amph Positives, 2001 (Jan-May)	Quest Amph Positives, 2002 (Jan-May)	Quest Amph Positives, 2003 (Jan-May)	Quest Amph Positives, 2004 (Jan-May)	Quest Amph Positives, 2005 (Jan-May)	Quest Amph Positives, 2006 (Ja n-Ma y)	% Change 2005-2006
RI	0.30%	0.33%	0.44%	0.35%	0.37%	0.57%	0.43%	-24.01%

Rhode Island Data Roundup

Rhode Island, which has enjoyed low numbers of methamphetamine laboratory incidents, did not implement any methamphetamine precursor controls before the Combat Meth Act took effect September 30th 2006. In the last four years, the State has reported one laboratory incident to the DEA. Workplace drug testing results showed a 24% decrease in positive tests for amphetamine, measuring the first five months in 2006, compared to the same period one year earlier.

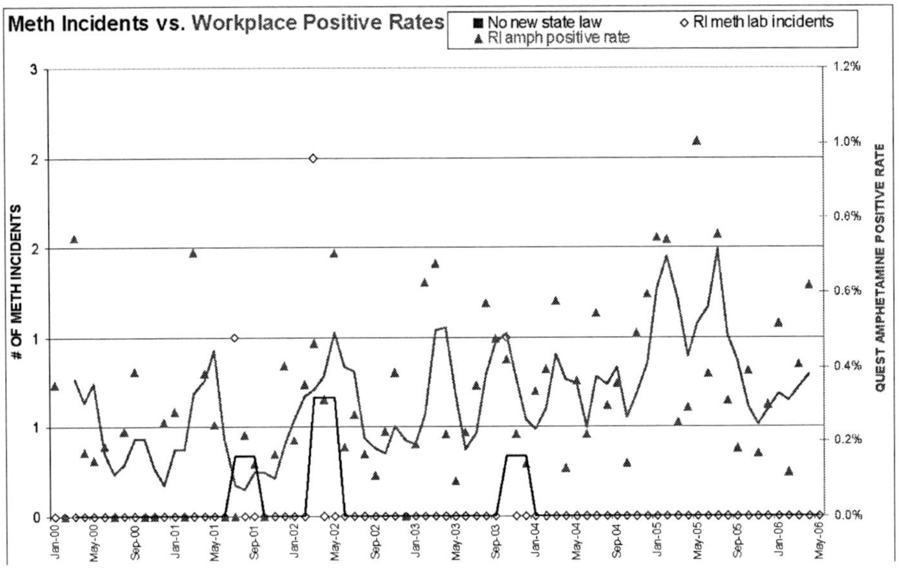

South Carolina

meth lab incident data not yet available positive amphetamine workplace tests: -9.1%

Federal Standard: The United States Combat Methamphetamine Act		**South Carolina State Law: Less Strict than Federal Standard**	
Effective Dates:	4/8/2006	*Effective Date:*	Nov 4th, 2006
	9/30/2006	Meth lab reduction:	unavailable
Sales locations limited to pharmacies?	**No**	**Sales locations limited to pharmacies?**	**No**
Behind the counter/locked cabinet?	**Yes**	**Behind the counter/locked cabinet?**	**Yes**
All listed chemicals?	**Yes**	**All listed chemicals?**	**EPH, PSE**
Daily sales limits:	**3.6 g**	*Transaction limit:*	*3 pkg/9 g*
***30-day purchase limit*:**	**9 g**	*30-day purchase limit:*	*None*
Identification/logbook requirement?	**Yes**	**Identification/logbook requirement?**	**Yes**

"Listed chemicals" means any productcontaining ephedrine (EPH), pseudoephedrine (PSE), or phenylpropanolamine (PPA).Items in bold indicatethe controlling standard in the state. Items in *italics* indicatethat the provision is trumped by a stricter standard.

Summary

South Carolina's methamphetamine precursor law went into effect on November 4th 2006. The South Carolina law is less strict than the CMEA in most respects.

South Carolina's law applies to single-entity and multi-active products containing pseudoephedrine or ephedrine. The law places a 9 gram limit on daily purchases, which is less strict than the Federal CMEA's 3.6 gram limit, and is thus largely irrelevant. There is an identification and logbook requirement in South Carolina. The State does not limit sales of products containing methamphetamine precursor chemicals like pseudoephedrine to pharmacies, and does not classify products containing those chemicals as Schedule V drugs under the State scheduling scheme.

State	Quest Amph Positives, 2000 (Ja n-Ma y)	Quest Amph Positives, 2001 (Jan-May)	Quest Amph Positives, 2002 (Jan-May)	Quest Amph Positives, 2003 (Jan-May)	Quest Amph Positives, 2004 (Jan-May)	Quest Amph Positives, 2005 (Jan-May)	Quest Amph Positives, 2006 (Ja n-Ma y)	% Change 2005-2006
SC	0.23%	0.34%	0.33%	0.38%	0.43%	0.54%	0.49%	-9.13%

South Carolina Data Roundup

Methamphetamine laboratory incidents in South Carolina have generally been on a downward trend since April 2005. However, the new State law, like the Federal CMEA law, is too recent to measure its impact. Workplace drug testing results showed a 9.1% decrease in positive tests for amphetamine, measuring the first five months in 2006, compared to the same period one year earlier.

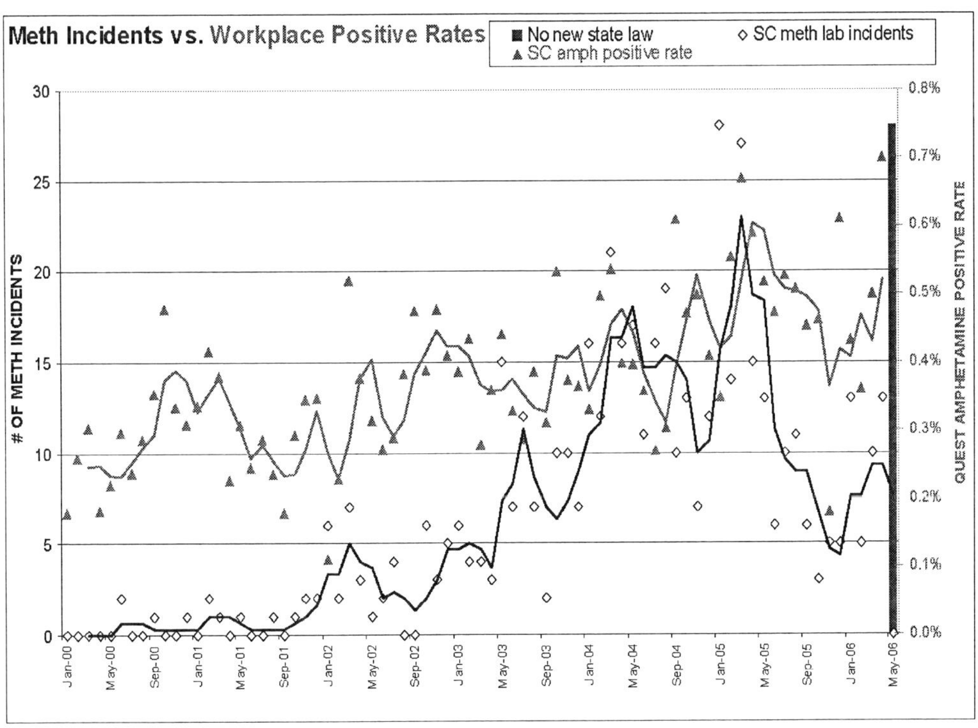

South Dakota

data not yet available positive amphetamine workplace tests: +7.7%

Federal Standard: The United States Combat Methamphetamine Act		**South Carolina State Law: Less Strict than Federal Standard**	
Effective Dates:	4/8/2006 9/30/2006	*Effective Date:* Meth lab reduction:	Nov 4th, 2006 n/a
Sales locations limited to pharmacies?	**No**	**Sales locations limited to pharmacies?**	**No**
Behind the counter/locked cabinet?	**Yes**	*Behind the counter/locked cabinet?*	*Some*
All listed chemicals?	**Yes**	**All listed chemicals?**	**EPH, PSE**
Daily sales limits:	*3.6 g*	**Transaction sales limit:**	**2 pkg**
***30-day purchase limit*:**	**9 g**	**30-day purchase limit:**	**9 g**
Identification/logbook requirement?	**Yes**	**Identification/logbook requirement?**	**Yes**
"Listed chemicals" means any productcontaining ephedrine (EPH), pseudoephedrine (PSE), or phenylpropanolamine (PPA).Items in bold indicatethe controlling standard in the state. Items in *italics* indicatethat the provision is trumped by a stricter standard.			

Summary

South Dakota's methamphetamine precursor law, SB 207, went into effect July 1st , 2006. The South Dakota Law is slightly less strict than the CMEA.

South Dakota's law applies to both single-entity and multi-active products containing pseudoephedrine or ephedrine. The law requires these products to be kept behind a store counter, in a locked container, or anywhere in the store if an electronic anti-theft system is used. (This last provision is not allowed under the Federal CMEA, so this option is presumably not being utilized.) The current purchase limits 2 packages daily or 9 grams monthly. South Dakota has an identification and logbook requirement. South Dakota does not limit sales of products containing methamphetamine precursor chemicals like pseudoephedrine to pharmacies, and does not classify products containing those chemicals as Schedule V drugs under the State scheduling scheme.

State	Quest Amph Positives, 2000 (Ja n-Ma y)	Quest Amph Positives, 2001 (Jan-May)	Quest Amph Positives, 2002 (Jan-May)	Quest Amph Positives, 2003 (Jan-May)	Quest Amph Positives, 2004 (Jan-May)	Quest Amph Positives, 2005 (Jan-May)	Quest Amph Positives, 2006 (Ja n-Ma y)	% Change 2005-2006
SD	0.22%	0.22%	0.26%	0.43%	0.29%	0.50%	0.53%	7.68%

South Dakota Data Roundup

South Dakota' methamphetamine precursor law went into effect on July 1st , 2006, and the law is too recent to measure its impact. In the last four years, 121 methamphetamine laboratory incidents were reported in South Dakota. Workplace drug testing results showed a 7.7% increase in positive tests for amphetamine, measuring the first five months in 2006, compared to the same period one year earlier.

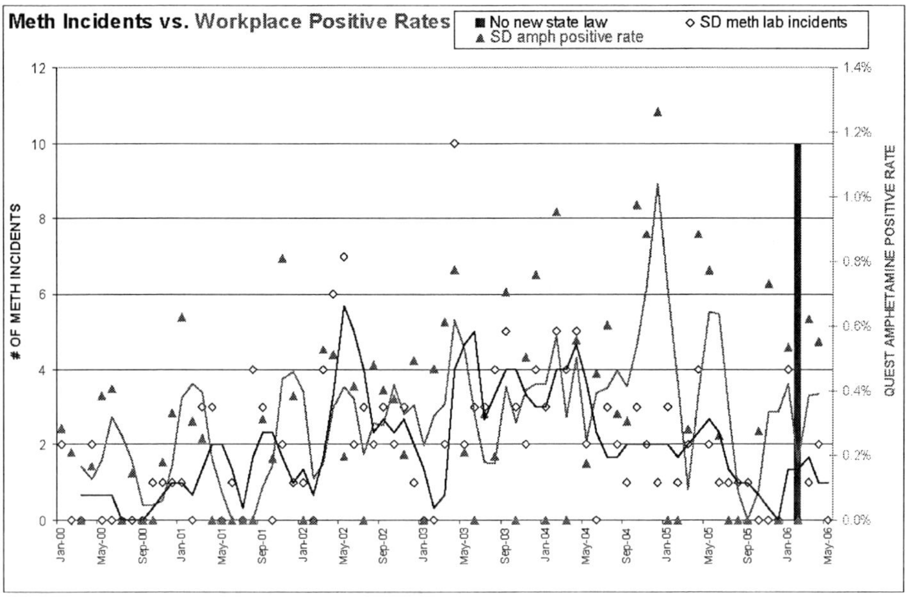

TENNESSEE

56% decline in meth lab incidents positive amphetamine workplace tests: +1%

Federal Standard: The United States Combat Methamphetamine Act		Tennessee State Law: Stricter than Federal Standards	
Effective Dates:	4/8/2006 9/30/2006	*Effective Date:*	March 31, 2005
		Meth lab reduction:	56%
Sales locations limited to pharmacies?	*No*	**Sales locations limited to pharmacies?**	**Yes**
Behind the counter/locked cabinet?	**Yes**	**Behind the counter/locked cabinet?**	**Yes**
All listed chemicals?	**Yes**	**All listed chemicals?**	**Yes**
Daily sales limits:	**3.6 g**	*Daily sales limits:*	*none*
30-day purchase limit:	**9 g**	**30-day sales limit:**	**3 pkg/9g**
Identification/logbook requirement?	**Yes**	**Identification/logbook requirement?**	**Yes**

"Listed chemicals" means any productcontaining ephedrine (EPH), pseudoephedrine (PSE), or phenylpropanolamine (PPA).Items in bold indicatethe controlling standard in the state. Items in *italics* indicatethat the provision is trumped by a stricter standard.

Summary

Tennessee's methamphetamine precursor law went into effect March 31st 2005 , and on April 29, 2005. The Tennessee law is stricter than the CMEA.

Tennessee's law applies to any product (both single entity and multi-active) containing pseudoephedrine, ephedrine, or phenylpropanolamine, and limits sales of those products to pharmacies (as of March 31, 2005). The law also requires that these products be kept behind pharmacy counters or in a locked container within view of and 25 feet of the counter, that the purchaser show identification and sign a logbook, and limits sales of the products to three packages or nine grams per transaction.

State	Quest Amph Positives, 2000 (Ja n-Ma y)	Quest Amph Positives, 2001 (Jan-May)	Quest Amph Positives, 2002 (Jan-May)	Quest Amph Positives, 2003 (Jan-May)	Quest Amph Positives, 2004 (Jan-May)	Quest Amph Positives, 2005 (Jan-May)	Quest Amph Positives, 2006 (Ja n-Ma y)	% Change 2005-2006
TN	0.20%	0.20%	0.27%	0.29%	0.37%	0.40%	0.40%	0.98%

Tennessee Data Roundup

In Tennessee, methamphetamine laboratory incident seizures declined by 56% after the State's methamphetamine precursor control law went into effect, with the State reporting 645 seizures from March 31st, 2005 to April 30th, 2006, compared to 1461 over the same time period one year earlier. Workplace drug testing results showed a 1% increase in positive tests for amphetamine, measuring the first five months in 2006, compared to the same period one year earlier.

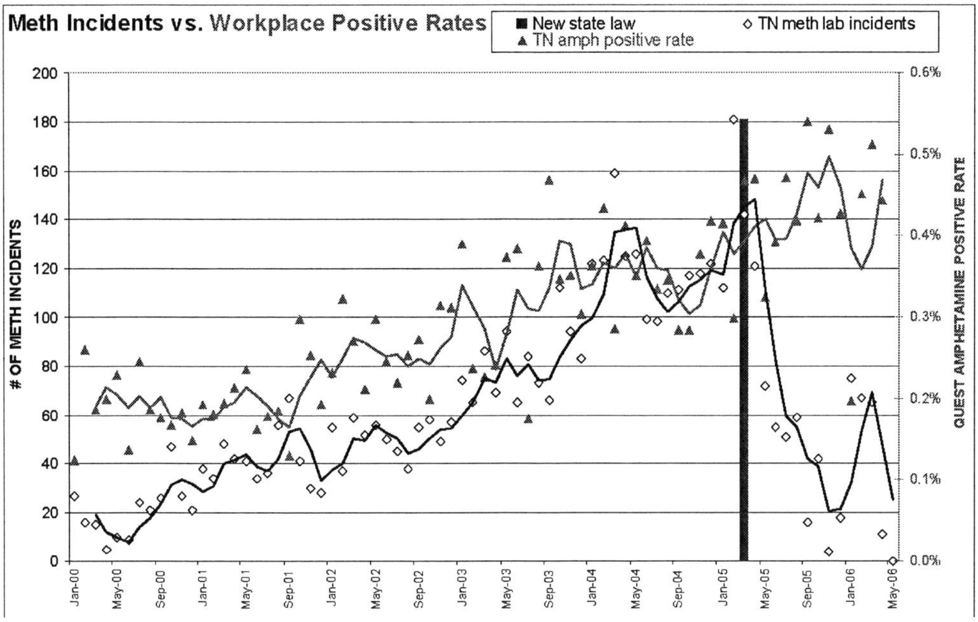

TEXAS

62% decline in meth lab incidents positive amphetamine workplace tests: -14.8%

Federal Standard: The United States Combat Methamphetamine Act		**Texas State Law: Similar to the Federal Standard**	
Effective Dates:	4/8/2006	*Effective Date:*	September 1, 2005
	9/30/2006	Meth lab reduction:	62%
Sales locations limited to pharmacies?	**No**	**Sales locations limited to pharmacies?**	**No**
Behind the counter/locked cabinet?	**Yes**	**Behind the counter/locked cabinet?**	**Yes**
All listed chemicals?	**Yes**	**All listed chemicals?**	**EPH, PSE**
Daily sales limits:	**3.6 g**	*Transaction sales limit:*	*2 pkg/6 g*
30-day purchase limit:	**9 g**	*30-day purchase limit:*	*None*
Identification/logbook requirement?	**Yes**	**Identification/logbook requirement?**	**Yes**

"Listed chemicals" means any productcontaining ephedrine (EPH), pseudoephedrine (PSE), or phenylpropanolamine (PPA).Items in bold indicatethe controlling standard in the state. Items in *italics* indicatethat the provision is trumped by a stricter standard.

Summary

Texas' methamphetamine precursor law went into effect August 1st 2005. The Texas law is stricter in some respects that the CMEA, but less strict in others.

Texas' law applies to products containing pseudoephedrine or ephedrine. It does not expressly put a sales or purchase limit on these products, but instead indicates that authorized sellers must take "reasonable steps" to ensure that sales do not exceed 2 packages or 6 grams. (This is trumped in Texas by the Federal CMEA, which has a 3.6 gram purchase limit). Sales are limited to either pharmacies or any business authorized to sell the products by the Department of State Health Services, and products must be placed behind the counter or within 30 feet of the counter and within the direct line of sight of the employee monitoring the counter. Texas law contains an identification and logbook requirement.

State	Quest Amph Positives, 2000 (Ja n-Ma y)	Quest Amph Positives, 2001 (Jan-May)	Quest Amph Positives, 2002 (Jan-May)	Quest Amph Positives, 2003 (Jan-May)	Quest Amph Positives, 2004 (Jan-May)	Quest Amph Positives, 2005 (Jan-May)	Quest Amph Positives, 2006 (Ja n-Ma y)	% Change 2005-2006
TX	0.21%	0.28%	0.35%	0.38%	0.51%	0.61%	0.52%	-14.79%

Texas Data Roundup

In Texas, methamphetamine laboratory incident seizures declined by 62% after the State's methamphetamine precursor control law went into effect, with the State reporting 109 seizures from August 1st , 2005 to April 30th, 2006, compared to 285 over the same time period one year earlier. Workplace drug testing results showed a 14.8% decrease in positive tests for amphetamine, measuring the first five months in 2006, compared to the same period one year earlier.

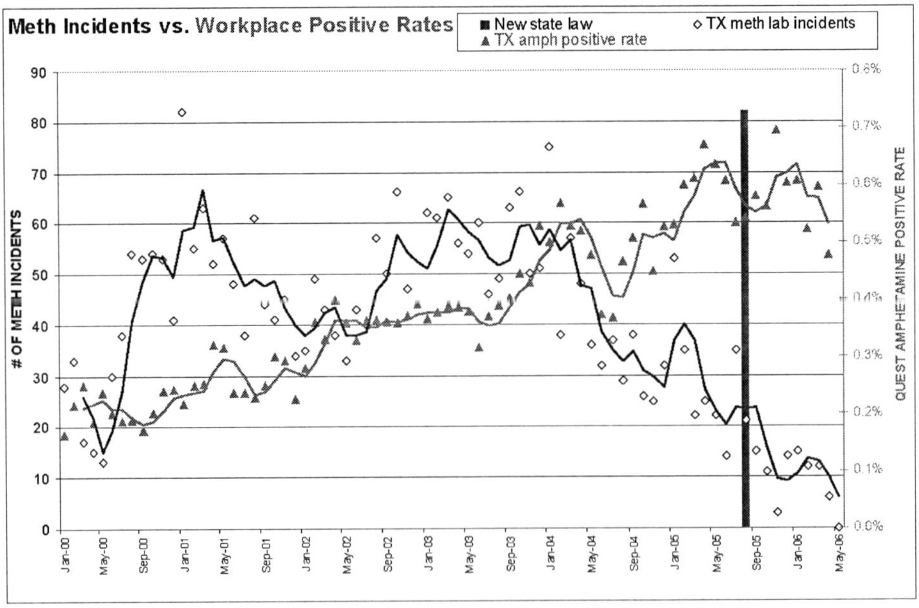

UTAH

no state law positive amphetamine workplace tests: -2.4%

Federal Standard: The United States Combat Methamphetamine Act		Utah State Law: No state law, only CMEA applies	
Effective Dates:	4/8/2006	*Effective Date:*	May 1, 2000
	9/30/2006	Meth lab reduction:	10%
Sales locations limited to pharmacies?	No	Sales locations limited to pharmacies?	No
Behind the counter/locked cabinet?	**Yes**	*Behind the counter/locked cabinet?*	*No*
All listed chemicals?	**Yes**	*All listed chemicals?*	*No*
Daily sales limits:	**3.6 g**	*Daily sales limits:*	*12 g*
30-day purchase limit:	9 g	*30-day purchase limit:*	*12 g*
Identification/logbook requirement?	**Yes**	*Identification/logbook requirement?*	*No*
"Listed chemicals" means any productcontaining ephedrine (EPH), pseudoephedrine (PSE), or phenylpropanolamine (PPA).Items in bold indicatethe controlling standard in the state. Items in *italics* indicatethat the provision is trumped by a stricter standard.			

Summary

Other than a 12-gram limit on the possession of pseudoephedrine or ephedrine enacted in 2000, Utah did not implement any methamphetamine precursor controls before the Combat Meth Act took effect September 30th 2006. In other words, the CMEA is the controlling standard in Utah. It also means that the State does not limit sales of products containing methamphetamine precursors like pseudoephedrine to pharmacies, and does not classify these products as Schedule V drugs under the State's scheduling scheme.

State	**Quest Amph Positives, 2000 (Ja n-Ma y)**	**Quest Amph Positives, 2001 (Jan-May)**	**Quest Amph Positives, 2002 (Jan-May)**	**Quest Amph Positives, 2003 (Jan-May)**	**Quest Amph Positives, 2004 (Jan-May)**	**Quest Amph Positives, 2005 (Jan-May)**	**Quest Amph Positives, 2006 (Ja n-Ma y)**	**% Change 2005-2006**
UT	0.41%	0.35%	0.36%	0.51%	0.66%	0.62%	0.60%	-2.43%

Utah Data Roundup

Utah did not implement any state-level methamphetamine precursor control legislation, and it is premature to measure the impact of the CMEA in Utah. There was a 10% increase in amphetamine workplace Positives from 2005 to 2006. Workplace drug testing results showed a 2.4% decrease in positive tests for amphetamine, measuring the first five months in 2006, compared to the same period one year earlier.

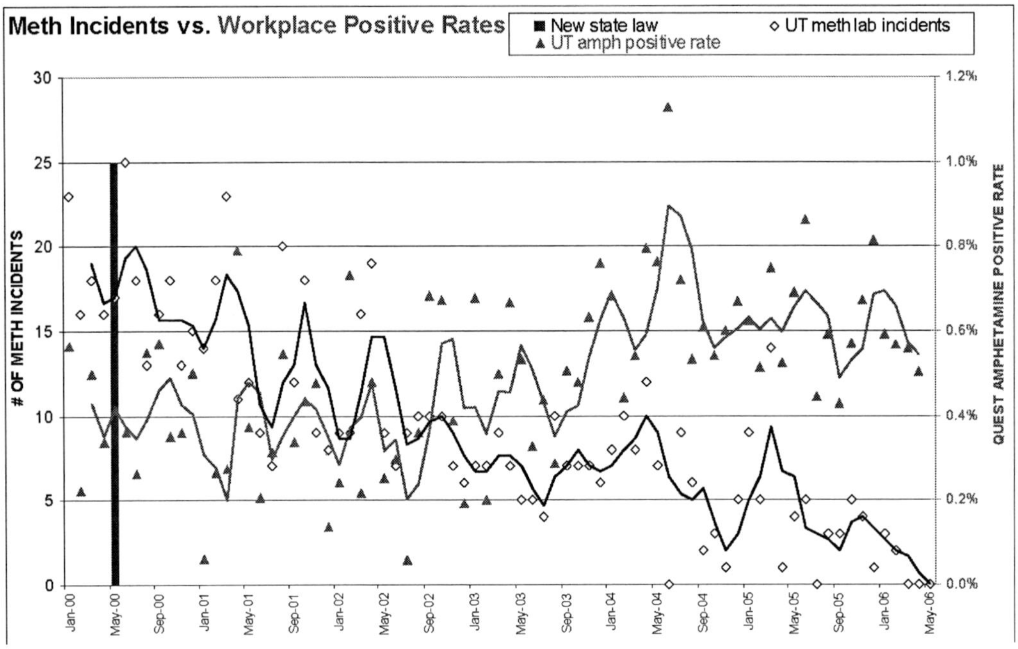

VERMONT

data not yet available/historically low lab numbers positive amphetamine workplace tests: -79.5%

Federal Standard: The United States Combat Methamphetamine Act		**Vermont State Law: Similar to the Federal Standards**	
Effective Dates:	4/8/2006	*Effective Date:*	September 30, 2006
	9/30/2006	Meth lab reduction:	n/a
Sales locations limited to pharmacies?	**No**	**Sales locations limited to pharmacies?**	**No**
Behind the counter/locked cabinet?	**Yes**	**Behind the counter/locked cabinet?**	**Yes**
All listed chemicals?	**Yes**	**All listed chemicals?**	**Yes**
Daily sales limits:	**3.6 g**	**Daily sales limits:**	**3.6 g**
30-day purchase limit:	**9 g**	*30-day purchase limit:*	*none*
Identification/logbook requirement?	**Yes**	**Identification/logbook requirement?**	**Yes**

"Listed chemicals"means any productcontaining ephedrine (EPH), pseudoephedrine (PSE), or phenylpropanolamine (PPA).Items in bold indicatethe controlling standard in the state. Items in *italics* indicatethat the provision is trumped by a stricter standard.

Summary

Vermont's methamphetamine precursor law went into effect September 30th 2006 – the same day as the Federal CMEA. The Vermont Law is fairly similar to the CMEA, putting a daily sales limit of 3.6 grams on products containing pseudoephedrine, ephedrine, or phenylpropanolamine, and requiring that these products be kept behind store counters or in a locked case or cabinet. Although there is not an explicit identification and logbook requirement in the State law, the Federal CMEA contains one, and the State law directs the Department of Health to develop a brochure explaining, among other things, the importance of retailers keeping a logbook of purchases. Vermont does not limit sales of products containing methamphetamine precursor chemicals like pseudoephedrine to pharmacies, and does not classify products containing those chemicals as Schedule V drugs under the State scheduling scheme.

State	Quest Amph Positives, 2000 (Ja n-Ma y)	Quest Amph Positives, 2001 (Jan-May)	Quest Amph Positives, 2002 (Jan-May)	Quest Amph Positives, 2003 (Jan-May)	Quest Amph Positives, 2004 (Jan-May)	Quest Amph Positives, 2005 (Jan-May)	Quest Amph Positives, 2006 (Ja n-Ma y)	% Change 2005-2006
VT	0.00%	0.51%	0.30%	0.20%	0.40%	0.63%	0.13%	-79.51%

Vermont Data Roundup

Vermont's methamphetamine precursor control law went into effect on September 30th, 2006, so it is premature to measure the impact of the State's law. Additionally, the State has historically enjoyed low levels of methamphetamine laboratory incidents, with only two incidents reported to the DEA over the last four years. Workplace drug testing results showed a 79.5% decrease in positive tests for amphetamine, measuring the first five months in 2006, compared to the same period one year earlier.

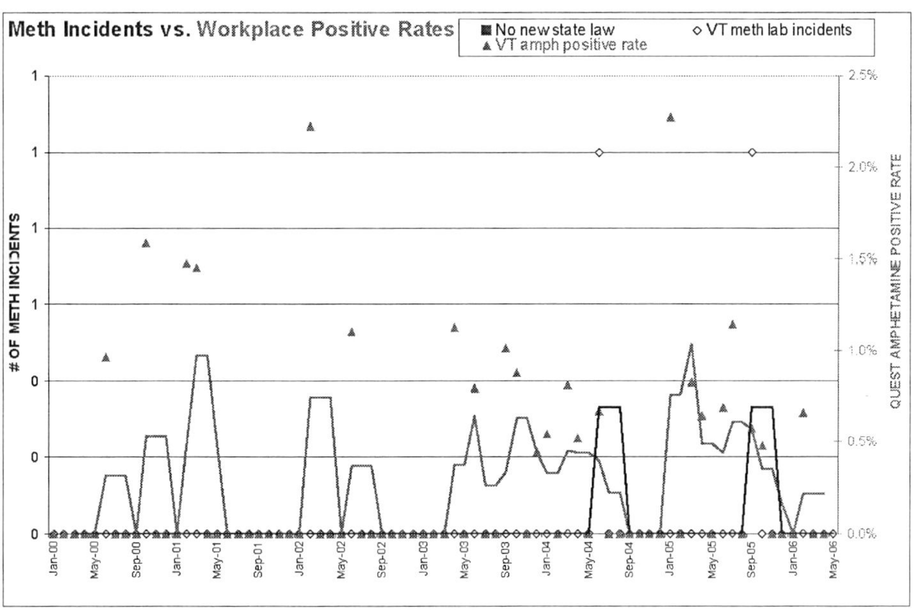

VIRGINIA

76% decline in meth lab incidents positive amphetamine workplace tests: -16.4%

Federal Standard: The United States Combat Methamphetamine Act		**Virginia State Law: Similar to Federal Standard**	
Effective Dates:	4/8/2006 9/30/2006	*Effective Date:*	August 30, 2006
		Meth lab reduction:	76%
Sales locations limited to pharmacies?	**No**	**Sales locations limited to pharmacies?**	**No**
Behind the counter/locked cabinet?	**Yes**	**Behind the counter/locked cabinet?**	**Yes**
All listed chemicals?	**Yes**	**All listed chemicals?**	**Yes**
Daily sales limits:	**3.6 g**	**Daily sales limits:**	**3.6 g**
30-day purchase limit:	**9 g**	*30-day purchase limit:*	*none*
Identification/logbook requirement?	**Yes**	**Identification/logbook requirement?**	**Yes**

"Listed chemicals"means any productcontaining ephedrine (EPH), pseudoephedrine (PSE), or phenylpropanolamine (PPA).Items in bold indicatethe controlling standard in the state. Items in *italics* indicatethat the provision is trumped by a stricter standard.

Summary

Virginia's methamphetamine precursor regulations went into effect October 1st , 2005. These were temporary, and by September 30th 2006, the State adopted provisions similar to the Federal CMEA.

Virginia law does not restrict the sale of products containing pseudoephedrine, ephedrine, or phenylpropanolamine to pharmacies, and does not classify products containing these chemicals as Schedule V drugs. Until June 30th , 2006, products containing only pseudoephedrine, ephedrine, or phenylpropanolamine (single-entity) had to be kept behind a store counter or in a locked container or case; products containing these chemicals in multi-active with other chemicals (multi-active products) had a slightly more lenient standard, allowing video surveillance or anti-theft devices as options. Now, with the Federal CMEA in effect (and Virginia law expressly adopting most of the CMEA), single-entity and multi-active products are treated the same.

Until June 30th , 2006, there was a nine-gram retail transaction limit for these products. Now, Virginia law contains a 3.6 gram retail transaction limit, like the CMEA. Virginia law now also contains an identification and logbook requirement.

State	**Quest Amph Positives, 2000 (Ja n-Ma y)**	**Quest Amph Positives, 2001 (Jan-May)**	**Quest Amph Positives, 2002 (Jan-May)**	**Quest Amph Positives, 2003 (Jan-May)**	**Quest Amph Positives, 2004 (Jan-May)**	**Quest Amph Positives, 2005 (Jan-May)**	**Quest Amph Positives, 2006 (Ja n-Ma y)**	**% Change 2005-2006**
VA	0.17%	0.20%	0.21%	0.26%	0.25%	0.40%	0.34%	-16.43%

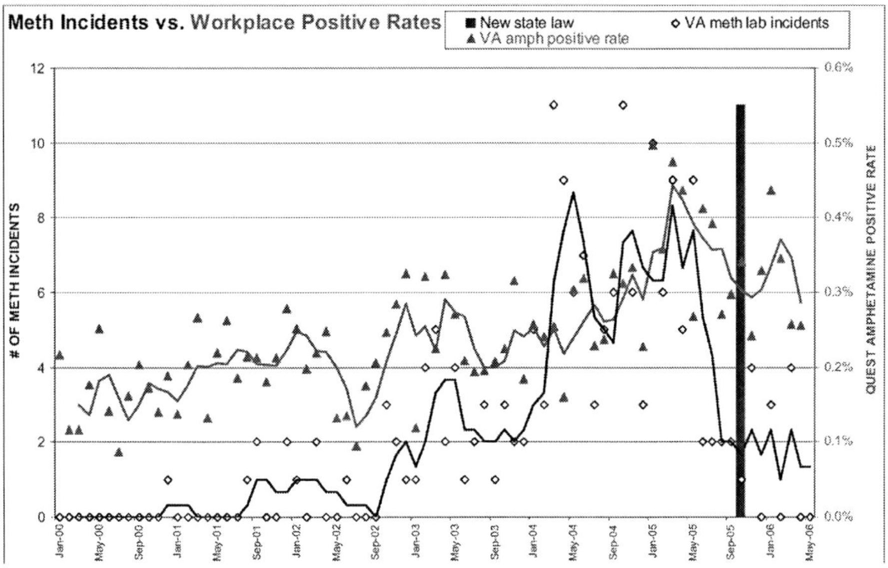

Virginia Data Roundup

In Virginia, methamphetamine laboratory incident seizures declined by 76% after the State's methamphetamine precursor controls went into effect, with the State reporting 12 seizures from October 1st , 2005 to April 30th, 2006, compared to 50 over the same time period one year earlier. Workplace drug testing results showed a 16.4% decrease in positive tests for amphetamine, measuring the first five months in 2006, compared to the same period one year earlier.

WASHINGTON

71% decline in meth lab incidents positive amphetamine workplace tests: -10.2%

Federal Standard: The United States Combat Methamphetamine Act		**Washington State Law: Stricter than the Federal Standard**	
Effective Dates:	4/8/2006 9/30/2006	*Effective Date:*	July 24, 2005
		Meth lab reduction:	71%
Sales locations limited to pharmacies?	No	**Sales locations limited to pharmacies?**	**Some**
Behind the counter/locked cabinet?	Yes	**Behind the counter/locked cabinet?**	Yes
All listed chemicals?	Yes	**All listed chemicals?**	Yes
Daily sales limits:	**3.6 g**	**Daily sales limits:**	**2 pkg/6 g**
30-day purchase limit:	**9 g**	**30-day purchase limit:**	--
Identification/logbook requirement?	Yes	**Identification/logbook requirement?**	Yes

"Listed chemicals"means any productcontaining ephedrine (EPH), pseudoephedrine (PSE), or phenylpropanolamine (PPA).Items in bold indicatethe controlling standard in the state. Items in *italics* indicatethat the provision is trumped by a stricter standard.

Summary

Washington State's' methamphetamine precursor law went into effect in several stages. Most provisions went into effect on July 24th 2005. The sales limits went into effect on January 1, 2006. The Washington law is slightly stricter than the CMEA in several respects.

Washington's law limits sales of any product containing pseudoephedrine, ephedrine or phenylpropanolamine to pharmacies or stores registered with the Washington State Department of Health. The law limits sales of these products to 3 grams or less within a single transaction or 24-hour period – slightly stricter than the federal 3.6 gram limit for single transactions. There is no monthly limit on purchases under the state law, although the Federal law limits it to 9 grams. There is an identification and logbook requirement.

Washington law does not restrict the sale of products containing pseudoephedrine or ephedrine to pharmacies, although it comes somewhat close by requiring that retailers register with the Department of Health in order to sell these products. Washington does not classify these products as Schedule V controlled substances.

State	Quest Amph Positives, 2000 (Ja n-Ma y)	Quest Amph Positives, 2001 (Jan-May)	Quest Amph Positives, 2002 (Jan-May)	Quest Amph Positives, 2003 (Jan-May)	Quest Amph Positives, 2004 (Jan-May)	Quest Amph Positives, 2005 (Jan-May)	Quest Amph Positives, 2006 (Ja n-Ma y)	% Change 2005-2006
WA	0.47%	0.44%	0.42%	0.46%	0.53%	0.66%	0.60%	-1 0.23%

Washington Data Roundup

In Washington, methamphetamine laboratory incident seizures declined by 71% after the State's methamphetamine precursor control law went into effect, with the State reporting 193 seizures from July 24th, 2005 to April 30th, 2006, compared to 677 over the same time period one year earlier. Workplace drug testing results showed a 10.2% decrease in positive tests for amphetamine, measuring the first five months in 2006, compared to the same period one year earlier.

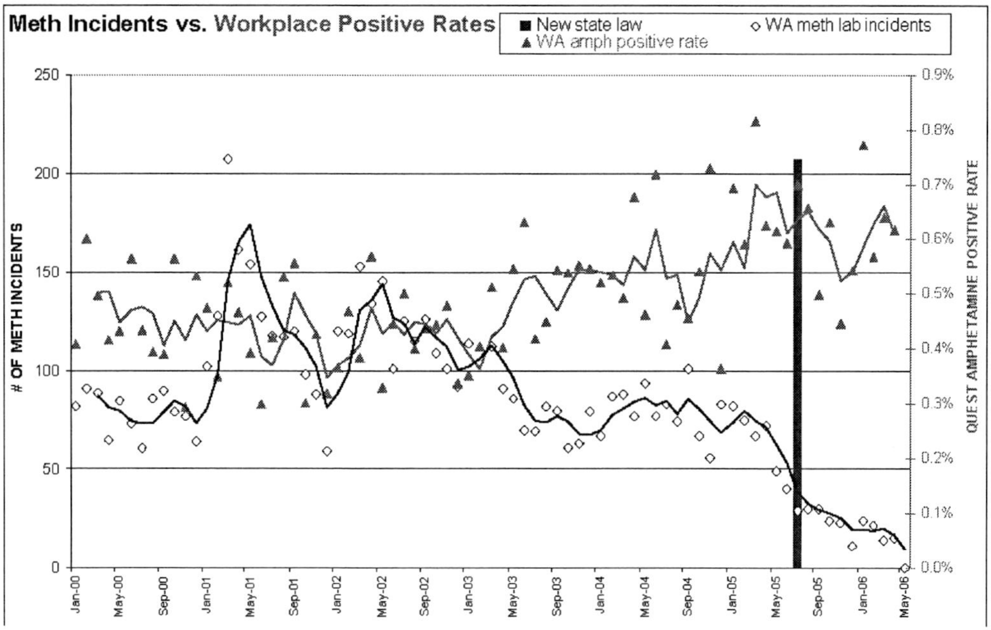

WASHINGTON, D.C.

No District law/historically low lab numbers positive amphetamine workplace tests: +115.24%

Federal Standard: The United States Combat Methamphetamine Act		Washington DC State Law: No Law in Place, CMEA Controls	
Effective Dates:	4/8/2006	*Effective Date:*	None
	9/30/2006	Meth lab reduction:	n/a
Sales locations limited to pharmacies?	**No**	*Sales locations limited to pharmacies?*	*No*
Behind the counter/locked cabinet?	**Yes**	*Behind the counter/locked cabinet?*	*No*
All listed chemicals?	**Yes**	*All listed chemicals?*	*No*
Daily sales limits:	**3.6 g**	*Daily sales limits:*	*None*
30-day purchase limit:	**9 g**	*30-day purchase limit:*	*None*
Identification/logbook requirement?	**Yes**	*Identification/logbook requirement?*	*No*
"Listed chemicals"means any productcontaining ephedrine (EPH), pseudoephedrine (PSE), or phenylpropanolamine (PPA).Items in bold indicatethe controlling standard in the state. Items in *italics* indicatethat the provision is trumped by a stricter standard.			

Summary

Washington, D.C., which has enjoyed low numbers of methamphetamine laboratory incidents, did not implement any methamphetamine precursor controls before the Combat Meth Act took effect September 30th 2006. In other words, the CMEA is the controlling standard in the District of Columbia. It also means that the District does not limit sales of products containing methamphetamine precursors like pseudoephedrine to pharmacies, and does not classify these products as Schedule V drugs under the State's scheduling scheme.

State	Quest Amph Positives, 2000 (Ja n-Ma y)	Quest Amph Positives, 2001 (Jan-May)	Quest Amph Positives, 2002 (Jan-May)	Quest Amph Positives, 2003 (Jan-May)	Quest Amph Positives, 2004 (Jan-May)	Quest Amph Positives, 2005 (Jan-May)	Quest Amph Positives, 2006 (Ja n-Ma y)	% Change 2005-2006
DC	0.00%	0.11%	0.08%	0.13%	0.09%	0.09%	0.20%	115.24%

Washington D.C. Data Roundup

The District of Columbia did not implement methamphetamine precursor control legislation prior to the effective date of the CMEA. Since January of 2000, Washington has reported just one methamphetamine laboratory incident seizure to the DEA. Workplace drug testing results showed a 115.2% increase in positive tests for amphetamine, measuring the first five months in 2006, compared to the same period one year earlier.

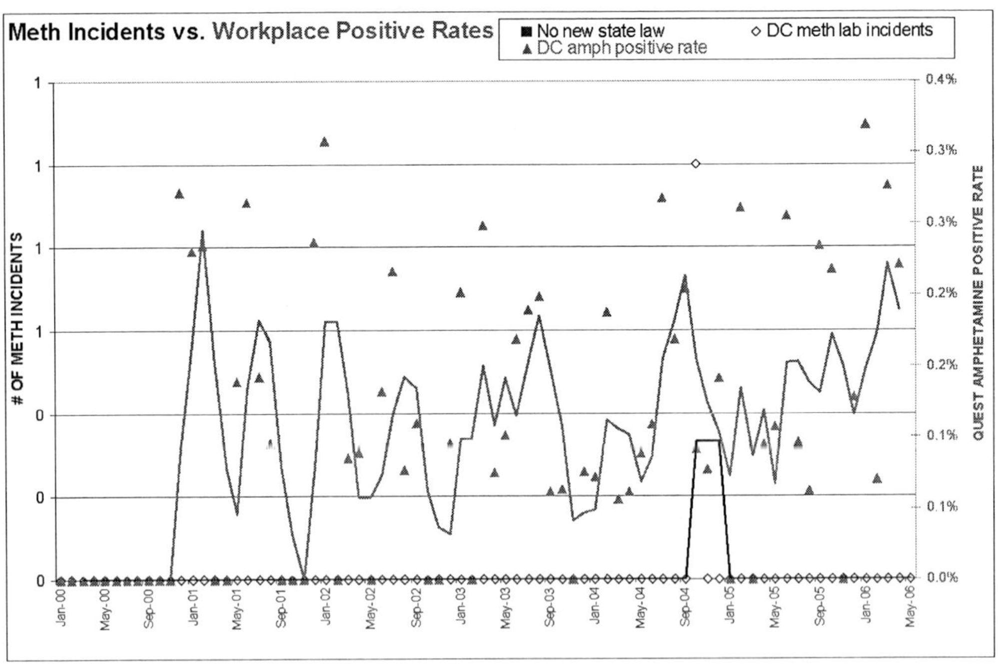

WEST VIRGINIA

54% decline in meth lab incidents positive amphetamine workplace tests: -34.8%

Federal Standard: The United States Combat Methamphetamine Act		**West Virginia State Law: Different from the Federal Standard**	
Effective Dates:	*4/8/2006* 9/30/2006	*Effective Date:*	August 5, 2005
		Meth lab reduction:	54%
Sales locations limited to pharmacies?	*No*	**Sales locations limited to pharmacies?**	**Some**
Behind the counter/locked cabinet?	**Yes**	**Behind the counter/locked cabinet?**	**Yes**
All listed chemicals?	**Yes**	*All listed chemicals?*	*single-entity only*
Daily sales limits:	**3.6 g**	**Daily sales limits:**	--
30-day purchase limit:	**9 g**	**30-day purchase limit:**	**3 pkg/9 g**
Identification/logbook requirement?	**Yes**	**Identification/logbook requirement?**	**Yes**

"Listed chemicals"means any productcontaining ephedrine (EPH), pseudoephedrine (PSE), or phenylpropanolamine (PPA).Items in bold indicatethe controlling standard in the state. Items in *italics*indicatethat the provision is trumped by a stricter standard.

Summary

West Virginia's methamphetamine precursor law went into effect July 8th , 2005.The West Virginia law is stricter than the CMEA in that it limits sales of products containing pseudoephedrine, ephedrine or phenylpropanolamine to pharmacies, but less strict in that it does not apply to multi-active products (products that contain these chemicals in addition to other active ingredients).

West Virginia's law classifies products containing only pseudoephedrine or ephedrine as Schedule V controlled substances. This limits the sale of these products to pharmacies, and requires placement of these products behind pharmacy counters. There is a 9 gram limit on monthly purchases and a requirement that the purchaser show identification and sign a logbook, as with the Federal CMEA standard.

State	Quest Amph Positives, 2000 (Ja n-Ma y)	Quest Amph Positives, 2001 (Jan-May)	Quest Amph Positives, 2002 (Jan-May)	Quest Amph Positives, 2003 (Jan-May)	Quest Amph Positives, 2004 (Jan-May)	Quest Amph Positives, 2005 (Jan-May)	Quest Amph Positives, 2006 (Ja n-Ma y)	% Change 2005-2006
WV	0.11%	0.30%	0.20%	0.21%	0.29%	0.50%	0.33%	-34.82%

West Virginia Data Roundup

In West Virginia, methamphetamine laboratory incident seizures declined by 54% after the State's methamphetamine precursor control law went into effect, with the State reporting 88 seizures from July 8th, 2005 to April 30th, 2006, compared to 193 over the same time period one year earlier. Workplace drug testing results showed a 34.8% decrease in positive tests for amphetamine, measuring the first five months in 2006, compared to the same period one year earlier.

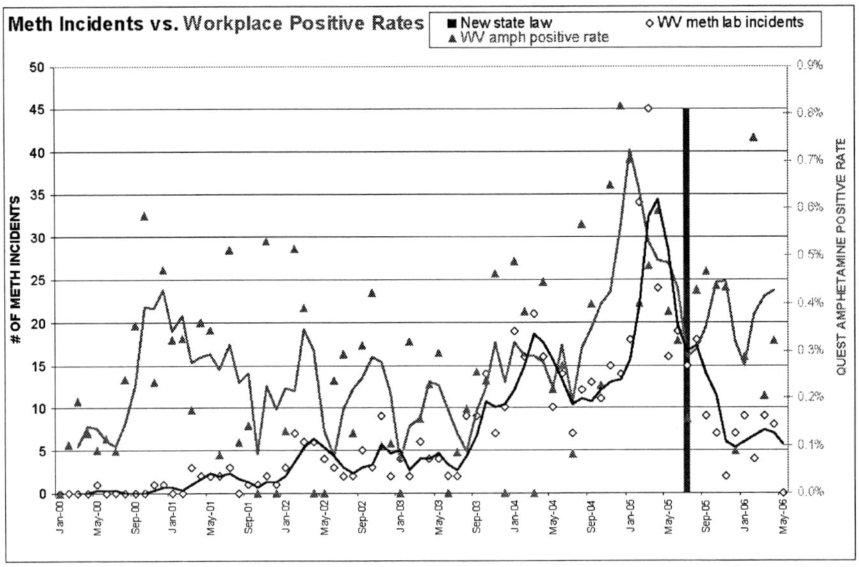

WISCONSIN

26% decline in meth lab incidents positive amphetamine workplace tests: +31.1%

Federal Standard: The United States Combat Methamphetamine Act		**Wisconsin State Law: Stricter than the Federal Standard**	
Effective Dates:	4/8/2006	*Effective Date:*	June 22, 2005
	9/30/2006	Meth lab reduction:	26%
Sales locations limited to pharmacies?	*No*	**Sales locations limited to pharmacies?**	**Yes**
Behind the counter/locked cabinet?	**Yes**	**Behind the counter/locked cabinet?**	**Yes**
All listed chemicals?	**Yes**	**All listed chemicals?**	**PSE**
Daily sales limits:	**3.6 g**	**Sales limit:**	**4 oz/48 hrs**
30-day purchase limit:	**9 g**	**30-day purchase limit:**	**7.5 g**
Identification/logbook requirement?	**Yes**	**Identification/logbook requirement?**	**Yes**

"Listed chemicals"means any productcontaining ephedrine (EPH), pseudoephedrine (PSE), or phenylpropanolamine (PPA).Items in bold indicatethe controlling standard in the state. Items in *italics*indicatethat the provision is trumped by a stricter standard.

Summary

Wisconsin's methamphetamine precursor law went into effect in two stages: Most provisions went into effect on June 22nd 2005. The provisions that classify products containing pseudoephedrine as a Schedule V controlled substance under the State's scheduling scheme went into effect on October 1, 2005.

The Wisconsin law is stricter than the CMEA. Other than those products in liquid and gelatin form, any product containing pseudoephedrine may be sold only at pharmacies and by a pharmacist. There is a 7.5 gram 30-day purchase limit, which is moderately stricter than the CMEA 9-gram limit. Purchasers must present photo identification and the pharmacist must record the information. Interestingly, Wisconsin's law does not appear to directly require placement behind a counter or in a locked container, but because the products are classified as a Schedule V controlled substance, the practical effect is to require placement behind pharmacy counters.

State	Quest Amph Positives, 2000 (Ja n-Ma y)	Quest Amph Positives, 2001 (Jan-May)	Quest Amph Positives, 2002 (Jan-May)	Quest Amph Positives, 2003 (Jan-May)	Quest Amph Positives, 2004 (Jan-May)	Quest Amph Positives, 2005 (Jan-May)	Quest Amph Positives, 2006 (Ja n-Ma y)	% Change 2005-2006
WI	0.18%	0.25%	0.26%	0.33%	0.35%	0.42%	0.55%	31.11%

Wisconsin Data Roundup

In Wisconsin, methamphetamine laboratory incident seizures declined by 26% after the State's methamphetamine precursor control law went into effect, with the State reporting 39 seizures from June 22nd, 2005 to April 30th , 2006, compared to 53 over the same time period one year earlier. Workplace drug testing results showed a 31.1% increase in positive tests for amphetamine, measuring the first five months in 2006, compared to the same period one year earlier.

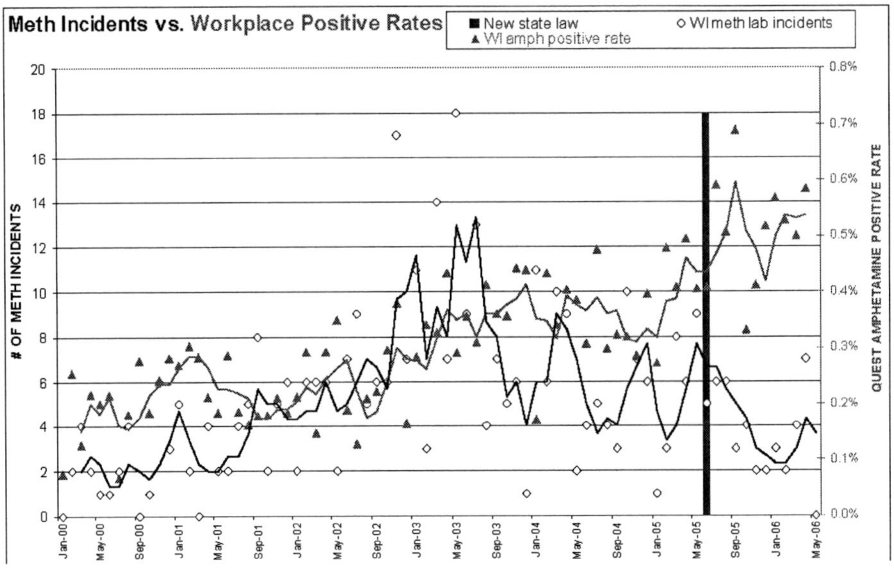

WYOMING

data not yet available positive amphetamine workplace tests: +6.0%

Federal Standard: The United States Combat Methamphetamine Act		Wyoming State Law: Less strict than Federal Standard	
Effective Dates:	4/8/2006	Effective Date:	August 1, 2005
	9/30/2006	Meth lab reduction:	data not yet available
Sales locations limited to pharmacies?	**No**	**Sales locations limited to pharmacies?**	**No**
Behind the counter/locked cabinet?	**Yes**	**Behind the counter/locked cabinet?**	**Yes**
All listed chemicals?	**Yes**	**All listed chemicals?**	**Yes**
Daily sales limits:	**3.6 g**	**Transaction limit:**	**2 pkg**
30-day purchase limit:	**9 g**	**30-day purchase limit:**	--
Identification/logbook requirement?	**Yes**	*Identification/logbook requirement?*	*No*

"Listed chemicals" means any product containing ephedrine (EPH), pseudoephedrine (PSE), or phenylpropanolamine (PPA). Items in bold indicatethe controlling standard in the state. Items in *italics* indicate that the provision is trumped by a stricter standard.

Summary

Wyoming's methamphetamine precursor law went into effect August 1st 2005.The Wyoming law is less strict than the CMEA, meaning that the CMEA standards are controlling in Wyoming in most respects. Wyoming's law applies to products containing only pseudoephedrine, ephedrine, or phenylpropanolamine, and limits sales of these products to 6 grams per transaction. This, of course, is trumped by the Federal CMEA's 3.6 gram standard.

State law also requires the products be placed in a secure area (behind a counter, in a locked case, or in the direct line of sight of an employee, et cetera). However, this provision also appears less strict than the CMEA, so the CMEA is controlling. Wyoming law does not contain an identification or logbook requirement, although it is required by the CMEA in Wyoming and all other states.

Wyoming does not limit sales of products containing methamphetamine precursor chemicals like pseudoephedrine to pharmacies, and does not classify products containing those chemicals as Schedule V drugs under the State scheduling scheme.

State	Quest Amph Positives, 2000 (Ja n-Ma y)	Quest Amph Positives, 2001 (Jan-May)	Quest Amph Positives, 2002 (Jan-May)	Quest Amph Positives, 2003 (Jan-May)	Quest Amph Positives, 2004 (Jan-May)	Quest Amph Positives, 2005 (Jan-May)	Quest Amph Positives, 2006 (Ja n-Ma y)	% Change 2005-2006
WY	0.14%	0.09%	0.43%	0.44%	0.43%	0.68%	0.72%	5.98%

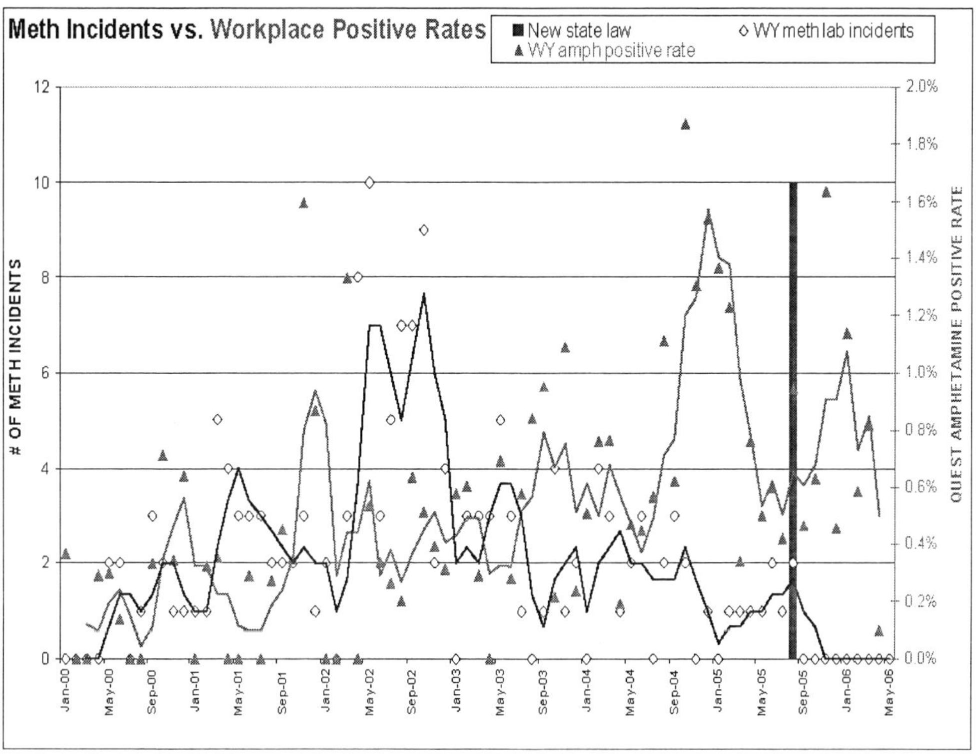

Wyoming Data Roundup

In Wyoming, there were about 111 methamphetamine laboratory incident seizures reported to the DEA over the last four years. Although no laboratory incident seizures have been reported since the law went into effect, it is unclear whether this is due to reporting trends or an actual absence of methamphetamine laboratories. Workplace drug testing results showed a 6% increase in positive tests for amphetamine, measuring the first five months in 2006, compared to the same period one year earlier.

End Notes

[1] The Federal CMEA has been in effect for two months prior to this publication, which is not sufficient time to measure the impact of the law. This chapter summarizes, rather than exhaustively details, each State law. Retailers and other individuals or organizations interested in compliance with these State laws, and with the Federal law, should consult the actual statute, any related regulations, and legal authorities as appropriate. Also note that this document intentionally omits minor differences between State laws and the Federal CMEA, and does not discuss provisions of the CMEA or State laws that apply to mail or Internet orders.

In: Methamphetamine: Background, Controls and Issues ISBN: 978-1-60692-548-5
Editor: Andrea S. Sandoval

Chapter 6

BREAKING THE METHAMPHETAMINE SUPPLY CHAIN: LAW ENFORCEMENT CHALLENGES

United States Senate

Washington, DC.

The hearing was convened, pursuant to notice, at 10:04 a.m., in room SD–215, Dirksen Senate Office Building, Hon. Charles E. Grassley (chairman of the committee) presiding.

Present: Senators Baucus and Lott.

OPENING STATEMENT OF HON. CHARLES E. GRASSLEY, A U.S. SENATOR FROM IOWA, CHAIRMAN, COMMITTEE ON FINANCE

The Chairman. Thanks to everybody for coming this morning. And particularly we have had panelists come from Iowa and Montana, which is a long ways away, Montana obviously much further away than Iowa. You have come to share your insights into this growing epidemic of methamphetamine use across the country. We thank you very much.

It is no longer a secret that methamphetamine abuse and the disastrous effects of its manufacture have reached crisis levels in many areas of the country, and I'll quote from a survey by the National Association of Counties, released in July, that found "county law enforcement officials across 44 States reported that meth- amphetamine remains the number-one drug problem in this country," with 48 percent of their counties reporting that meth is the primary drug problem. This was more than the number who reported cocaine, marijuana, and heroin all combined.

Whereas methamphetamine production and use may once have been geographically limited, this survey, as well as other reports, indicates that it appears to be moving steadily into most of the country.

I am encouraged by Congress's recognition of the need to control this crisis. Earlier this year, Congress passed the Combat Meth Act, which limits sale of meth precursor drugs like pseudo- ephedrine, and mandates that a log be kept of each sale.

A number of States have already enacted similar restrictions on the availability of meth precursor drugs, and this appears to have made a very major impact on the number of small toxic labs in those States, as well as indicated by the great decrease in the number of local lab seizures in most of those States that have such laws.

It is reasonable to expect a comparable reduction of the number of small toxic labs in all the States when the Federal legislation becomes effective September 30, this month.

The challenges before us, however, are not reduced because of this legislation. They are still very substantial. One of the results of a decrease in small toxic meth labs in those States that have restricted access to precursor products has been, sadly, an increase in the importation of meth by large, sophisticated drug cartels based primarily in Mexico.

These smuggling organizations import a purer version of meth, employ smuggling techniques that are difficult to uncover and track, and are now operating in most parts of the country. They are also engaged in repatriating large amounts of money in their home bases, laundering it through a variety of methods, and often through legitimate business channels.

The Drug Enforcement Administration estimates that the illegal money laundering drug trade is almost $50 billion a year. It is also believed that a large portion of that money is smuggled out of the country in bulk across our borders.

Under these new circumstances, it is clear that a priority has to be placed on cooperation between the numerous Federal agencies that are engaged in combatting the meth traffic, and, of course, State and local law enforcement agencies that are on the ground in our local communities.

So our hearing today is about this issue. We will be hearing testimony from State and local officials deeply engaged in the effort to close down meth traffickers, and from Federal officials equally deeply engaged in the effort at the Federal level.

We not only want to hear about their efforts at their respective levels and what we in Congress might do to help, but also about their cooperation and what we can do to help that cooperation more effectively.

I would call on Senator Baucus for two reasons now. One, to give any opening comments he has, and also to introduce the two constituents he has here and should introduce.

OPENING STATEMENT OF HON. MAX BAUCUS, A U.S. SENATOR FROM MONTANA

Senator Baucus. Well, thank you very much, Mr. Chairman.

Methamphetamine is a personal fight for me. I have seen it firsthand. I am mentoring a couple of kids in schools who come from dysfunctional families, because a mother or a father is on meth- amphetamine. It is a big cause for me to stamp out, as much as possible, methamphetamine, certainly in our State of Montana, and in the country.

More than 4 out of 10 Montana teens report that meth is easy to get. I ask for a show of hands at high school assemblies and middle schools, and it is astounding, the number of hands that go up when I ask, can you get meth or do you know somebody who is on meth? It is astoundingly high. Those 4 out of 10 teens report that meth is easy to get, second only to marijuana.

Montana police officers tell me that meth is their number-one law enforcement problem. Methamphetamine is the number-one illegal drug problem for nearly half of the counties in the United States. Nationwide, nearly 4 in 10 local law enforcement agencies have identified meth as the drug that poses the greatest threat to their area.

In April, this committee held a hearing on the effects of meth on the child welfare system and how it is hurting kids and parents alike. In July, the Senate passed the Improving Outcomes for Children Affected by Meth Act of 2006, and that is a bill which includes provisions to enhance the safety of children affected by meth abuse and addiction.

We reauthorized the Promoting Safe and Stable Families program. That bill targets an available $40 million—that is an increase—in mandatory funding for meth-related services that include family treatment. Two-thirds of the children who come into the child welfare system in Montana come in because meth has destroyed their families.

We are working to help protect children and protect families from the dangers of meth. Today we will focus on a new angle, that is, how to break the meth supply chain through law enforcement. We are working on the problem. We now have improved law enforcement techniques and measures to monitor the chemicals that are used to make meth. One example is the Combat Meth Act of 2005, which I am proud to have co-sponsored.

That Act requires that medicines containing pseudoephedrine be relocated behind the counter, and that law establishes a pharmacy log book registry for purchases of these cold products.

In our State of Montana, we passed this law earlier. We passed it in July of 2005. The Yellowstone County Drug Task Force told me that this makes a difference, it is helping. Now it is very difficult for small, mom-and-pop meth producers to obtain the chemicals that can be used to produce meth.

As a result, the meth production in Montana and elsewhere in our country appears to be decreasing. That is not to say that meth demand is decreasing. Demand is still, I am told, about as high as it was before these laws were passed to put the precursors behind the counter.

But production of meth in Mexico, largely in super-labs controlled by drug trafficking organizations, has picked up. The biggest link in the meth supply chain is now at the southwest border. It is now estimated that 80 percent of meth consumed in the United States originates in Mexico and is smuggled into the country.

Today we will examine where to put our resources to most effectively break the meth supply chain. We will hear from Lt. Dan Springer, commander of the Missouri River Drug Task Force, headquartered in Bozeman.

We are proud that you are here, Dan. I am proud of the work the task force is doing. Investigations in Bozeman are critical to stem the tide of national and international drug organizations that are preying on Montanans.

That task force and others around the country need the dollars to fight meth. They need the resources. They need the resources to locate and clean up the labs, and the resources to put criminals making and dealing with meth behind bars where they belong.

I am eager to hear from Lt. Springer about changing meth hot spots and the challenges that law enforcement officers now face.

Carl Venne, welcome. Chairman Venne is the chairman of the Crow Nation in Montana, and an advisory council member of the Montana Meth Project. Chairman Venne will be testifying here today on meth abuse as it particularly affects reservations, and it is devastating.

I look forward to hearing Chairman Venne's perspective on tribal efforts and tribal strategies to combat meth, as well as meth law enforcement resources for reservations.

Education, prevention, and treatment are vital. Our law enforcement officers are stepping up to meet the challenge, and I am doing all I can to help out. I very much look forward to our testimony today.

We have to break the meth supply chain. Let us do so for the health and safety of Montanans, and all Americans. Thank you, all three of you, very, very much for taking the time and effort to come and, jointly together, help us out to solve this problem.

Thank you.

[The prepared statement of Senator Baucus appears in the appendix.]

The Chairman. Yes. Before I introduce the panel, I will call on Senator Lott.

OPENING STATEMENT OF HON. TRENT LOTT, A U.S. SENATOR FROM MISSISSIPPI

Senator Lott. Mr. Chairman, I will be very brief. I just want to thank you for following through on the legislation we passed earlier and to look at the continuing and even growing problem and try to find ways to break this chain of supply.

I think to have the local panel of people dealing with it where it really happens, and then of course the Federal panel, will be extremely interesting and helpful. I am glad we did get the Combat Meth Act done.

I think it is appropriate we follow up and see what is happening, how is it working, how are the local officials dealing with it. So, I am looking forward to reviewing the testimony of the witnesses.

Thank you, Mr. Chairman.

The Chairman. Yes. And thank you, Senator Lott. Thank you, Senator Baucus. Senator Baucus introduced two of the first panel, so joining Lt. Springer and Chairman Venne is a constituent of mine, a person who has had experience both at the State level and at the local level in the issue of combatting drugs.

Once before we called Sean McCullough before us to testify three or 4 years ago. We enjoyed his testimony then. He has moved up the ladder now to be special agent in charge of the Iowa Division of Narcotics Enforcement, so he is going to share testimony.

We thank you all for coming, and particularly thank you, Sean, for your coming out here from Iowa to testify before me once again.

So we will start with Lt. Springer, then Chairman Venne, then Special Agent McCullough.

Lt. Springer? By the way, if you have longer statements than the 5 minutes that you were allotted, they will be included in the record as you submit them. So whatever you want to say now, you can say it any way you want to.

Lt. Springer?

STATEMENT OF LT. DAN SPRINGER, COMMANDER, MISSOURI RIVER DRUG TASK FORCE, BOZEMAN, MT

lt. Springer. Good morning, Mr. Chairman, Senator Baucus, and members of the committee. It is my great pleasure to be here today.

In 1992, the Missouri River Drug Task Force was established in Montana as a regionally proactive enforcement response designed to aggressively combat the increasing effects of dangerous drug use and distribution occurring within seven specific jurisdictions of concern.

The Missouri River Drug Task Force has nine full-time investigators and covers an area of approximately 17,000 square miles; New Jersey, Connecticut, and Massachusetts combined do not equal the size of our jurisdiction. Financial allocations received from the Byrne Memorial Grant served as the fiscal catalyst behind the jurisdictional alignment.

Operating beneath this collaborative investigation premise, the Missouri River Drug Task Force investigations, in conjunction with Federal, State, and local authorities, have been instrumental in the identification, disruption, and dismantling of drug trafficking organizations.

Narcotics officers across the country are facing multiple challenges regarding methamphetamine. The largest challenge is the fight itself. We are working with decreased funding, limited resources, a growing epidemic, and vicious drug-related crimes.

Forty-two percent of law enforcement agencies recognize meth- amphetamine as the number-one drug concern within their jurisdiction, and there is no close second. When I started as a patrol deputy 10 years go, it was extremely rare to find even personal use methamphetamine on the street. Today it is not only common, but it is the norm, and often in larger quantities than personal use.

Meth hit our area like a freight train, and we have seen nothing but a steady increase in the supply and the demand over the last 10 years. If your area has not been hit by this epidemic, be very thankful, but prepare yourselves for something that you have never seen before.

With this increase in drug activity, there has been an increase in crime. However, the primary funding source of the Missouri River Drug Task Force, the Byrne Memorial Grant, has decreased by 62 percent over the past 5 years.

Due to significant cuts in Federal funding, the number of investigators needed to combat this epidemic has stagnated to a point where we are just maintaining rather than conducting proactive, hard-hitting investigations.

The advantage of the Byrne Memorial Grant has been the ability to use the money in multiple ways. The Byrne Grant allows us to use the money for salaries, overtime, vehicles, drug buy money, informant payments, and many other areas.

I would ask for a consistent and stable form of funding that does not keep agencies hanging in the balance from year to year. A funding source of this nature would allow for extended planning and extended expectations.

The Montana State legislature has recently passed precursor laws, limiting access to items used in the making of methamphetamine. These laws have apparently been highly effective, and we have seen a dramatic decrease in the number of mom-and-pop meth labs. However, we have seen a dramatic increase in the importation of methamphetamine.

The meth imported to Montana is primarily coming from Washington, Oregon, California, Utah, and Idaho, and eventually Mexico. The super-labs of Mexico supply the majority of the meth for the United States. The factories that make pseudoephedrine are now shipping pseudoephedrine to Mexico in extremely large quantities.

Directly linking meth to other crimes is not easy to do. Very few defendants admit to committing the crime, let alone committing that crime while using meth, or in an attempt to purchase meth. One thing we do know is, meth is no longer the cheap drug used only by those who cannot afford other drugs.

In our area, meth is currently twice the price of cocaine. With the increase in price and the addictive nature of this drug, the pursuit of methamphetamine has increasingly become a criminal motive for violent and weapons-related criminal acts.

Through my very small window of the world, I see individuals getting killed over drugs. I see people losing family members to drugs. I see family members and friends being torn apart by these drugs. But, most importantly, I see the productive citizens of our communities becoming victims of crime due to drugs, and primarily methamphetamine.

Money alone cannot solve the methamphetamine issue in Montana. However, without a sustainable source of financial support, the success and momentum of these historically complex and effective efforts will inevitably falter.

Local enforcement efforts are arguably the first and last line of defense in the war on methamphetamine. And, while our communities cannot afford to lose the battle, the Missouri River Drug Task Force cannot afford to wage the war alone. Thank you for your time.

The Chairman. Thank you, Lt. Springer.

[The prepared statement of Lt. Springer appears in the appendix.]

The Chairman. Now, Chairman Venne?

Statement of Carl Venne, Crow Tribal Chairman; Tribal Leaders Council Chairman; and Advisory Member, Montana Meth Project, Crow Agency, MT

Mr. Venne. Mr. Chairman, good morning. Honorable committee members, it is an honor for me to provide testimony today on very important issues for the Crow people, and for all Native American populations. I thank you for this opportunity.

The Crow reservation is about 2.5 million acres, about the size of Rhode Island. It is one of the poorest counties in the whole United States, according to the last census. Meth use on our reservation is at epidemic stages, not only on my reservation, but all the reservations in Montana. I am also the chairman of the Tribal Leaders Council, and we have discussed this quite a bit.

One of the biggest problems we have in controlling meth is, we have three different jurisdictions on Indian reservations. We have our local BIA, the FBI, and the county. None of them are working together to fight this problem.

If you look at the whole picture and what is going on in America today and how we are fighting the war in Iraq, you know the bullets in Iraq do not say, you are Indian or you are a non-Indian. That is the way I look at law enforcement in Indian country. We are all constituents of you Senators from America. We are all constituents of the government of the State of Montana.

Why do we not fight this together with our resources instead of saying, because this is a reservation line we cannot cross it, we do not have jurisdiction? No longer can we act that way. We are all Americans in fighting this, I call it the devil.

What it is doing to our younger kids today—you know, there is an increase of suicides, increase in major crimes. But yet, when I approach the DEA or the FBI, they say, well, we want to get the big guys, so they do not look at what is going on within the reservations. We should be able to do that, not saying, because I am the FBI, I go for the big guys in Mexico and the cartels and stuff. What is their jurisdiction in Indian tribes? What are the jurisdictions of the local county sheriffs when they should be doing something? We are taxpayers of that county, so they need to provide services to our tribe. Those are the kinds of things Indian tribes are up against today.

We talk about meth labs. We had a meth lab. You know, we have a housing shortage. When you go in and knock down a house, how do we replace it? The insurance will not cover that type of stuff. There are a lot of things.

Take the social problems that it is creating. What type of prevention programs do we have in our local schools? None. What control do we have? None. We need to work together by building bridges, not burning them, between communities and between races.

I think those are the types of things I am looking at as a tribal leader in Indian country and what we are faced with today. It is very important that we realize one thing: we are all Americans. We need to fight everything together. That is how important it is to me and my people.

My people live in poverty. Our annual income is only $6,000 to $7,000 a year. We need to do something today. No longer can I stand by as an Indian leader and not talk about these things. I need to let you know: you need to help me. We need to come together as a country. Too much has divided us because of politics, but today I beg you people to help us in Indian country. Thank you.

The Chairman. Thank you, Chairman Venne.

[The prepared statement of Mr. Venne appears in the appendix.] The CHAIRMAN. Now, Special Agent McCullough?

STATEMENT OF SEAN MCCULLOUGH, SPECIAL AGENT IN CHARGE, IOWA DIVISION OF NARCOTICS ENFORCEMENT, DES MOINES, IA

Mr. McCullough. Mr. Chairman, committee members, I have been involved in drug enforcement in Iowa on the State level for the past 17 years. Since the early 1990s, Iowa has been plagued by methamphetamine. Methamphetamine could be found in Iowa before the 1990s, but not in large quantities like we had after 1990.

The majority of methamphetamine at that time was imported from Mexico and the southeast region of the United States. The people in Iowa, those involved in methamphetamine, soon found that it was easy to manufacture methamphetamine on their own, and then they did not have to deal with the dangers of the organized crime groups that were involved in the importation of meth- amphetamine.

We then saw a rise in meth labs in Iowa. Processing these labs was very time-consuming and expensive for law enforcement. Then law enforcement found themselves fighting methamphetamine on two fronts, the methamphetamine manufacturing in clandestine labs, and the meth imported into our State.

In 1993, my agency, the Division of Narcotics Enforcement, or DNE, seized two methamphetamine labs. Each year following 1993, meth labs in Iowa grew to epidemic proportions. By the year 2004, Iowa law enforcement officials seized over 1,500 meth labs in Iowa.

In 2004, the DEA recorded that Iowa had the third highest number of methamphetamine laboratories. Approximately 97 percent of these meth labs seized in Iowa produced only 1-gram to 1- or 2- ounce quantities of methamphetamine.

The Iowa law enforcement agencies found ourselves spending 80 percent of our resources on 20 percent of the meth problem. We then wanted to reduce the number of meth labs in our State so we could concentrate our efforts and resources towards the importation of meth into our State.

In May of 2005, Iowa passed one of the Nation's strongest nonprescription pseudoephedrine laws. This law restricted the sale of pseudoephedrine, which is a main ingredient in the illegal manufacture of methamphetamine. The law had an immediate and significant impact on the methamphetamine manufacturing problem in Iowa.

Law enforcement's purpose behind the law was to reduce the number of meth labs which were taking up the resources, allowing the agencies to dedicate their efforts towards reducing the amount of imported meth brought in by these organized crime groups. Since the law was enacted in May of last year, methamphetamine laboratories in Iowa have declined 72 percent.

In 2004, the University of Iowa hospitals and clinics spent approximately $2.7 million to treat patients with methamphetaminerelated injuries. In 2005, after Iowa passed the pseudoephedrine law, University of Iowa hospitals and clinics spent a little over $200,000 on methamphetamine laboratory-related injuries. This equals a savings of approximately $2.5 million.

Iowa's pseudoephedrine law has also caused a reduction in total methamphetamine laboratory costs, which involve the costs of the personnel, salaries, clean-up, and so forth. After the law was passed, costs dropped to approximately $1.5 million, and before that it was $2.5 million. These figures equal a savings of a little over $1 million.

Even though Iowa's clandestine methamphetamine laboratory seizures have declined, drug trafficking organizations continue to dominate the State's illicit trade. Most of the methamphetamine in Iowa is coming across the southwest border from Mexico.

Along with increased seizures of methamphetamine in Iowa from imported meth, the drug purity rate has also increased. This pure form of methamphetamine is also known as crystal methamphetamine. The purity rate in Iowa in 2002 was approximately 27 percent. In 2004, it rose to approximately 54 percent pure meth- amphetamine.

Law enforcement in Iowa continues to work proactively against those individuals and groups involved in trafficking methamphetamine into Iowa. I think Iowa is lucky in that all the agencies get along together, local, State, and Federal. We all work together to combat the problem, and I think that is what is important and key to addressing the methamphetamine problem.

The methamphetamine problem is transient, it is moving. It is spreading across our country, and the key is that we all work together to fight the problem and continue the dialogue that we share here today to find answers. Thank you.

The Chairman. Yes. Thank you, Sean.

[The prepared statement of Mr. McCullough appears in the appendix.]

The Chairman. I think I am going to lead in with my first question where you left off, because it is my guess that most drug investigations begin at the local level with the arrest or seizure of drugs.

So this cooperation that you referred to in Iowa—I am going to ask several questions, but they all lead to the same general discussion. So, rather than going question by question, I will just lay these out and let you deal with them. Maybe Lt. Springer would want to join in, too, from his experience.

Explain how meth cases you initiate are adopted at the Federal level or with Federal agencies. How and when, for instance, do DEA and others get involved? Do you know what criteria they use, and why, to get involved?

What is your involvement at your level after an initial arrest or seizure? More specifically, do you continue to be involved after the case is taken up by Federal officials, and do you get feedback on cases that are adopted by Federal law enforcement?

Mr. McCullough. In Iowa, most of the cases are initiated by my agency or local law enforcement agencies' drug task forces that work together. We usually initiate the investigation, work up the case, and, if it looks like it has a nexus into the Federal system—and those variables are the criminal history of the people involved in trafficking the drugs, the drug quantities, if there is an interstate nexus to the case—if some of those factors exist, we then contact usually the Drug Enforcement Administration, which we have a very good working relationship with.

I think their issue is, there are just not very many DEA agents in Iowa, so their resources are limited. Usually we work the investigation up, contact the DEA to see if they are interested in working with us on the investigation, and then we go ahead and work it. We do have several—in fact, I think the figure is seven—DNE agents assigned to DEA task forces throughout the State also, which helps.

The Chairman. So you are involved pretty much throughout the entire case then, but mostly because of the lack of the number of Federal people to help you to carry it on.

Mr. McCullough. Yes. DEA has limited resources in Iowa, not enough agents.

The Chairman. Sure.

Mr. McCullough. We usually work up the cases. Also, at DNE we are fortunate that we have agents spread throughout the State, in both the metro areas and the rural areas, and the DEA agents are housed out of the——

The Chairman. Have you had a different experience, Lt. Springer?

Lt. Springer. It is a fairly similar experience. It is kind of like throwing darts. You start on the outside, and eventually you will hit a bulls-eye and take a case beyond the local or State level and up into the Federal level.

What we see, though, is we do not have a DEA agent within 160 miles of our task force, so what will happen with our cases, in starting the case, you never know if it is going to go Federal until you are kind of into the case a little ways.

At some point it looks like it may be going, so you call the DEA— for us it is down in Billings—and get their authorization. They have the title 21 authority that we do not have to take a case to a Federal level. We get their, kind of, permission, they sort of sign off on it, at which point we run the case. So, we basically become the Federal agent running the case.

At some point when we finish the case, if it gets outside of our State or goes down to California, we will certainly pass that off to an agent somewhere else. But if it stays within our State or somewhere nearby, we will continue with it. At some point, we will call the DEA agent and they will then run it up through the U.S. Attorney's Office.

The problem is you will inevitably lose something in the translation because they are not there from the ground level and all the way through the case; they are getting a briefing of the case, at which point then they are trying to explain it to the Attorney's Office. So, it is difficult that way.

We have had great relationships with the DEA. Most recently, the IRS—Senator Baucus has helped us with that—has assigned some agents to help us when need be, and currently they are helping us right now.

The Chairman. By implication, I think you answered my next concern. That is if, as a member of a task force, you are treated as an equal partner. Do you have access to the same information and intelligence that the Federal agency does? I assume the answer to that is yes, because you supply that information.

Lt. Springer. If you ask, yes. We supply the information when it is our case. Now, there are times where cases are coming——

The Chairman. Well then, if it comes from the top down, are you treated equally with access to all the information that the Federal agency has?

Lt. Springer. Most of the time. It depends on the relationship between the agent and the investigators. We have very good relationships, so they will end up talking to each other all the time. If that relationship is not there, then there may be an issue.

The Chairman. Senator Baucus?

Senator Baucus. Thank you, Mr. Chairman.

Dan, what do you need to do an even better job? You talked about Byrne money being cut, for example. I know we had to struggle with HIDTA money and other resources. But just the basic question. When you and your colleagues get together and say, this is what we really need if we are going to get these guys, what do you need?

Lt. Springer. Bodies. The only way work gets done is by people beating the street, and that takes money, and getting money that can be used in multiple ways. A lot of times, like HIDTA, money and things are very specific for training and overtime and those issues.

But salaries, support staff salaries, drug buy money, all these things—which have been beneficial with the Byrne Grant—that is what has been the most effective for us.

The other thing we need is a Federal agent locally, a DEA agent locally. Bozeman, obviously, has become a growing town. Helena is becoming a growing town. Right now, Bozeman has no title 21 authority outside of two FBI agents, but they are working mostly homeland security at this point.

So I would say, at this point, we need bodies. As bodies increase, then equipment becomes more of an issue, and those things. But we need the people on the street, at the local level.

Senator Baucus. All right.

Now, just being reasonable here, what percent increase in resources will this Byrne Memorial money, or whatever, without asking for the moon, will get the job done?

Lt. Springer. The decrease of 62 percent in the last 5 years, even getting a third of that back would help us add another investigator to our task force, or two. I certainly understand there are fiscal problems everywhere and everyone has their own issues, but getting back to where we were would be a significant help.

We have been backtracking for the last 5 years. If we can just kind of get us back up even to where we were a few years ago, it would be beneficial, 20 percent, 30 percent.

Senator *Baucus.* And how many Federal personnel are there, whether DEA, FBI, or whatnot, available in Montana so you can federalize the case?

Lt. Springer. I am sorry. How many Federal agents?

Senator *Baucus.* How many Federal agents are there in Montana?

Lt. Springer. I do not know the total number, but there is ICE, there is ATF, there is DEA.

Senator Baucus. But are they responsible for and assigned to take drug cases?

Lt. Springer. I believe there are probably six to eight DEA agents in the State of Montana. I may be off on those numbers. I know there are six out of Billings, and I believe there are a couple up in Great Falls, and maybe in Missoula. Now, like I said, for the most part we deal strictly with Billings.

Senator Baucus. Now, how important is it to federalize? I ask because, when I talk to some people at home, they tell me that some of these pushers know that, if it is a State system only, they will get a deferred sentence or they will not get put in jail, there is not enough room in the jails, and so forth.

But if it is federalized, then the accused starts to get serious and starts to cooperate a little more, particularly in trying to go up the chain and trying to find the next higher level of people.

Lt. Springer. The criminals do not like being charged Federally, and they know that they will be going to prison. They spend, I think, 95 percent of their sentence, versus quite a bit less at the State system.

If they know they are going to the State system, chances are they are not going to help us. But the Federal system, they know they are going away for a long time and they will help us significantly.

Senator Baucus. Is that true in Iowa, too, Mr. McCullough?

Mr. McCullough. Yes, it is. The drug traffickers do not want the case to go to the Federal level. Usually they receive a lot more time Federally than they do in State court. I believe Iowa ranks 43rd, too, in the number of Federal agents.

Senator Baucus. All right.

Chairman Venne, the unique problems of the reservation, it seemed, listening to you, relate to inadequate coordination among law enforcement agencies. To what degree is that the problem? To what degree is it insufficient resources? Just generally, again, the same question I asked Lt. Springer. What do we need to do on reservations? What do we need?

Mr. Venne. Well, if you look at our reservation, it is about the size of Rhode Island, and some nights there is only one officer patrolling the whole reservation. The Bureau of Indian Affairs is the one who handles all law enforcement on the reservation.

We have a total amount of 14 officers and 2 investigators. That is probably half of what they need. I looked at some statistics where they are supposed to have 23 officers and four investigators, when they cannot meet the funding of it. Then probably they need a lot of training, surveillance equipment, prevention efforts, and alternative sentencing.

I think the part you are talking about, the different sentences, that is very important. They need to be harsh. They need to be going to Federal court instead of State court.

Senator Baucus. So what does it take, to use this awful word, to federalize on reservations? Does BIA involvement necessarily——

Mr. Venne. Mostly all our drug cases go to the BIA, then on up to Federal court or some local things we are taking care of.

Senator Baucus. All right.

Mr. Venne. So the biggest thing is, we started a Safe Trails Task Force with DEA, FBI, and the Colstrip Sheriff's Department to put a team together with both the northern Cheyenne and the Crow

Tribe, putting a team together and starting to fight this meth problem that we have.

Senator Baucus. One more question, Mr. Chairman.

If there are insufficient resources in law enforcement personnel, say, in our States, Montana, Iowa, or other rural States, how well is that known among drug pushers? Do they, therefore, say, hey, there is not a lot of FBI, not a lot of Federals in Montana someplace, so that is where we are going to go? I mean, is that an issue or not an issue? Anybody can address that.

Mr. McCullough. I do not think they are cognizant of it. When I talk to some of these people, they mainly say, hey, I just thought I was never going to get caught. I just do not think they think about it. They are involved in the methamphetamine trade, making money. They just think it is never going to happen to them. I do not think they actually sit down and think about the Federal issue.

Senator Baucus. Lt. Springer?

Lt. Springer. What they like to do, in Montana they know they can make a lot of money. They are doubling their money out of Spokane, buying an ounce for half the price that they can sell it for in Montana. So that is what is driving them into Montana: the price, the demand.

Senator Baucus. I was stunned to hear you say it was twice the cost of cocaine. That must be a change.

Lt. Springer. It is a change. We did not see cocaine a year ago. We are starting to see quite a bit more cocaine. The price was so much lower, I think that it ended up as kind of a simple economics course for them.

Senator Baucus. All right.

But you need resources. You need dollars, you need people, basically.

Lt. Springer. We need bodies. Yes, sir.

Senator Baucus. Both State and Federal. Thank you very much.

Mr. Chairman, I think it is an outrage. It is an outrage that Byrne Memorial funds have been cut as much as they have. Those grants go a long, long ways to fight. Money for drug law enforcement makes a huge difference, and we just have to find some way to do that.

The Chairman. And I hear that from every level of law enforcement in my State as well. Yes.

Sean, I assume that your agents are trained to investigate and gather information with a goal of breaking down larger criminal organizations other than just local users or dealers and trying to move that information to getting people higher up in the chain.

I assume that your agents then collect data and interview suspects, keeping in mind they can get higher-ups in the drug trafficking. If you collect such intelligence, and I assume you do, what happens to it?

Mr. McCullough. That goes to our Intelligence Bureau for the Iowa Department of Public Safety. They house all the intelligence information for DPS, and then they keep that in Des Moines and they try to forward that on to other task forces around the State.

The Chairman. If you just do it within the State of Iowa, though, that information does not move to Federal officials to make use of it?

Mr. McCullough. It does. One of the vehicles is through HIDTA. We send our intelligence information down to our HIDTA, which is headquartered out of Kansas City, then that information gets funneled out.

The Chairman. And do you feel that it is effectively used, the information that you send?

Mr. McCullough. I think so. It is getting better. We had a meeting last week about this issue in Kansas City at the HIDTA office, about intelligence sharing and putting more information out to other areas of the Nation. I think it is working and it is getting better.

To go back to something we talked about earlier, with DEA, we do know a lot of their intelligence information from our people assigned to the DEA task forces. So, information flow is both ways, from our agency and from DEA, through our designated task force officers at the DEA.

The Chairman. And Chairman Venne, you spoke about the complications due to sovereignty. Do you know if there have been efforts, other than the August 22, 2006 agreement that you spoke about, either through formal Memoranda of Understanding or informal agreements through which tribes work together with non- tribal law enforcement to combat the meth problem occurring in tribal communities?

Mr. Venne. I do not know if there are any other ones, but that is the only one in Montana right now.

The Chairman. And it is obviously too soon to know if it is working.

Mr. Venne. Yes, it is too soon.

The Chairman. Chairman Venne, you spoke about the lack of exchange of information or intelligence. Do you have suggestions of what can be done to help improve that situation?

Mr. Venne. Yes, I do. All of us have to realize, usually they talk about, well, we do not have jurisdiction here or we do not have jurisdiction there. All it takes is people to step up to the plate, create agreements between agencies or governments to handle this problem. To me, that is fairly simple. It is a matter of people just stepping up to the plate, wanting to do something.

The Chairman. So one of your main criticisms is that there is a lack of willingness to do that?

Mr. Venne. Yes.

The Chairman. And is that something that you sense all over the country, or just between law enforcement agencies and tribes?

Mr. Venne. It is between, probably, law enforcement agencies, the different law enforcement agencies we have in the State. People like to protect their own little areas and be the boss of that.

The Chairman. Yes. We run into that all the time.

Senator Baucus. Yes. It never happens here.

Mr. Venne. That is the problem.

The Chairman. Yes. All right.

Well, I am done asking questions. We did not have all of our members here today, so you may get questions from other members for answer in writing. We would appreciate your cooperation on that. Thank you all.

Senator Baucus. One more, Mr. Chairman.

The Chairman. Sure. You can have more time.

Senator Baucus. Chairman Venne, can you tell us a little bit about the Seven Hills Healing Center, and how is that working?

Mr. Venne. That is working excellent. What we did was, a year and a half ago, in 1 week, we had six deaths, all related to alcohol and drug use. I finally said, we have to do something. The tribe owns a ranch of about 28,000 acres out by the mountains, so we developed this program.

It is a culture program, in what we, as Indians, believe in, the different types of religious practices we do. We bring our people and show them, to let them appreciate who they are and where they are from, and to educate them in the Crow way of life. We have been doing that for the past year and a half. We have been very successful. We probably have a 70-percent success rate out of that. We take women and men. We alternate them, though.

It is not that great of a building and ranch stuff, but we have been doing a lot of fixing up on our own and trying to get that going, bringing them back to what we believe in as people. It is working out pretty well, Senator.

Senator Baucus. This is kind of a wild idea, it just occurred to me. There is a warrior culture in Native Americans, that is, when a warrior falls, the warrior is honored and a lot of tribal songs are sung to warriors.

Mr. Venne. Sure.

Senator Baucus. Fallen warriors. The thought is, if somehow we could convert that so warriors are also fighting meth like they are fighting other armies, fighting other enemies. I do not know if that is possible or if it makes any sense, but it was just a thought that occurred to me.

Mr. Venne. We have been attacking it just like that. We go on long marches and walks with our young kids in school, starting prevention-type projects in our schools against meth. They need to know that we support them as an administration and we do care for them and participate in what they do.

Senator Baucus. What works best in preventing or lowering teenaged suicides? How much of that is meth-related, dysfunctional families, and whatnot?

Mr. Venne. Usually on my reservation there are no suicides. In the last year, we have had five suicides because of meth. A prime example is, three of them walked straight into a moving train. Things like that are happening.

But I think it takes the community working together with everybody to really put a stop to it, and prevention-type programs. I think the community is the answer.

Senator Baucus. All right. Thank you very much. I deeply appreciate the time you have taken to come here and help out. It means a lot to all of us. Thank you.

The Chairman. I thank you as well. If you want to stay, you are welcome to stay.

I would call the second panel now. I am going to introduce the second panel as they come, so please come, all of you.

We have Joseph T. Rannazzisi, Deputy Assistant Administrator, Office of Diversion Control, Drug Enforcement Administration; Mr. Robert Patton, Chief, Mexico-Central American Section, Office of

Financial Operations, DEA. Mr. Patton will not make a statement, but is here to answer any questions that may arise about DEA's financial investigations.

We have Gregory Passic, Director of the Office of Drug Interdiction, U.S. Customs and Border Protection; and, finally, Mr. Andre′ Martin, Director, Operations Policy and Support, of the IRS Criminal Investigation Division.

I have introduced you in the same order that I will call on you to testify. So we will wait until you get ready, Mr. Rannazzisi, then we will start with you.

Also, for all of you, your statements, if they are longer than your 5 minutes, will be included in the record as you submit them.

STATEMENT OF JOSEPH T. RANNAZZISI, DEPUTY ASSISTANT ADMINISTRATOR, OFFICE OF DIVERSION CONTROL, DRUG ENFORCEMENT ADMINISTRATION, WASHINGTON, DC; ACCOMPANIED BY ROBERT T. PATTON, SECTION CHIEF, MEXICO-CENTRAL AMERICA SECTION, OFFICE OF FINANCIAL OPERATIONS, DRUG ENFORCEMENT ADMINISTRATION, ARLINGTON, VA

Mr. Rannazzisi. Thank you, sir, and good morning. Chairman Grassley, Ranking Member Baucus, distinguished members of the committee, on behalf of DEA's Administrator, Karen P. Tandy, thank you for the opportunity to testify here today regarding DEA's efforts to break the methamphetamine supply chain.

I am joined by Mr. Robert Patton of DEA's Office of Financial Investigations, who will respond to any questions regarding our financial investigations related to methamphetamine.

Methamphetamine poses a significant threat to the United States. Through our law enforcement partnerships across the country and around the world, DEA is actively engaged in attacking criminal organizations responsible for trafficking methamphetamine, the precursors utilized in its production, and their illicit proceeds.

DEA's efforts to address the methamphetamine drug problem have been ongoing for decades. Methamphetamine production requires no specialized skill or training, and its recipes are readily available on the Internet. Its precursor chemicals also have been historically easy to obtain and inexpensive to purchase.

The unique nature of this synthetic drug warrants a targeted response. In 2006, the Administration released the Synthetic Drug Strategy, which provides a framework for DEA and contributing agencies to continue ongoing efforts and to chart new milestones in achieving domestic and international progress against meth- amphetamine and other synthetic drugs.

Methamphetamine consumed in the U.S. originates from two principal sources. Most methamphetamine found in the U.S. is produced by Mexico- or California-based traffickers whose organizations control super-labs. Current data suggest that roughly 80 percent of the methamphetamine consumed in the U.S. comes from these large labs, which are increasingly found in Mexico.

When we talk about super-labs, those are labs that produce approximately 10 pounds or more of methamphetamine in a 24-hour production cycle.

The second source of methamphetamine is small toxic labs, or STLs, which produce relatively small amounts of methamphetamine and are generally not affiliated with major trafficking organizations. It is estimated that these labs are responsible for approximately 20 percent of the methamphetamine consumed in the United States.

In response, DEA is taking its fight to the organizations responsible for this menace. We have initiated successful investigations that have disrupted and dismantled significant methamphetamine trafficking organizations and have also taken an active role in fighting the diversion of ephedrine and pseudoephedrine through both enforcement operations and international agreements.

It is noteworthy that law enforcement efforts have been aided by both State and Federal legislation. As you well know, the Combat Methamphetamine Epidemic Act of 2005 has provided additional tools to enhance our efforts, both domestically and internationally.

DEA's efforts, coupled with these legislative tools, have already resulted in a substantial reduction in the amount of precursor chemicals entering the United States. DEA has also stepped up its efforts to focus on the financial side of drug trafficking organizations.

Our financial enforcement strategy is mission-driven, focusing on the flow of money back to international sources of drug supply. There is little doubt that the sole reason people sell drugs is for financial gain; therefore, attacking the financial infrastructures of traffickers plays a key role in our enforcement strategy.

Our objective is to identify and halt the flow of drug proceeds by focusing on bulk currency smuggling and the remission of drug money through U.S. wire transfers. DEA works closely with our other law enforcement counterparts to address these initiatives. DEA has mandated that all drug investigations include a financial investigation component, which our financial investigations teams help carry out.

A key element in combatting methamphetamine is international cooperation, particularly in the area of precursor chemical control. DEA and DOJ have facilitated and played a leadership role in several recent meetings of the international community.

These meetings, such as the National Methamphetamine Chemical Initiative Strategy Conference, where the Attorney General announced several new anti-methamphetamine initiatives, have helped increase awareness around the world and resulted in agreements to monitor and track key precursor chemicals. Several nations, most notably Mexico, also have taken independent steps to control methamphetamine precursors.

DEA will continue to fight methamphetamine on all fronts by targeting both the trafficking organizations and the financial proceeds they generate. We are fully committed to meeting this international threat by working in a cooperative effort with other agencies and nations.

Chairman Grassley, Ranking Member Baucus, and members, I thank you again for this opportunity to testify. I would be happy to answer any questions you may have. Thank you.

The Chairman. Thank you.

[The prepared statement of Mr. Rannazzisi appears in the appendix.]

The Chairman. Now, Mr. Passic?

STATEMENT OF GREGORY PASSIC, DIRECTOR, OFFICE OF DRUG INTERDICTION, U.S. CUSTOMS AND BORDER PROTECTION, WASHINGTON, DC

Mr. Passic. Chairman Grassley and Ranking Member Baucus, thank you for your personal attention to this. I know, by talking to your staffs, you really want to do something about this problem.

I sense that this is a very busy committee, and for you to take this on, I laud you for your efforts. I hope that what we can present today will move in the direction of your challenge.

I could not help but be moved by the prior panel about how devastating methamphetamine is in their communities. In my humble opinion this is a weapon of mass destruction introduced from Mexican criminal organizations into this country, and as such demands that we in Customs and Border Protection pay attention to it and team up with the members sitting here at this table to do something about it.

We were looking at two specific areas that we think we can challenge and meet that contribution that you are looking for. The first one is along the border, along the line. The southwest border is responsible for 80 percent of the meth and other drugs that enter this country. It is a tough challenge. We will be adding 6,000 to 8,000 Border Patrol Agents along that border.

As the Border Patrol Agents and National Guard are deployed, we have noticed a shift into the ports of entry, so we cannot ignore that. We have to have better technology. We have to have an increased effort also at vehicles smuggling traps and individuals entering the country through the ports.

To do that, we need DEA's help. We have to not only seize more meth on its way to the U.S. market, but we have to make smart seizures. A seizure of outbound currency or drugs coming in is significant in that we might deny funds to trafficking groups and meth from hitting the street, but more importantly, we feel that is a starting point for an investigation. We feel we need to couple with DEA's active meth investigations, if they share their data with us—and there is every indication they are doing that.

We have a team coming in tomorrow from Los Angeles, DEA agents and analysts, who are going to be meeting with our people to talk about precursor controls directly to include sharing our systems with them. And if we can couple the gears in the government machinery, we go way beyond cooperation—this thing requires collaboration.

It requires teaming in a fashion that we have never done before. As other members of your panel mentioned earlier, we can do a better job of coordinating and teaming that effort.

Smart interdiction also allows us to provide to DEA evidence in drug conspiracies. If they have wire taps, informants, or undercover operations running into meth groups and we can make a seizure from one of those couriers, that is added value to DEA's attempts to arrest and prosecute major traffickers. It also provides leads that go back into Mexico, where we have to have impact on the Mexican organizations that are the root of the problem.

The second area we in Customs and Border Protection are concentrating on is the control of precursors. We are working very closely with DEA to identify companies, brokers, and transshippers that are sending ephedrine and pseudoephedrine to and through the United States, primarily to those laboratories mentioned before in Mexico, the super-labs.

This challenge also involves engaging the Mexican authorities, and we laud DEA's efforts to build that task force down in Mexico, because we feel, until we are able to impact the super-labs and the principals that are engaged in those, that our impact will be somewhat limited.

We also feel that by denying precursors to the super-labs, that we can impact their ability to produce high-quality methamphetamine that is introduced into the United States now.

My written statement actually goes into specifics of the game plan. I also met with your staffs. We are looking forward to working with them to continue to be challenged and really do something about this problem. Thank you for the opportunity of being here.

The Chairman. Thank you.

[The prepared statement of Mr. Passic appears in the appendix.]

The Chairman. Now, Mr. Martin?

Mr. Martin. Good morning.

The Chairman. Good morning.

Statement of C. Andre ′ Martin, Director, Operations Policy and Support, IRS Criminal Investigation, Washington, DC

Mr. Martin. Chairman Grassley, Ranking Member Baucus, and members of the committee, I appreciate the opportunity to appear before you today to discuss the Internal Revenue Service Criminal Investigation Division's role in combatting money laundering and narcotics trafficking.

These are serious national problems that erode our economy and destroy thousands of lives each year. The mission of the Internal Revenue Service Criminal Investigation Division is to serve the American public by investigating potential criminal violations of the Internal Revenue Code and related financial crimes in a manner that fosters confidence in the tax system, in compliance with the law.

This includes the investigation of complex tax and money laundering cases, covering a broad range of crimes, from tax evasions, to corporate fraud, to sophisticated narcotics trafficking organizations.

Our approximately 2,800 criminal investigators are in demand throughout the law enforcement community because of our unique financial investigative skills. The Attorney General recently communicated to IRS Commissioner Everson, "The agents of the Internal Revenue Service Criminal Investigation are among the most important resources we can bring to bear in connection with the complex financial investigations that are critical to our success."

Our core mission at IRS is tax administration. Our country de-pends on a sound tax system. This fact was reinforced by Judge William Webster, who was commissioned by the IRS in response to concerns raised by this committee in 1998, to direct an independent review of IRS CI.

Judge Webster concluded that we suffered from a mission drift away from investigating core mission tax cases. He specifically attributed demands placed on CI by other law enforcement entities to participate in narcotics investigations as a primary cause of the drift away from the investigation of criminal violations of the Internal Revenue Code and those financial crimes that have a nexus to tax enforcement.

He correctly pointed out that IRS CI must investigate tax violations arising out of title 26 of the U.S. Code because no other Federal law enforcement agency has the authority or responsibility, or similar mission.

At the same time that CI has sharpened its focus on tax investigations, we have carefully monitored our narcotics work to ensure we are focusing our scarce resources on those narcotics cases that bring the most value to the government's counter-drug efforts. With the tax gap estimated at over $300 billion, CI's focus on tax investigations must remain our top priority.

As part of the larger law enforcement community, we recognize that IRS CI's role is broader than tax administration. We contribute our efforts in many areas, including money laundering, counter-terrorism, and public corruption.

Tracing the money is often the key to conviction and to disgorging assets. In fact, we view money laundering violations as tax evasion in progress because the offenders are essentially trying to hide their dirty money from the government.

We recognize that drug trafficking organizations are motivated by greed, money, and assets. Therefore, the objective of our narcotics program is to dismantle and/or disrupt the highest level narcotics organizations, as designated by the Department of Justice, through the Organized Crime Drug Enforcement Task Force program, or OCDETF.

Some of our OCDETF efforts include cases such as Operation North Star, Operation Brain Drain, Operation Snow Globe, and Operation Ice Storm.

While our narcotics program does not focus on specific types of illegal drugs, it does conform to the qualitative framework established by the OCDETF program. It places emphasis on conducting financial investigations of each case, with an aim toward the elimination of the drug organization's infrastructure and permanently removing their profits.

In conclusion, regardless of the type of drug threat, whether it's methamphetamine, cocaine, heroin, or marijuana, IRS CI will continue to support this effort by strategically targeting and dismantling the financial infrastructure of the most significant drug trafficking organizations.

The women and men of IRS CI carry on an 87-year tradition of solving financial crimes by following the money trail, and we do that in a spirit of cooperation with all of our law enforcement partners.

Mr. Chairman, I thank you for this opportunity to appear before this distinguished committee, and I would be happy to answer any questions you and Senator Baucus may have.

[The prepared statement of Mr. Martin appears in the appendix.]

The Chairman. All right. To any and all of you on this first question. We get reports about increasing amounts of drug seizures and we get other reports about decreasing numbers, not going up, so we do not really know where we are.

So could you clarify whether seizures of meth at the southwest border are increasing or decreasing? Could you explain why there may be differing reports about seizures at the border? Lastly, is there an effort being made to have a uniform standard of reporting or collecting this information?

Mr. Passic. We have noticed an increase of 11 percent at the ports of entry, and a slight decrease, actually, between the ports of entry with our Border Patrol people.

The reason that we have two different statistics or numbers is that, the old system had a threshold on the amount of drugs that could be issued a Federal identification number by EPIC, and if you did not meet the threshold, your smaller seizures did not get into the system. That has been rectified. Our people now can put in all of our seizures along the border, regardless of the amount.

The other thing is, DEA was collecting seizure data from State and local task forces along the border, in other words, meth shipments that had already made it across our line, so that made the numbers different.

But hopefully our people are being trained how to do input into the new EPIC system out there, and the next time we are up here, hopefully we can say that thing has been fixed.

The Chairman. Does anybody else want to add to that?

Mr. Rannazzisi. If I may just add, sir, I think we have learned our lesson from the clandestine lab seizure system. A couple of years ago, people were looking at the lab seizure system and they noticed a dramatic drop. That was not a drop because there was a lack of lab seizures, it was a drop because of reporting. The reporting was consistently late. It is just a problem.

Right now, we are looking at clandestine lab numbers from 2005. We could definitely say that, in 2005, we had approximately 12,500 incidents. We cannot look at the 2006 numbers because those numbers change every day.

It is a lack of timely reporting as well, and I think that is why the numbers fluctuate. We think it is premature to talk about any numbers until well towards the end of the year or into the following year.

The Chairman. Is there an effort to bring some uniformity?

Mr. Rannazzisi. Well, it is difficult. With the lab seizure system, there is no requirement to.

The Chairman. I guess my question, though, as I look back at it, was more directed towards smuggling across the southwest border than the clandestine labs that you are speaking about.

Mr. Passic. Yes. I think that has been addressed.

The Chairman. All right.

Mr. Passic. The DEA came up with the fix, and we have agreed that that is the best place to do it. We are working with the people out at EPIC to implement that.

The Chairman. All right.

On another question, Mr. Rannazzisi, I am referring to Mr. McCullough's statement how finding a decreasing number of small toxic labs has enabled the people in Iowa to be more proactive in initiating cases involving smuggling by sophisticated drug organizations.

What criteria would the DEA use to become involved in cases that may be initiated at the State level, using Mr. McCullough as an example, but not necessarily commenting on what he said?

Generally, what is the criteria that DEA uses in placing agents and resources in different cities and areas? How often is this placement of resources reevaluated and redistributed?

Mr. Rannazzisi. Let me answer the last question first. I think we go through a regular assessment of our resources, where our personnel are deployed, and we measure that as compared to the drug threat. As an agency, we have a finite number of resources. Manpower is our most significant resource. We have to go and concentrate where the major drug threats are.

If you will remember, we go after the larger organizations. We try to go after the organizations that are putting the most meth- amphetamine out on the street nationwide, the ones that are multi- jurisdictional and international in scope. That does not mean that we do not assist State and local agencies.

The Chairman. Well, he did not criticize you.

Mr. Rannazzisi. No, no. And I understand that. But we built our reputation on working with State and local agencies. Our task force program has been operational since the early 1970s, and we are proud of that fact.

As a task force group supervisor, we would look at every case that the State and local agency would bring to us and we would work them. Obviously there are no criteria. It's just what the supervisor and the case agent who reviews the case, where they think they can take the case with their State and local counterparts. So there are really no criteria involved.

The Chairman. Senator Baucus?

Senator Baucus. Thank you, Mr. Chairman.

I am concerned about the precursors and the countries that manufacture them, and what is being done to stop the precursors that are manufactured to be used for methamphetamine.

Could you name the major suppliers, either countries or companies, of precursors that are used for meth, that is, for illegal purposes?

Mr. Rannazzisi. Well, if you are looking at ephedrine and pseudoephedrine, in India there are probably, I would say, seven to nine manufacturing operations that produce pseudoephedrine or ephedrine. I do not have their names handy, but obviously there is Lahore, India, Malladi, a lot of the large ones.

Senator Baucus. So India is a major source?

Mr. Rannazzisi. Yes. India is a large source.

The Chairman. And those are companies——

Mr. Rannazzisi. That manufacture pseudoephedrine and ephedrine.

The Chairman. But they are companies that have sprung up in India? They are not companies from America that went over there, or have any relationship to companies that are multinational, or anything like that?

Mr. Rannazzisi. No. Well, I am sure at least one or two of those companies might have a U.S. component in the United States, but for the most part, yes, they are Indian corporations.

The Chairman. All right. Go ahead.

Mr. Rannazzisi. They are all legitimate.

Senator Baucus. Sure.

Mr. Rannazzisi. I mean, these are legitimate companies.

Senator Baucus. They are legitimate companies, but I suspect they have an idea, when they make a big shipment to Mexico, what it is going to be used for.

Mr. Rannazzisi. Well, yes and no. If I could continue on the other countries, I will get back to it.

Senator Baucus. Sure.

Mr. Rannazzisi. Germany. Their largest producer is BASF Germany. Then China. It is a little more problematic in China because we are not sure how many companies produce in China. But that is the third largest. Out of the three largest, they are a very large producer of pseudoephedrine and ephedrine.

Senator Baucus. Are there any producers in Mexico?

Mr. Rannazzisi. No.

Senator Baucus. So it is all imported into Mexico?

Mr. Rannazzisi. Yes, sir. And just to say that, well, why can India not just tell us where the pseudoephedrine is going in Mexico, it is not that easy.

Senator Baucus. Yes.

Mr. Rannazzisi. The traffickers adapt to chemical control regulations. They are not going to ship right into Mexico, especially since COFEPRIS,* the Mexican regulatory authority, has cut import limits to 70 metric tons from 150 metric tons previous to year 2005.

It does not go into Mexico, it goes into Africa, Central and South America, Europe. It goes through a system of brokers. It is not being shipped. Somewhere along the transportation line, the transit line, it is diverted out of that line and into the hands of smugglers who smuggle it in.

Senator Baucus. So what is the answer here? I mean, better data? More data? More reporting of shipments of goods, especially precursors?

Mr. Rannazzisi. That is the question we ask all the time. I think the answer is, better cooperation with our international counterparts.

Now, the International Narcotics Control Board, Precursor Unit, basically controls all of the chemicals trafficked throughout the world. They do that under the authority of the 1988 Vienna Convention. The INCB, and recently the Commission on Narcotic Drugs, the CND, passed a resolution that now is basically encour-aging countries to report all shipments of precursor chemicals to the INCB.

Now, before, tablet shipments, pharmaceutical preparations, were not reportable. They could ship out millions and millions of tablets and they did not have to be reported to the INCB.

Senator Baucus. Now, did these companies in India have to report?

Mr. Rannazzisi. They did not, but India has. India started reporting, I believe, late in 2005, early in 2006, and they started reporting all tablets.

Senator Baucus. Then why does that not stop Indian manufacturing of precursors going to Mexican meth labs?

Mr. Rannazzisi. Because India will export tablets to a broker, say, in Europe or in Africa. Once it gets to that broker, we have lost it out of the chain.

Senator Baucus. What about the organization you mentioned. Should there not be reporting there, too, that is, to a broker?

Mr. Rannazzisi. Yes. Well, yes. If it is a legitimate organization operating under the rules of the country that it is operating in, absolutely. But what we find is, down the chain, some companies are just illegitimate, they are shell companies that trick the regulatory boards in that country into agreeing to allow the shipment or the import to occur.

Senator Baucus. So, if you could wave a magic wand, you are the man to solve this thing, what would you do? You have carte blanche. Whatever you say, you are the man.

Mr. Rannazzisi. Well, what I would require is all countries to abide by the 1988 convention and the CND resolution that everybody signed onto in March of 2006.

Senator BAUCUS. And what does it take to get those countries to comply?

Mr. Rannazzisi. Well, since it is a voluntary compliance they could sign on, but the fact is, when it comes time to do the reporting, it becomes diplomatic. A lot of diplomatic efforts need to be exercised in order to do this.

Senator Baucus. Yes. I see my time is almost up. Very briefly, Mr. Chairman.

Mr. Martin, so what tools do you have for solving this part of the tax gap?

Mr. Martin. Well, you had mentioned earlier, or asked, and I know the first panel talked about this, but in terms of how we get involved with State and local law enforcement, that vehicle, for the most part, is through the auspices of the grand jury, so we are talking about U.S. Attorneys' offices.

Being able to get formally into the game with State and local law enforcement, for us, the vehicle has been the U.S. Attorney's office. We take our cue from them, and also our partnerships with DEA, for the most part, when you are talking about the narcotics program.

Once we are able to get the intelligence, because I know we are talking about a resources issue here, a concern, particularly out in Bozeman, is we are going to take whatever information is given us, whether that be from State and local law enforcement, directly from the U.S. Attorney's Office, or from other Federal law enforce-ment agencies—for instance, DEA—and we are going to evaluate that against the OCDETF standards. Again, similar for us with limited resources, we are looking to focus in on the most significant drug trafficking organizations.

If the intelligence that we evaluate takes us in that direction, then we will be prepared to commit resources, and we have, to significant narcotics investigations, and that includes methamphetamine investigations.

Senator Baucus. The same question. What needs to be done? Again, Mr. Martin, you are the man again. How are you going to find the money? What do you need to find the money?

Mr. Martin. At whatever level Congress wants us to be involved in addressing this problem——

Senator Baucus. No. We want you to solve it. You are supposed to tell us what you would need, what you would do, or tell the executive, whatever. Based on what you know, what is the best and most efficient way to have an efficient money trail to crack down and catch these guys?

Mr. Martin. You have to have resources involved.

Senator Baucus. You want more resources then.

Mr. Martin. You have to have resources in order to be able to do it. We have the expertise. That is there. So whatever resources——

Senator Baucus. Resources where?

Mr. Martin. We have 30 field offices across the country. And just to put it in perspective for you, as far as our resource commitment to the narcotics program, if you go back to 1996, at that time we committed about 22 percent of our Special Agent resources at that time to the narcotics program.

Fast forward to fiscal year 2006, right now. We are right at about 9 percent commitment of our resources to the narcotics program. That has been driven, between 1996 and now, by whatever we have been budgeted, and we work from that vantage point.

Senator Baucus. Thank you very much. I went way over my time. Thank you very much.

The Chairman. I want to follow on with something Senator Baucus brought up. I suppose it is because of some of the things you said, Mr. Rannazzisi. That is, I would like to get kind of a corporation's attitude towards our efforts.

Now, you have made it very clear that it is difficult once it leaves corporate manufacturing, that it could go through all sorts of shenanigans to avoid finding out that it is going to Mexico. But I would be interested in knowing—for instance, let us use BASF as one, because we all know that company.

Either your agency or an agency in Europe goes to them on this problem and says, we want some help on where these precursors go because some of them are going to be used for methamphetamine. Do they have a healthy attitude towards helping us?

Mr. Rannazzisi. Absolutely. BASF, we work very closely with.

The Chairman. All right.

Mr. Rannazzisi. While we do see product that potentially is from BASF, it is not a lot. Again, a lot of times when we see bulk precursor, it is difficult to determine the origin of that bulk precursor. But I can tell you that the European authorities and BASF U.S. have been very cooperative in dealing with our issues and our investigations without any problem.

The problem is, again, we could only act on the information that is available to us in the international community. The INCB has a system set up to monitor all chemicals that are trafficked internationally.

The INCB stops shipments probably on a weekly basis. The INCB is stopping shipments. They have that authority to tell a competent authority, say in India, we do not think this shipment can go through. We cannot verify on the other end if the company is legitimate or not. They do that. But like everyone else, the INCB has resources that are stretched, and they cannot catch everything.

The Chairman. On another issue—and again, to you—would it be fair for me to assume, even though we have passed these good State laws, and now the Federal law that is going into effect— which you could not say for the Federal law yet, but at least for the State laws—that that probably has not affected the workload of the DEA much at all? It probably has affected the workload of local and State law enforcement people, but probably has not changed your workload at all.

Mr. Rannazzisi. Well, not necessarily. We do have active lab teams. But in States like Oklahoma, Iowa, Oregon, Missouri, and Kansas, States that have passed that Schedule 5 or Schedule 5- type legislation, Illinois, those States that do have lab teams, we are looking at the fact that those lab teams are not as active because the lab numbers have dropped considerably.

So what we are doing now is, instead of those lab teams going back to work in general drug investigations, we have now told them to focus their efforts on meth organizations. If you are not looking for labs because the labs just are not there any more, you had better be looking at meth organizations, large organizational targeting.

The Chairman. All right. So those funds that would have gone for lab clean-up now can be used for further law enforcement.

Mr. Rannazzisi. Well, yes. The funds that are available right now—I do not know if you are familiar with the container program, but we are using some of those funds to fund these container programs, these hazardous waste container programs, that started in Kentucky, and now we have expanded it to four or five other States, and we will continue to expand.

That helps States so the officers are not on the lab sites for long periods of time. They can do the clean-up at the lab site, move it to a container program, and then a hazardous waste contractor will come and clean up the container rather than at the lab site.

The Chairman. Also, what is the level of cooperation between Customs and Border Protection and the Drug Enforcement Administration, and do you share intelligence with Customs and Border Protection? What is the basis for sharing information protocols, for instance?

Mr. Rannazzisi. Well, I can tell you that our relationship with CBP is probably the best it has ever been. We have a couple of joint projects working right now. We share information on a regular basis. We are in the process of creating—and Greg could tell you better because he is more hands-on with this—a port program that really is going to be a dynamic program.

Do you want to add?

Mr. Passic. Yes. As I mentioned before, this thing requires collaboration. Cooperation does not work. We have to have all the intelligence that DEA has, and any other agencies, on license plates from vehicles that are potential couriers, money movers, individuals. We have to be able to get that to the front line somehow if our interdiction on outbound cash and meth coming back is going to be effective.

They have to trust us, if they are going to give us that type of detailed information from active methamphetamine cases involving undercover agents, that we do not just hit every car that comes back across that border and look at interdiction as being the end game. We have to do that in cooperation with them, which means we have to co-locate our resources with DEA offices and task forces along that border, and we also have to have DEA analysts and diversion investigators located with our port people. All of that is going on right now. We are very pleased with the cooperation and the candid sharing that we have received from DEA.

The Chairman. Well, now is that cooperation based on Memoranda of Understanding? Do they exist? Do they explain the protocols? If so, do you seem to have avoided confusion and ensured safety?

Mr. Passic. No, it does not involve a protocol and an MOU.

The Chairman. It is very informal, is what you are saying.

Mr. Passic. It involves the good will of agents on both sides of that aisle that want to do something about this. The exchange of information goes way beyond what either one of us is required by MOU to do, and we prefer to keep it that way. We see ourselves as working as an integrated team, not as one agency sharing something with another.

The Chairman. Well, then let me ask my staff something.

[Pause.]

The Chairman. This would be to all of you. Would you describe the level of interaction between your agency and the Office of National Drug Control Policy, if any?

Mr. Rannazzisi. I personally have almost daily contact with ONDCP. As a policy arm, we are continually discussing different issues. They sit on the Methamphetamine Task Force and, with the Department of Justice and HHS, form the Synthetic Drug Interagency Working Group that establishes policy and actually put out the Synthetic Drug Strategy.

The Chairman. So that would be an example of guidance that you see from them?

Mr. Rannazzisi. Policy guidance. Yes. Again, policy is developed with agencies such as CBP and DEA getting together with DOJ and looking at issues and developing policy. It is not just one agency.

The Chairman. Do they provide any assistance in coordinating with other agencies on narcotics-related issues?

Mr. Rannazzisi. Yes. Absolutely. Yes. That is absolutely correct. The CHAIRMAN. Do any of the other two witnesses have anything to add to that?

Mr. Martin. At the IRS, we do have one Grade 15 analyst who is assigned to the staff at ONDCP here in Washington, DC.

Mr. Passic. We participate in the same working groups that DEA does, basically.

The Chairman. All right.

In regard to bulk cash smuggling, it is my understanding it is on the rise on the southwest border. How is your agency addressing the rise of this form of money laundering, and how are you working together with other agencies to approach this evolving problem?

Mr. Patton. If I may, Mr. Chairman.

The Chairman. You sure can.

Mr. Patton. Yes. From DEA's standpoint, we have initiated a number of strategic initiatives, such as our bulk currency initiative, whereby we ask our agents to work directly with the 700,000 State and local counterparts and other Federal counterparts throughout the Nation when a bulk currency seizure is made along the Nation's highways or on the Nation's jetways, and so on, where we try to share the intelligence from that seizure.

For example, cell phone information or scraps of paper with information in the perpetrator's pockets, or other information related to that seizure, we try to tie that back to existing investigations, either to where the money may be going or to where the money may be coming from.

We have other initiatives, such as our concealed trap initiative, our National trucking initiative, and our money trail initiative, where we try to tie financial investigations into different investigations where we are attacking the command-and-control structure of the drug trafficking organizations utilizing their communications systems. So, we are proceeding and realizing that bulk currency smuggling is the main threat pertaining to methamphetamine distribution.

The Chairman. Mr. Martin, obviously your agency, through criminal investigators, has a great deal of expertise, so I was kind of wondering how it is being called upon.

What percentage of your agents are working on these types of cases? Are there requests for assistance that you have turned down due to the lack of manpower? Then I will have a follow-up.

Mr. Martin. Unfortunately, we have had to turn down investigations across the country. The criteria that we have tried to use, again, is to evaluate the information and assess whether or not it rises to the level of what we call an OCDETF-quality type investigation. If it does, then we commit resources to that investigation.

For fiscal year 2006, we have a goal of between 9 and 11 percent of our direct investigation time that we will commit to the narcotics program, including OCDETF investigations. But once we are in, we are focused in a number of different respects with different initiatives, including the bulk currency initiative.

We do have initiatives in six field offices where we are taking on a similar approach. It is not just enough to seize with regard to bulk currency stops. As a matter of fact, it is particularly important, with State and local law enforcement, particularly State troopers, we rely so much on them with these initiatives because they are in the position to actually make the stops, and not just with regard to cash, but also the intelligence. We cannot say enough how important it is to take the intelligence and run with that.

So we are particularly interested in getting that kind of information through the six initiatives we started about a year ago, and we are going to continue that focus with the bulk currency initiative as well.

We have other initiatives, such as Suspicious Activity Report (SAR) review teams. We have about 80 SAR review teams around the country. Again, they are focused on analyzing information under the Bank Secrecy Act.

That is particularly important in terms of enabling us to be able to follow the money, if you will, through our analytical work, through working with other law enforcement agencies, again, including State and local.

The Chairman. Are you in any way, through your agency, able to help train law enforcement agencies in dealing with these issues as well?

Mr. Martin. Absolutely. That is something we have been very committed to. We have 30 field offices around the country. The relationship part of it is something that we focus on.

However we are able to provide resources, we put on financial investigation training for State and local law enforcement. We have done that in a number of our field offices around the country, and we will continue to do that. We consider that to be very important.

That includes our SAR review teams. They have an outreach component. That outreach component means that you pull in the financial and regulatory community, as well as State and local law enforcement, to work together on issues that are common in that particular geographical area for SAR review teams.

The Chairman. We have spent all of our time—I think most of the time—referring to Mexico as being the source of entry into this country. Do we have to be concerned about any other countries getting product from that country into this country, or maybe the meth being made in another country transshipped into the United States through Mexico?

In other words, are there other countries out there other than Mexico where this is being manufactured that are a real problem? If they are not a real problem, then do not worry about it.

Mr. Rannazzisi. Yes. In this region, Mexico would be a primary- source country for the United States. There are manufacturing operations in Canada, but it is very small for methamphetamine.

The Far East. Many countries in the Far East produce huge amounts of methamphetamine, but it is for consumption in the Far East. We rarely see methamphetamine, the Yabba tablets or meth- amphetamine, from Far East countries in the U.S. or domestically.

The Chairman. In my State, at my town meetings, the perception of constituents that bring up the issue of illegal immigrants would also most likely associate it as a source of methamphetamine getting into the United States and into our State. Is that a correct perception that my constituents might have, or not correct?

Mr. Rannazzisi. I think that whenever you have a transient population, migrant workers, you will have traffickers that basically blend into the community and distribute. The problem is, traf-fickers hide very well and adapt to whatever community they are in.

The Chairman. So, illegal or legal, it does not make much difference? In other words, it is not a case of the sophistication of the cartel that they would be more apt to use legal people coming into the country as opposed to illegal people coming into the country as a source of trafficking.

Mr. Rannazzisi. As couriers.

The Chairman. Yes. Couriers.

Mr. Rannazzisi. Or transportation routes. Both legal and illegal. The CHAIRMAN. Just so long as they get it in the country, it does not matter.

Mr. Rannazzisi. Yes. And since they are using established trafficking routes for cocaine and heroin, they are using the same couriers.

Mr. Passic. Mr. Chairman, if I might offer this from our perspective: illegal drug traffickers in this country are definitely a problem. Both the Mexican and Colombian organizations deploy workers in the form of traditional cells, very similar to intelligence cells.

They are hired for a specific purpose. They are deployed for a specific purpose. They provide that service to the trafficking organization and will return, often to Mexico or Colombia, once law enforcement heats them up or their tour of duty has ended.

We have seen recent shifts in drug smuggling patterns based on the priority put on the southwest border, where the Mexican organizations are looking back again at an end run around that border.

The Colombian organizations that were very comfortable in moving drug loads from Mexico, are back in the Caribbean, with significant shipments. So we want to look ahead, also. We are looking at Colombia as a potential meth problem.

The Chairman. On another issue, to what extent are you getting cooperation from foreign banks and nations in battling money laundering?

Mr. Patton. Through our offices, through our Financial Investigative Team (FIT) teams, we do receive cooperation from Mexico, through our office in Mexico City and the other related offices throughout the country. We try to work closely and develop a rapport with the Mexican banking officials and the Mexican banking system.

The Chairman. Well, do you feel that it is full cooperation? Is it something you have to work at all the time or are they interested in solving the problem as much as you are?

Mr. Patton. Well, I mean, it is a case by case basis. But we do believe that there are certain people there that really do believe that they can solve the problem and will help us do so.

The Chairman. Are there any banks in Mexico that you know are in cahoots with drug trafficking and the cartels?

Mr. Patton. No, sir, I do not.

The Chairman. I think I have asked all my questions. You have been very cooperative, and I appreciate it very much. I have a closing statement that I want to put in the record.

[The prepared statement of Senator Grassley appears in the appendix.]

The Chairman. The hearing is adjourned. Thank you all very much for your cooperation.

[Whereupon, at 11:41 a.m., the hearing was concluded.]

APPENDIX: ADDITIONAL MATERIAL SUBMITTED FOR THE RECORD

Committee On Finance

Max Baucus, Ranking Member

Opening Statement of U.S. Senator Max Baucus (D-Mont.)
Breaking the Methamphetamine Supply Chain: Law Enforcement Challenges

Thank you, Mr. Chairman, for calling this hearing.

Meth is a personal fight for me. I've seen firsthand how it can ruin lives. I've seen what it does to young people. I've gone to high schools in Montana and talked with kids about meth.

More than four out of ten Montana teens report that meth is easy to get. That's second only to marijuana.

And Montana police officers tell me that meth is their number one law enforcement problem.

The National Association of Counties found that methamphetamine is the number one illegal drug problem for nearly half of the counties in the United States. Nationwide, nearly four in ten local law enforcement agencies have identified meth as the drug that poses the greatest threat to their area.

In April, the Finance Committee held a hearing on the effects of meth on the child welfare system and how it is hurting kids and parents alike.

And in July, the Senate passed the Improving Outcomes for Children Affected by Meth Act of 2006, which includes provisions to enhance the safety of children affected by meth abuse and addiction.

We reauthorized the Promoting Safe and Stable Families Program, which is the largest source of child welfare funding dedicated to services for children and families, and targets an available $40 million dollar increase in mandatory funding for meth-related services that include family treatment.

We are working to help protect children and families from the dangers of meth abuse. Today, we will focus on a new angle: how to break the meth supply chain through law enforcement.

We're working on the problem. We now have improved law enforcement techniques and measures to monitor the chemicals that are used to make meth. The Combat Meth Act of 2005, which I am proud to have co-sponsored, was a major step forward in preventing diversion of medicines containing pseudoephedrine, an ingredient found in many over-the-counter common cold and allergy medicines, into meth.

The Combat Meth Act requires that medicines containing pseudoephedrine be relocated behind the counter on or after September 30, 2006, and establishes a pharmacy logbook registry for purchasers of these cold products. Putting the meth precursor chemicals "behind the counter" is meant to disrupt supply.

In Montana, we placed these medicines behind the counter by passing a similar law in July 2005. The Yellowstone County Task Force told me that this is a step in the right direction. Because now it is very difficult for the small, 'mom and pop' meth producers to obtain the chemicals that can be used to produce meth.

And as a result, meth production in Montana and elsewhere — by both small and large-scale laboratories — appears to be decreasing.

Even though meth production for both small and large-scale laboratories is decreasing in the United States, production of meth in Mexico, largely in "superlabs" controlled by drug trafficking organizations, has picked up.

The biggest "link" in the meth supply chain is at the southwest border. It is now estimated that 80 percent of meth consumed in the United States originates in Mexico and is smuggled into the country.

What Benjamin Franklin once said is true of meth as well: "An ounce of prevention is worth a pound of cure." In order to make our prevention efforts more effective, we need to know where to put our resources to break the meth supply chain.

Today we will hear from Lt. Dan Springer, Commander of the Missouri River Drug Task Force, headquartered in Bozeman, Montana.

I am proud of the work that the Task Force is doing. The investigations in Bozeman are critical to stem the tide of national and international drug organizations that are preying on Montanans.

And the Missouri River Task Force and other task forces around the country need the dollars to fight meth — to locate and clean up meth labs and put criminals making and dealing meth behind bars where they belong.

I am eager to hear from Lt. Springer about the changing meth "hot spots" and the challenges that law enforcement officers now face as a result of the shift in meth production.

Carl Venne, the Crow Tribal Chairman and an Advisory Council Member of the Montana Meth Project, will also be testifying here today. Meth abuse is particularly devastating on the reservations, which are experiencing an increase in drug trafficking. I look forward to hearing Chairman Venne's perspective on Tribal efforts and strategies to combat meth, as well as meth law enforcement resources for reservations.

Education, prevention and treatment are vital in the fight against this growing threat to the welfare of our kids. Our law enforcement officers are stepping up to meet this challenge. And I am working to help them in their efforts.

I look forward to the testimony of our witnesses. We must do everything that we can to support our law enforcement officers. We must break the meth supply chain. We must do so the health and safety of Montanans and all Americans. And we must do so for our children.

U.S. SENATE COMMITTEE ON

Finance

SENATOR CHUCK GRASSLEY, OF IOWA - CHAIRMAN

http://finance.senate.gov

Statement of Chairman Grassley
Senate Finance Committee Hearing: "Breaking the Methamphetamine Supply Chain: Law Enforcement Challenges," Tuesday, September 12, 2006

I want to thank you for joining us today. I especially want to thank our panelists from Iowa and Montana for making the trip to Washington to share with us their insights on the growing epidemic of meth use across our country. It's no longer a secret that methamphetamine abuse and the disastrous effects of its manufacture have reached crisis levels in many areas of our country. The National Association of Counties released a survey in July that found that "county law enforcement officials across 44 states reported that methamphetamine remains the number one drug problem in their county," with forty-eight percent of their counties reporting that meth is the primary drug problem. This was more than the number that reported cocaine, marijuana and heroine combined. Whereas meth production and use may once have been geographically limited, this survey, as well as other reports, indicate that it appears to be moving steadily into most of the country.

I am encouraged by Congress' recognition of the need to control this crisis. Earlier this year, Congress passed the *Combat Meth Act*, which limits sales of meth precursor drugs like pseudoephedrine, and mandates that a log be kept of each sale. A number of states have already enacted similar restrictions on the availability of meth precursor drugs, and this appears to have had a major impact on the number of small toxic labs in those states as indicated by the great decrease in the number of local lab seizures in most of those states. It is reasonable to expect a comparable reduction in the number of small toxic labs in all states when the federal requirements become effective September 30th this year.

The challenges before us are still substantial. One of the results of the decrease in the small toxic meth labs in those states that have restricted access to the precursor products is an increase in the importation of meth by large, sophisticated drug cartels based primarily in Mexico. These smuggling organizations import a purer version of meth, employ difficult to uncover and track smuggling techniques, and are now operating in most parts of the country.

They are also engaged in repatriating large amounts of money to their home bases, laundering it through a variety of methods and often through legitimate business channels. The Drug Enforcement Administration estimates the illegal money laundering drug trade to be almost 50 billion dollars a year. It is also believed that a large portion of that money is smuggled out of our country in bulk across our borders.

Under these new circumstances, it is clear that a priority has to be placed on cooperation between the numerous federal agencies that are engaged in combating the meth traffic and the state and local law enforcement agencies that are on the ground in our local communities.

Our hearing today will hear testimony from state and local officials deeply engaged in the effort to close down meth traffickers and from federal officials equally deeply engaged in the effort at the federal level. We not only want to hear about their efforts at their respective levels and what we in the Congress might do to help them, but also about their cooperation and what we can do to help that cooperation become more effective.

WRITTEN TESTIMONY OF
C. ANDRE' MARTIN
DIRECTOR OF OPERATIONS, POLICY AND SUPPORT
CRIMINAL INVESTIGATION
INTERNAL REVENUE SERVICE
BEFORE THE
SENATE FINANCE COMMITTEE
ON
BREAKING THE METHAMPHETAMINE SUPPLY CHAIN: LAW ENFORCEMENT CHALLENGES
SEPTEMBER 12, 2006

Chairman Grassley, Ranking Member Baucus, and Members of the Committee, I appreciate the opportunity to discuss the Internal Revenue Service's Criminal Investigation Division's (CI) role in combating money laundering and narcotics trafficking. These are serious national problems that erode our economy and destroy thousands of lives each year.

CI Mission

The fundamental mission of the Criminal Investigation Division, or CI, is to serve the American public by detecting and investigating criminal violations of the Internal Revenue Code and related financial crimes. Nearly 2,800 of our 4,330 workforce in CI are federal criminal investigators who have accounting or business backgrounds. Through a process of rigorous training and years of experience, we shape our agents into law enforcement professionals adept at investigating the most sophisticated financial crimes whether they involve tax evasion, corporate fraud or narcotics trafficking. Our highly skilled special agents follow the money in tax and related investigations that involve sophisticated schemes and complex transactions that span the globe.

Many of the "badges of fraud" our agents pursue in tax investigations are identical to those in money laundering investigations. These include the extensive use of nominees, currency, multiple bank accounts, layering of financial transactions through multiple entities, and the movement of funds offshore. Therefore, the same financial investigative skills required to conduct complex tax cases can be readily adapted to money laundering investigations. This is especially true in intricate financial investigations involving the movement of funds associated with organized criminal enterprises. CI's statutory authority for money laundering, coupled with the financial expertise of its special agents, has made it possible to disrupt and dismantle criminal organizations employing complex financial transactions to launder illegal proceeds.

These unique skills place our special agents in high demand throughout the law enforcement community. The Attorney General recently communicated to IRS Commissioner Everson, "The agents of the Internal Revenue Service-Criminal Investigation (IRS-CI) are among the most important resources we can bring to bear in connection with the complex financial investigations that are critical to our success."

Strategic Priorities

The IRS Criminal Investigation strategic plan is comprised of three interdependent programs: Legal Source Tax Crimes; Illegal Source Financial Crimes; and Narcotics Related Financial Crimes. Within these three programs, our special agents utilize all statutes within IRS-CI's jurisdiction, the grand jury process, multi-agency task forces and various enforcement techniques to combat tax, money laundering and currency crime violations.

Managing the Strategic Priority Balance

Tax Administration

The tax administration system in our country depends on voluntary compliance. Our core mission at the IRS *is* tax administration. This fact was reinforced by Judge William Webster who was commissioned by the IRS in response to concerns raised by this committee in 1998 to direct an independent review of IRS-CI and assess our effectiveness in accomplishing our mission as the Service's criminal enforcement arm. Judge Webster concluded that IRS-CI suffered from a "mission drift" away from investigating core mission focused tax cases. Judge Webster specifically attributed "demands placed on CI by other law enforcement entities to participate in narcotics investigations" as a primary cause of the drift away from the investigation of criminal violations of the Internal Revenue Code. Thus, CI's *primary* focus is criminal investigations involving legal source tax crimes and those financial crimes that have a direct nexus to tax enforcement.

More importantly, IRS-CI must investigate violations arising out of the Internal Revenue Code (or Title 26 of the USC) because no other federal law enforcement agency has the authority or responsibility to do so. Without a criminal investigation component, voluntary compliance would be seriously compromised. At the same time that IRS CI has sharpened its focus on tax investigations, we have carefully monitored our narcotics work to ensure we are focusing our scarce resources on those narcotics cases that bring the most value to the government's counterdrug efforts. With the tax gap estimated at over $300 billion, CI's focus on tax investigations must remain our top priority.

IRS-CI's Role in the Law Enforcement Community

As part of the larger law enforcement community, we recognize that IRS-CI's role is broader than tax administration. We contribute our financial investigative expertise to many areas including money laundering, counterterrorism and public corruption. When traditional law enforcement investigative tools cannot solve a crime, IRS-CI can often make the connection between the crime and the criminal through a financial investigation. Tracing the money is often the key to a conviction. The broader financial linkage of multiple participants in criminal activity is also effective in dismantling criminal enterprises. IRS-CI works with other Federal, state and local law enforcement agencies because the unique skills we bring to the collaborative investigative effort cannot be easily duplicated.

State and Local Law Enforcement Support

IRS-CI supports cooperative efforts with Federal, state and local law enforcement agencies through task force participation under the auspices of each United States Attorney Office across the country. In particular, IRS-CI has consistently provided resource support to the following Federal, state and local joint initiatives, including but not limited to:

- High Intensity Drug Trafficking Areas (HIDTA)
- High Intensity Financial Crime Areas (HICFA)
- The OCDETF Fusion Center (OFC)
- DEA Special Operations Division (SOD)
- Suspicious Activity Report (SAR) Review Teams
- Bulk Currency Project
- Joint Terrorism Task Forces (JTTF)
- USAO Anti-Terrorism Advisory Councils (ATACs)
- El Paso Intelligence Center (EPIC)
- Interpol

IRS-CI Narcotics Program

IRS-CI's narcotics enforcement program works under the principal that drug trafficking organizations are motivated by greed, money, and assets – as are the financial and other professionals who assist drug traffickers and their organizations. Our ability to remove profits and identify all conspirators is often accomplished through in-depth financial investigations. In this respect, IRS-CI agents are important and logical additions to any investigative team when following the money helps piece together an intricate puzzle. This has proven true since our very first IRS narcotics investigation in 1920 when an opium grower failed to report the income earned from his product.

The objective of the IRS-CI narcotics-related financial investigation program is to leverage its financial investigative expertise to disrupt and ultimately dismantle the highest level drug trafficking and drug money laundering organizations that pose the greatest threat to Americans and American interests. We accomplish this in two ways. First, we foster compliance and confidence in the tax system through the investigation of unreported and "untaxed" proceeds (legal or illegal). Second, IRS-CI special agents trace the path of illicit drug proceeds and help prosecute drug and money laundering organizations by identifying the financial linkages among their members, associates, and all other co-conspirators. In fact, IRS-CI views money laundering violations as "tax evasion in progress" because the offenders are essentially trying to hide their dirty money from the government.

Historically, money launderers used legitimate businesses to "launder" their illegal proceeds. Now money launderers use more sophisticated schemes, computer technology, and international borders to conceal their income and/or assets. The leaders and lieutenants of criminal drug organizations go to great lengths to conceal their illicit income and its sources.

Department of Justice

IRS-CI focuses its narcotics program investigative resources on the highest level investigations as designated by the Department of Justice through the Organized Crime Drug Enforcement Task Force (OCDETF) Program. An indication of this type of quality investigation focus can be seen in the continually high prosecution recommendation acceptance rate by the Department of Justice -- which has been 100% for the last three years. Examples of methamphetamine investigations meeting this OCDETF significant case standard and to which IRS-CI has committed investigative resources include Operation Northern Star; Operation Brain Drain; Operation Snow Globe; and Operation Ice Storm.

Our narcotics enforcement strategy does not focus on specific types of illegal drugs; rather, our targeting efforts conform to the qualitative framework established by the Department of Justice. In this respect, the OCDETF program places emphasis on conducting financial investigations as an integral part of each investigation to eliminate the infrastructure of drug organizations and to permanently remove the profits enjoyed by drug traffickers. As a result, all OCDETF-approved investigations must include a financial investigation, beyond merely the seizure of cars or other personal property of the main defendants.

Conclusion

In conclusion, regardless of the type of drug threat, whether it is methamphetamine, cocaine, heroin, or marijuana, IRS-CI will continue to support the Department of Justice through its OCDETF program in strategically targeting and dismantling the most significant drug trafficking organizations. The women and men of IRS-CI—the most skilled financial investigators in federal law enforcement—carry on an 87-year tradition of solving financial crimes by following the money trail. We also carry a proud tradition of working in a spirit of cooperation with our law enforcement partners in the Department of Treasury, Department of Justice, Department of Homeland Security and the state and local law enforcement community.

Mr. Chairman, I thank you for this opportunity to appear before this distinguished committee and I will be happy to answer any questions you and the other committee members may have.

Questions for the Record From C. André Martin
Senate Finance Committee Hearing
Breaking the Methamphetamine Supply Chain
September 12, 2006

Senator Grassley

Q1. Do you find that you receive the cooperation that you need from foreign banks and nations in battling money laundering?

A1. International issues always add complexity to the investigative process. Our experience shows that criminal organizations are all too eager to exploit the soft spots in the international financial community. However, foreign banks, like U.S. banks, are governed by their country's financial regulations and statutes limiting the sharing of customer data. Therefore, their cooperation is in many instances dependent upon the U.S. requesting information pursuant to a Mutual Legal Assistance Treaty or through other formal channels. Overall, the level of cooperation from foreign countries for our investigations increased significantly over the past five years. This increase was the consequence of several initiatives, including:

- Internal Revenue Service Criminal Investigation (IRS-CI) works closely with other law enforcement agencies, the Department of State, and Treasury Department's Office of Foreign Asset Control (OFAC) and Financial Crimes Enforcement Network (FinCEN) to leverage all of our collective tools and skills most effectively.
- IRS-CI posted eight attachés in overseas locations to support our international investigations by enhancing cooperation with foreign countries. We also similarly have representatives assigned to FinCEN, OFAC and Interpol.
- IRS-CI is a permanent member of the U.S. delegation to the Financial Action Task Force Against Money Laundering (FATF) and several of its regional-style bodies such as its Caribbean equivalent (CFATF). The FATF, with assistance from the United States delegation revised and updated its 40 recommendations that set the standards for best practices to be adopted by countries to combat money laundering. In addition, FATF led a concerted international effort to increase international cooperation in combating money laundering and terrorism financing.
- IRS-CI participated in the assessments of numerous Middle Eastern, South American, and European countries' anti-money laundering laws, policies, and procedures.
- IRS-CI participated in anti-terrorism and anti-money laundering training with the FBI in countries such as Saudi Arabia, Thailand, Egypt, Pakistan, United Arab Emirates, Oman, Qatar, Bahrain, and others. This work helped these countries be in a better position to respond to our requests for cooperation.

Additionally, IRS-CI was a contributor to the "2006 International Narcotics Control Strategy Report (2006 INCSR)" released by the U.S. State Department's Bureau for International Narcotics and Law Enforcement Affairs in March 2006. Volume II of this report contains a section titled "Major Money Laundering Countries" which provides an excellent overview of the various issues with the major money laundering countries.

However, the level of cooperation still has room for growth. To achieve this goal, IRS-CI supports FATF's new initiative to form a working group to address international cooperation issues. The U.S. is one of the co-chairs of this new working group.

Q2. Is there anything that Congress should do to enhance our abilities to track this money and seize the assts of criminal enterprises?

A2. IRS-CI is currently working to identify optimal means and measures to effectively investigate both the domestic and international money laundering aspects of criminal enterprises. IRS-CI appreciates Congress's desire to help law enforcement attack money laundering in all its forms. We intend to work closely with our Legal Counsel, Department of Treasury and law enforcement partners to identify areas where changes to the law would assist will assist our collective efforts.

Q3. Congress passed the Combat Meth Act as part of the reauthorization of the USA Patriot Act this year. Part of this legislation was written to help state and local law enforcement deal with the large number of "mom and pop" meth labs. What more can Congress do to help law enforcement put an end to this scourge? Are there other laws that need to assist you in your efforts?

A3. A few short years ago, there was a major epidemic of illegal meth laboratories in the United States. These labs not only produced hazardous drugs, they created significant hazardous waste, seriously endangering the health of the public and particularly law enforcement officers, and heavily taxed the already limited resources of law enforcement. The Combat Meth Act helped law enforcement make significant progress in reducing meth use and shutting down meth labs inside the United States.

As we testified at the hearings, methamphetamine is only one part of our overall enforcement responsibilities, and it competes with many of our other priorities, of which the major portion do not pertain to narcotics crimes. As far as additional legislation targeted specifically at methamphetamine, we have to respectfully defer to our law enforcement colleagues at DEA who have primary jurisdiction for narcotics violations.

Senator Baucus

Q1. We understand that money launders are using more sophisticated computer programs and cross-border transactions to hide their drug profits. Please describe some of the recent schemes IRS uncovered.

A1. As identified in the 2005 National Money Laundering Threat Assessment to which IRS-CI was a contributor, bulk cash smuggling is currently believed to be the most pervasive money laundering method used by drug traffickers to move their illicit proceeds across the U.S. border. Drug Trafficking Organizations (DTOs) frequently use the same couriers, vehicles, routes and methods to smuggle narcotics to the U.S. and return the resulting proceeds to Mexico, often in concealed compartments, or "traps" in vehicles. The DEA, Bureau of Immigration and Customs Enforcement (ICE) and IRS-CI have each instituted bulk currency initiatives stressing the importance of immediate notification to federal law enforcement for contemporaneous exploitation of leads. These initiatives stress the exploitation of information collected from courier debriefings and seized evidentiary documents for analysis and linkage to ongoing investigations and/or to initiate new investigations.

In support of law enforcement, FinCEN issued an advisory to U.S. financial institutions warning of the prevalence of bulk cash smuggling by DTOs (FinCEN Advisory 2006-A003). FinCEN, in conjunction with Treasury and other law enforcement agencies, identified several activities indicative of bulk cash smuggling in this advisory. These include:

- An increase in the sale of large denomination U.S. bank notes to Mexican institutions by U.S. banks;
- Small denomination U.S. bank notes smuggled into Mexico being exchanged for large denomination U.S. bank notes possessed by Mexican financial institutions;
- Large volumes of small denomination U.S. bank notes being sent from Mexican casas de cambio to their accounts in the U.S. via armored transport, or sold directly to U.S. banks;
- Multiple wire transfers initiated by casas de cambio that direct U.S. financial institutions to remit funds to jurisdictions outside of Mexico that bear no apparent business relationship with that casa de cambio (recipients include individuals, businesses, and other entities in free trade zones and other locations associated with Black Market Peso Exchange-type activities);[1]
- The exchange of small denomination U.S. bank notes for large denomination U.S. bank notes that may be sent to jurisdictions outside of Mexico, including jurisdictions associated with Black Market Peso Exchange-type activities;
- Deposits by casas de cambio to their accounts at U.S. financial institutions that include third-party items (including sequentially numbered monetary instruments); and
- Deposits of currency and third-party items by Mexican casas de cambio to their accounts at Mexican financial institutions and thereafter direct wire transfers to the casas accounts at U.S. financial institutions.

IRS-CI and other federal law enforcement agencies documented that Money Service Businesses (MSBs) are also exploited by drug traffickers for money laundering. A key finding of the 2005 National Drug Threat Assessment was that drug traffickers frequently use MSBs--particularly money transmittal, currency exchanges (casas de cambios), and check-cashing businesses--to launder drug proceeds. The BSA and PATRIOT Act, combined with the cooperation of banks and banking regulators, have made it more difficult for money launderers to pass large amounts of cash through the formal banking system thereby making other parts of the financial system attractive to them to accomplish their nefarious purposes.

Q2. The USA Patriot Act amended the Bank Secrecy Act and broadened the anti-money laundering system to more segments of the financial community. In IRS's experience, are money launders starting to use smaller banks or institutions, now that the Bank Secrecy Act tightened up the reporting rules?

A2. IRS-CI does not track financial institutions by size within its case management system. Since enactment of the USA PATRIOT Act, there has been a substantial increase in Suspicious Activity Report (SAR) filings by MSBs. Suspicious Activity Reports filed by MSBs for the fiscal years 2003, 2004 and 2005 were 122,018, 301,372 and 368,049, respectively. Though final numbers have not been received yet, SARs filed by MSBs in FY 2006 are expected to exceed 450,000. This substantial increase might be indicative of escalating money laundering activity at smaller financial institutions such as MSBs. It might however also be indicative of increased awareness by the MSB industry of their BSA obligations, more effective outreach to MSBs by law enforcement and regulators, or enhanced suspicious transactions detections systems and training on the part of the MSB industry.

Testimony of Sean McCullough

Special Agent in Charge,
Iowa Division of Narcotics Enforcement
Department of Public Safety

before the

Senate Finance Committee

Breaking the Methamphetamine Supply Chain

September 12, 2006
10:00 a.m.
215 Dirksen Building

BREAKING THE METHAMPHETAMINE SUPPLY CHAIN: LAW ENFORCEMENT CHALLENGES

My name is Sean McCullough and I am a Special Agent in Charge with the Iowa Division of Narcotics Enforcement (DNE). I have served the state of Iowa since 1989.

Since the early 1990's Iowa has been plagued by methamphetamine. Methamphetamine could be found in Iowa before the 1990's, but not in epidemic quantities. The majority of methamphetamine, found in Iowa during the early 1990's, was imported from Mexico and the southwest region of the United States. Those involved in the methamphetamine underworld soon found methods to manufacture this drug on their own to avoid dealing with the dangerous organized groups that were involved in the importation of methamphetamine into Iowa. Law enforcement was then faced with the daunting task of uncovering, seizing, and cleaning up these clandestine methamphetamine laboratories. Processing methamphetamine laboratories is very time consuming and expensive. Iowa law enforcement was combating the methamphetamine problem on two fronts: methamphetamine that was manufactured in clandestine laboratories, and imported methamphetamine.

In 1993 the DNE seized two clandestine methamphetamine laboratories. Each year following methamphetamine laboratories grew to epidemic proportions. By 2004 Iowa law enforcement officials seized 1,500 clandestine methamphetamine laboratories (ANNEX A). In 2004, according to the Drug Enforcement Administration, Iowa recorded the third highest number of methamphetamine laboratories as compared to any state in the United States. Approximately 97% of these methamphetamine laboratories seized produced only gram to one or two ounce quantities of methamphetamine. The DNE, and other Iowa law enforcement agencies, were spending approximately 80% of their resources on 20% of the problem.

Reducing the number of methamphetamine laboratories, which produce approximately 10-15% of Iowa's total methamphetamine, would allow DNE and other Iowa agencies to concentrate enforcement efforts on the mid to upper level drug trafficking organizations that are responsible for importing about 85-90% of methamphetamine into Iowa.

In May of 2005, Iowa passed one of the nations strongest non-prescription pseudoephedrine laws (ODCP). This law restricted the sale of pseudoephedrine, which is the main ingredient in the illegal manufacture of methamphetamine. The law had an immediate and significant impact on methamphetamine manufacturing in Iowa. Law enforcement's purpose behind the law was to reduce the number of methamphetamine labs, which were taking most of their resources, to allow agencies to dedicate their efforts toward reducing the amount of imported methamphetamine. Since the law was enacted, methamphetamine laboratories have declined 72% (ODCP) (ANNEX B).

In 2004 the University of Iowa Hospitals and Clinics spent approximately $2,798,726 to treat patients with methamphetamine related injuries (Van Haaften). In 2005, after the passage of Iowa's pseudoephedrine law, the University of Iowa Hospitals and Clinics spent approximately $262,329 on methamphetamine laboratory related injuries. These figures equal a savings of $2,536,397 (Van Haaften).

Iowa's pseudoephedrine law has also caused a reduction in total methamphetamine laboratory enforcement costs, which involve the cost of personnel, approximately $2,590,482 (Van Haaften). In 2005, costs dropped to $1,506,263 (Van Haaften). These figures equal a savings of $1,084,219.

Even though Iowa's clandestine methamphetamine seizures have declined, Mexican drug trafficking organizations continue to dominate the state's illicit drug trade. These Mexican drug trafficking organizations are highly sophisticated and organized. This follows the information from the National Drug Information Center's National Drug Threat Assessment 2006, which states: "Mexican drug trafficking organizations and criminal groups are the most influential drug traffickers in the United States, and their influence is increasing. They are the predominant smugglers, transporters, and wholesale distributors of cocaine, marijuana, methamphetamine, and Mexico produced heroin in the United States; they are expanding their control over the distribution of these drugs in areas long controlled by Colombian and Dominican groups, including areas of New York and Florida" (p.1). It's even more imperative that law enforcement agencies work collaboratively to be effective against these sophisticated groups.

Along with increased seizures of methamphetamine, the drug purity rate in Iowa is also increasing. This purer form of methamphetamine is termed crystal methamphetamine or "ice" (ODCP). The average purity was 27% in 2001, 33% in 2004, and 54% in 2005 (ODCP).

Iowa law enforcement continues to work proactively against those individuals and groups involved in methamphetamine, by passing the pseudoephedrine law and now concentrating efforts against the organized groups importing the drug. The working relationships in Iowa remain united among the federal, state, and local law enforcement is important for Iowa to reach out to other areas of the country that are confronted by methamphetamine as the drug crosses borders. To effectively combat methamphetamine, it's important to maintain these collaborative relationships.

Thank you for allowing me to address the Finance Committee about Iowa's response to the continuing methamphetamine problem. I am optimistic that we can find answers through continued dialogue about the challenges associated with

Works Cited

Governor's Office of Drug Control Policy. *Iowa METH Facts.* July 31, 2006.

National Drug Information Center. *National Drug Threat Assessment 2006.* United States Department of Justice. < http://www.usdoj.gov/ndic/pubs11/18862/strateg.htm#Top>.

Van Haaften, Marvin L. Director. Iowa Governor's Office of Drug Control Policy. *The Impact of Senate File 169on Meth Abuse in Iowa.* A report to the Legislature. January 17, 2006.

ANNEX A
LAB COUNT

2006 – 106 (DNE)
2006 – 146 (Locals)
Total for 2006 – 252 (as of 8/31/06)

2005 – 348 (DNE)
2005 – 420 (Locals)
Total for 2005 – 768

2004 – 644 (DNE)
2004 – 856 (Locals)
Total for 2004 – 1500

2003 – 671 (DNE)
2003 – 484 (Locals)
Total for 2003 - 1,155

2002 – 709 (DNE)
2002 – 300 (Locals)
Total for 2002 - 1009

2001 – 511 (DNE)
2001 – 253 (locals)
Total for 2001 - 764

2000 – 393 (DNE)
2000 - 267 (locals)
Total for 2000 – 660

1999 – 502

1998 – 321

1997 – 63

1996 – 31

1995 – 8

1994 – 4

1993 – 2

ANNEX B

Tracking Iowa Meth Lab Incidents

252

Reported to DNE as of 08-31-06

Total Labs for 2005-746

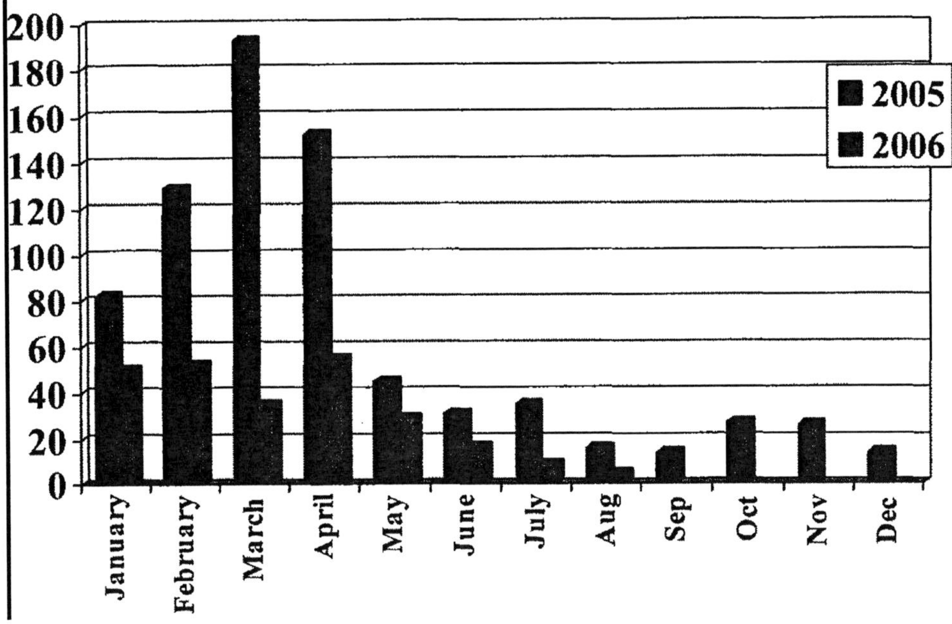

Thomas J. Vilsack
Governor
Sally J. Pederson
Lt. Governor

Kevin W. Techau
Commissioner

October 5, 2006

Charles E. Grassley
Chairman
Committee on Finance
Washington, DC 20510-6200

Dear Senator Grassley:

The following are my written responses to your follow-up questions concerning my testimony to the Senate Committee on Finance:

(1) You mentioned in your statement that your office has become more proactive and that the DEA has become more reactive due to increasing case load. Has the increased DEA case load affected their involvement in cases that your office is pursuing? If so, what has that effect been?

(A) The Iowa Division of Narcotics Enforcement (DNE) maintains a good working relationship with the Drug Enforcement Administration (DEA). DEA has a limited number of agents in Iowa. For example, when DNE is working an operation that requires personnel, oftentimes DEA can only send one or two people to assist. Additional DEA agents in Iowa would greatly help our efforts.

(2) In your statement, you said "it's even more imperative that law enforcement agencies work collaboratively to be effective against these sophisticated (drug smuggling) groups". On that point, how could your collaborative effort better address the smuggling problem?

(A) DNE has initiated a collaborative effort to address smuggling into and across Iowa with the Iowa State Patrol. DNE has 3 agents designated to assist the State Patrol after an interdiction stop has been made. These agents then work to gather investigative leads to the source of the drugs, as well as their destination. These agents are also responsible to provide proactive interdiction projects. Even though DNE has 3 dedicated interdiction agents, all agents participate in these types of investigations as well.

(3) Iowa was a state that took early action in moving the products that local meth makers use behind the counter, and this had the result of restricting these meth producers' access to those products. I am glad to hear that that law had its intended effect in reducing the number of small toxic labs in Iowa. Has the lower number of labs allowed you to reallocate resources? If so, how?

(A) The reduction in methamphetamine laboratories has allowed us to reallocate our resources, primarily personnel hours, toward individuals and groups trafficking methamphetamine in Iowa. Most of these investigations involve DNE agents working undercover to purchase drugs, conducting search warrants, surveillance, interviews, etc.

(4) You estimated the savings from the reduced number of meth lab clean-ups at more than one million dollars.

a. Do those savings accrue totally to your Agency?
b. Have those savings been reinvested in other Iowa law enforcement activities directed at combating the meth smuggling organizations that are bringing meth into Iowa?

(A) The savings from the reduction in methamphetamine laboratories are not attributed totally to DNE. Most of the money for laboratory clean-up came from federal funds. With the reduction of methamphetamine laboratories, federal funds from HIDTA and BYRNE have been reprogrammed to fund DNE's efforts against smuggling organizations. With DNE over 40 percent federally funded, HIDTA and BYRNE are critical in providing DNE the necessary funds to be effective in meeting our mission.

I appreciate your continued support in addressing the methamphetamine problem. Through continued dialogue and education, maybe we can find solutions. Please contact me if I can provide further assistance.

Sincerely,

Sean McCullough
Special Agent in Charge

Gregory Passic
Director, Office of Drug Interdiction
Customs and Border Protection
Department of Homeland Security

Regarding

"Breaking the Methamphetamine Supply Chain: Law Enforcement Challenges"

Before The

Senate Committee on Finance

September 12, 2006
Dirksen Senate Office Building
Washington D.C.

INTRODUCTION

Chairman Grassley, Ranking Member Baucus, and distinguished members of the Senate Committee on Finance, on behalf of Customs and Border Protection (CBP), I appreciate your invitation to testify today regarding the challenges that CBP and our law enforcement partners face in breaking the methamphetamine supply chain. The challenges are significant and those agencies confronting this threat must go beyond traditional cooperation if we are to be successful. Much of the methamphetamine used in the United States is manufactured in Mexico and smuggled across the border. Although Mexico has made significant regulatory changes in the past several months to reduce the amount of precursor chemicals that are diverted into illegal channels, more must be done to reduce precursor availability. Through seamless teaming among U.S. and Mexican Law Enforcement, along with several other international partners, it should be possible to disrupt the flow of precursors and thereby reduce the availability of methamphetamine. Disrupting the flow of drug cash smuggled to trafficking organizations will require new and creative ways of identifying transport vehicles and unprecedented intelligence sharing with CBP's front line. Intelligence-based interdictions will have to increase significantly to impact organizations smuggling drugs into U.S. Markets. By increasing our ratio of "Smart Interdiction," based on foreign and domestic investigative leads, we can provide valuable evidence for later criminal proceedings. Only by disrupting those key individuals who control illegal methamphetamine manufacturing, their suppliers of precursor chemicals, and the money that provides nourishment to their organizations, can we impact the availability of meth on our streets.

CBP's Interdiction efforts

Present seizure data and other Law Enforcement reporting indicates that the substantial majority of meth seized in the United States originates in Mexico. Small-scale domestic meth production has been replaced by "Super Labs" operated by criminal organizations often based in Mexico or with ties to Mexico, capable of producing more than 10 pounds of methamphetamine within a single production cycle. Major trafficking organizations have well established transportation routes and exercise significant control in many of the major drug markets in our major cities. Success means getting into the middle of an already well-established criminal network that is directed remotely from Mexico. Intelligence derived by our investigative partners on these organizations will drive better targeting of smugglers, their conveyances, and concealment methods.

Almost 90% of the drugs entering into our country cross through the Southwest Border. The Mexican Border remains a significant challenge for CBP. However, there are various initiatives underway to gain operational control of that vulnerability. Those initiatives include:

Ports of Entry:

- Continued improvement of non-intrusive inspection technologies

- Use of new technology that highlights less dense objects, such as drugs and currency

- Increase the use of canines along the border. Approximately 60% of all drug seizures at Ports of Entry result from Canine detection. For narcotics canines, training includes detection of methamphetamines

- Better radio connectivity among federal, state, local, and tribal agencies

- Closer teaming with the investigative agencies to identify and disrupt "spotters" deployed by traffickers on both the Mexican and U.S.-side of the border

- Improve the use, analysis, and dissemination of advanced information to identify drug smugglers, conveyances, and traps. Almost all of our present seizures result from "cold hits" (those instances in which drugs are seized in the absence of significant targeting). This includes responding to leads provided by ICE, DEA, and Mexican Law Enforcement.

- Continue working closely with DEA to identify shipments of precursors destined for clandestine labs in Mexico. This will include the teaming of CBP's predictive analysis unit with DEA's methamphetamine intelligence group. Also joint CBP/ICE/DEA field teams will be working together to identify suspect precursor shipments.

Between the Ports of Entry:

Efforts to secure the border through DHS's Secure Border Initiative (SBI) will have a positive impact on the effectiveness of our counter-drug efforts.

- Increase interdiction operations by adding Border Patrol Agents. The President has recommended the addition of between 6,000 and 8,000 Agents over the next three years.
- Develop and Deploy better Sensory and Surveillance capabilities under SBI.
- Enhance federal partnerships to include a closer working relationship with DEA, ICE, HIDTA's and established drug intelligence centers.
- Work with EPIC, DEA, and ICE to identify Mexican controllers or "Gatekeepers" that control smuggling "turf" along the Southwest Border.
- Co-locate DHS component agencies, such as CBP and ICE, and DEA resources in joint intel groups and existing inter-agency drug task forces to conduct post seizures analysis and ensure that leads flowing from those seizures are fully exploited. Provide feedback to the Field that enables future interdiction actions that can be coupled with on-going criminal investigations. This process would provide information to DEA and their Mexican Counterparts who can take disruptive action on Mexican based drug principals, to include methamphetamine

Hopefully the close working relationship between CBP and DEA will enable them to more effectively engage foreign counterparts in key countries to stem the flow of meth precursors to Mexico and other aspiring meth lab centers. Thank you again for this opportunity to testify. I would now be happy to answer any questions that you may have.

Senate Finance Committee Hearing
Questions Submitted for the Record
Mr. Gregory Passic
Breaking the Methamphetamine Supply Chain: Law Enforcement Challenges
September 12, 2006

Senator Grassley

1) What types of procedures are in place to assist CBP manage and process leads from other agencies? Do these procedures differ when the information relates to illegal narcotics at ports of entry or between ports of entry? If so, could you please explain why? Finally, are these protocols formalized in any formal memoranda of understanding?

Leads from other agencies are generally handled in the field on a case-by-case basis. If the lead requires action by more than one CBP element, or if it is general in nature, CBP Headquarters will coordinate through the Office of Drug Interdiction.

At the Ports of Entry, the principal method for handling information from other agencies is through the Treasury Enforcement Communications System (TECS). ICE uses TECS to create reports that link subject records to those reports. The subject records are essentially lookouts. When the person or vehicle crosses the border, CBP Officers will see the record and conduct the appropriate examination. Information received from other agencies is also entered into TECS.

Between the Ports of Entry (POEs), several Intelligence and Law Enforcement systems are used to receive and process intelligence and lead information from other agencies. Classified information is passed through secure systems including JWICS, SIPRNET/HSDN or secure telephone. Actionable information is then passed to the field at the appropriate classification level to assist in an operational response. Sensitive but Unclassified (SBU) information is passed via TECS, the Intelligence Reporting System (IRS), government e-mail and telephone. Due to the different working environment between the POE's, it is often more effective to pass leads through briefings, verbal or written "be on the lookout" alerts (BOLOs) and by disseminating intelligence reports directly to the agents.

Intelligence components within the Department of Homeland Security (DHS) and CBP are currently working on a policy that formalizes reporting protocols to receive and disseminate intelligence information. Field level intelligence components are in the process of collocating intelligence assets in many border locations.

2) I expect that, as part of the continuing unification and coordination of agencies in the Department of Homeland Security to improve efficiency and effectiveness, there has been some discussion as to streamlining the referral process regarding the seizure of illegal narcotics, such as one set of protocols and procedures that

would allow CBP, OFO and OBP to follow the same rules. Could you please share what has been discussed regarding this issue? If nothing has been discussed could you explain why not?

Within CBP the Offices of Field Operations (OFO) and Border Patrol (OBP) are reviewing present processes to establish common protocols and procedures. Immigration and Customs Enforcement (ICE) is CBP's primary investigative partner; however, OBP refers narcotic seizures to the Drug Enforcement Administration (DEA) as part of an existing MOU. Improving efficiencies with these partners in the drug arena is an important CBP goal. CBP management and the DHS Office of Counternarcotis Enforcement are currently reviewing means to enhance team coordination among the three partner agencies. By increasing connectivity with our ICE partners we have greater impact on the Drug organizations responsible for the drugs we seize at the border. Also, by increasing the ratio of intelligence-linked seizures DEA and ICE gain valuable evidence in their conspiracy cases. In addition to our primary role of interdicting drugs CBP's ultimate goal is integrating into a system that impacts major Drug Trafficking Organizations (DTOs) responsible for drugs entering the United States.

Following the creation of CBP and ICE within DHS, CBP met with ICE to negotiate standardized referral and/or notification procedures across the different components within CBP. Both CBP and ICE agreed that because of the uniqueness of OBP and OFO, separate agreements would be the most efficient and effective method of handling referrals. The flexibility offered by the differences in protocols and procedures is needed as it allows for tailored responses that meet the needs of components working under very different operating conditions and legal authorities.

OBP uses a variety of statutory authorities in order to interdict drugs; namely Title 8, 19, 21 and 31. Titles 19 and 31 require the government to demonstrate a direct and meaningful connection or nexus to the border. This requirement is easily met at the ports of entry, as their area of responsibility is generally limited to the actual border or functional equivalents. However, OBP's working environment does not always provide for a border nexus. Agents work in remote and vast areas as well as in interior locations, such as checkpoints, where interdictions may or may not involve people or cargo that can be readily tied to the border. Therefore, OBP places a greater reliance on its authorities under Title 21, which are delegated from DEA and do not require a nexus to the border. Both OBP and ICE receive delegated Title 21 authority from DEA who is the lead investigative agency for drugs. In the interests of promoting the strong and already existing working relationship with DEA, the Border Patrol will continue to refer drug cases to DEA in accordance with the existing MOU between CBP and DEA. However, when cases are encountered that have ties to ICE investigations, OBP notifies ICE of the arrest and/or interdiction. ICE and CBP share intelligence documents and have access to each other's intelligence systems.

3) I understand that there may be Memoranda of Agreement or Memoranda of Understanding between CBP and other agencies that detail or set out the rules, policies and procedures for case and information referrals when illegal narcotics

are seized. Please list those agencies and other law enforcement agencies with which CBP has agreements or MOAs/MOUs.

CBP presently has Drug MOAs/MOUs with DEA, ICE and FDA.

a. Please provide copies of each agreement.

Copies are provided.

b. Are CBP or DHS considering revising or rewriting any of these agreements in whole or in part? If so, which and why?

CBP is not currently considering revisions to the MOUs, but does conduct periodic reviews. From time to time, MOUs are further defined through addendums that help to further strengthen established alliances, clarify roles and responsibilities and ensure mission success.

c. Please explain if there are any withdrawal provisions in these agreements which would permit one party or another to withdraw without cause.

All CBP agreements have withdrawal agreements for either party with 30 days notice.

4) Can you please explain, briefly, what CBP does when it encounters and seizes meth at the border?

There are no special protocols for handling methamphetamine seizures at or between the Ports of Entry.

a. Who is notified and why?

At the Ports of Entry, the ICE duty agent is immediately contacted after the drugs are discovered. The potential for a controlled delivery is considered after interview of the smuggler. The Assistant U.S. Attorney is contacted to determine if the amount seized and any aggravating factors meet the local threshold for Federal prosecution. If a determination is made that there will not be a controlled delivery or Federal prosecution, CBP will then contact local law enforcement.

Between the Ports of Entry, the seizure is referred to DEA with an offer of "right of first refusal "in accepting the case. If DEA accepts the case, all evidence and suspects are turned over to their custody per existing MOU. If DEA declines the case local protocols are followed to engage state or local authorities.

b. Do Memoranda of Understanding exist that explain protocols and avoid confusion and ensure safety?

Yes, the previously mentioned MOUs outline protocols for notification and referrals. If ICE is able to conduct a controlled delivery to an interior location, an existing protocol is used to notify DEA and provide DEA with an operational plan.

When ICE and/or DEA are operating near the Border, local notification thresholds and protocols are used that consider their unique operational environments.

5) The Treasury Enforcement Communications System contains a tremendous volume of raw data on border crossings by vehicles. The information captured in the system includes the license plate numbers of most vehicles which have crossed the border. Does CBP, DEA or any other federal agency systematically provide state and local law enforcement officials with this raw data information on the tag numbers of vehicles crossing our borders so that those state and local officers can identify for the federal agents those vehicles that are locally known to be registered to or used by meth users or traffickers so that border lookouts can be placed on those vehicles? If not, why?

CBP does not systematically provide state and local law enforcement with raw data from TECS. CBP encourages those officials to enter the suspect plates into CBP's border lookout system, so that they may be informed of border crossings. In a pilot project underway with DEA, CBP is checking border crossing activity of their suspect vehicles. If that pilot is successful, CBP anticipates working further with DEA and their state and local drug partners to provide crossing data of value to their efforts. We welcome getting all suspect vehicle information into our lookout system and sharing the results.

CBP also has a program with Texas DPS, which is very advanced in the use of data from all highway seizures made in their state. Seizures made at the Texas ports of entry are also shared, allowing both agencies a better understanding of vehicle concealments, violator characteristics and patterns of drug and money movement.

6) Congress passed the Combat Meth Act as part of the reauthorization of the USA PATRIOT Act this year. Part of this legislation was written to help state and local law enforcement deal with the large number of "mom and pop" meth labs. What more can Congress do to help law enforcement put an end to this scourge? Are there other laws that need to assist you in your efforts?

CBP appreciates Congress's offer to help us attack this problem. We intend to work closely with our Law Enforcement partners to identify areas where changes in law would assist our collective efforts.

Senator Baucus

1. We understand that pseudoephedrine production takes place legally in about ten countries. Please discuss Customs and Border Protection's capability to track meth precursor shipments?

CBP tracks legitimate shipments of ephedrine and pseudoephedrine through its commercial databases. For substances that are legitimately imported, DEA approval is needed for the importation. The DEA approval and notification is handled electronically. CBP ensures that the foreign shippers and US importers are authorized to conduct these transactions. CBP conducts examinations to ensure that quantities and descriptions are accurate.

2. Regarding efforts to identify shipments of meth precursors diverted or destined for clandestine labs in Mexico, please describe the teaming of Customs and Border Protection's Predictive Analysis Unit with the Drug Enforcement Administration's meth intelligence group.

CBP primarily coordinates with DEA through its Office of Field Operations, supported by the Office of Drug Interdiction. OFO then engages various CBP components to review and analyze data from cargo manifests. The Predictive Analysis Group is instrumental in assisting in that effort. Intelligence on suspect shipments primarily flows through the Trend Analysis Group and Automated Targeting System program managers. The Trend Analysis Group has the ability to handle very large amounts of data from within CBP and from other law enforcement agencies. They will add value to the information provided by DEA, return additional investigative targets and create lookouts for the ports of entry.

The Automated Targeting System program will take DEA intelligence on precursor movements through the maritime environment and attempt to identify those shipments that may be entering the U.S. or transiting U.S. ports destined to Mexico or South America. In most cases, the shipments will be illegally described as some other commodity.

Joseph T. Rannazzisi
Deputy Assistant Administrator
Office of Diversion Control
Drug Enforcement Administration
U.S. Department of Justice

Regarding

"Breaking the Methamphetamine Supply Chain: Law Enforcement Challenges"

Before The

Senate Committee on Finance

September 12, 2006
Dirksen Senate Office Building
Washington D.C.

INTRODUCTION

Chairman Grassley, Ranking Member Baucus, and distinguished members of the Senate Committee on Finance, on behalf of the Drug Enforcement Administration (DEA), I appreciate your invitation to testify today regarding the challenges that DEA and our law enforcement partners face in breaking the methamphetamine supply chain. Doing what we do best, DEA, through our law enforcement partnerships across the country and around the world, is actively engaged in attacking the criminal organizations responsible for the trafficking in methamphetamine, the precursors utilized in its production, and the financial infrastructure these organization have established to feed and support their illicit activity.

METHAMPHETAMINE: AN OVERVIEW

The Administration's *2006 Synthetic Drug Control Strategy - A Focus on Methamphetamine and Prescription Drug Abuse* is a companion document to the President's *National Drug Control Strategy*. The unique nature of the illicit market for synthetic drugs, such as methamphetamine, warrants a targeted response as the illicit markets for synthetic drugs contain unique challenges and vulnerabilities. The *Synthetic Drug Control Strategy* also adheres to the format of the President's *National Drug Control Strategy* by setting goals, specifically for reducing synthetic drug use primarily of methamphetamine by 15 percent over three years and reducing domestic methamphetamine laboratories by 25 percent over the same period. The President's *National Drug Control Strategy* and the *Synthetic Drug Control Strategy* have established a framework on which DEA will continue to perform its mission in support of those strategic goals.

Methamphetamine poses a significant threat to the United States. Methamphetamine is unique from other common drugs of abuse in that it is a synthetic drug and its precursor chemicals have historically been easy to obtain and inexpensive to purchase. These factors have contributed to methamphetamine's rapid sweep across our nation.

Methamphetamine's addictive characteristics produce devastating effects on all of its victims. These victims are not only limited to those who choose to use this poison, but others who become part of what could be considered methamphetamine's "collateral damage." Those who suffer the "second hand" effects of meth include the victims of methamphetamine-related crimes, innocent children whose homes have been turned into toxic clandestine lab sites, law enforcement officers who work with the hazardous materials found at lab sites, and the environment from the approximately five pounds of toxic waste produced for every pound of methamphetamine cooked. Methamphetamine has not only left a mark on the United States, but continues to be a significant problem in Asia and is increasingly becoming a problem in other parts of the world.

Methamphetamine consumed in the United States originates from two general sources, controlled by two distinct groups. Most of the methamphetamine consumed in the United States is produced by Mexico-based and California-based Mexican traffickers. These drug trafficking organizations control "super labs" (a laboratory capable of producing 10 pounds or more of methamphetamine within a single production cycle) and have distribution networks throughout the United States, as well as access to drug transportation routes to smuggle the methamphetamine from Mexico into the United States. Current drug lab and seizure data suggest that the majority of the methamphetamine used in the United States comes from these larger labs, which are increasingly found in Mexico.

Many of these drug trafficking organizations are of a poly-drug nature and distribute large quantities of methamphetamine to the domestic market. These same Mexican criminal organizations control most wholesale, mid-level, and retail methamphetamine distribution in the Pacific, Southwest, and West-Central regions of the United States, as well as much of the distribution in the Great Lakes and Southeast regions.

The second source for methamphetamine used in this country comes from small, toxic laboratories (STLs) located throughout the United States. These STLs produce relatively small amounts of methamphetamine, are generally not affiliated with major trafficking organizations, and are responsible for approximately 20 percent of the methamphetamine consumed in this country. Initially found only in most Western States, over the past 10 years there has been an eastward expansion of STLs, peaking with over 17,000 lab incidents reported in the United States in 2004. A number of factors have served as catalysts for the spread, including the presence of "recipes" easily accessible over the Internet, ingredients needed to produce methamphetamine, which were available in many over-the-counter cold medications and common household products found at retail stores, coupled with the relatively simple process involved to manufacture methamphetamine. Thanks in large part to the legislative restrictions placed on the sales of methamphetamine precursor chemicals, DEA has seen a significant decrease in the number of STLs found in 2005.

The common denominator in targeting both STL's and foreign source methamphetamine is the control of methamphetamine's primary precursor chemicals: ephedrine, pseudoephedrine, and phenylpropanolamine. At DEA, we have taken an active role in fighting the diversion of these key methamphetamine precursors. These efforts, through both enforcement and international agreements, have resulted in a reduction in the amount of precursor chemicals entering the United States. However, with this success, we have seen an increase in the flow of these precursor chemicals to other areas and an increase in the trafficking of methamphetamine from foreign sources into the United States.

In response to the threat posed by methamphetamine, DEA has taken several steps to address this threat through both domestic and international enforcement efforts. Domestically, law enforcement efforts have been aided by State and Federal legislation placing restrictions on the sale of methamphetamine's precursor chemicals. Of note, the recent passage of the re-authorization of the USA PATRIOT Act (particularly Title VII, the "Combat Methamphetamine Epidemic Act of 2005") has provided important additional tools to enhance law enforcement efforts both domestically and internationally.

DEA has also stepped up its efforts to focus on the financial side of drug trafficking organizations. Drug money is the life blood of drug trafficking organizations, and denying this funding is at the core of any effective drug enforcement strategy. DEA's financial enforcement program and the philosophy behind it apply DEA resources in the most effective and efficient manner to accomplish our mission of stopping the supply of illegal drugs from reaching the American Public. DEA's financial enforcement strategy is mission-driven in that we are focused on the flow of money back to international sources of drug supply, because this is the money that is destined to finance the next cycle of illegal drugs that will target our consumer market.

Domestic Initiatives

With respect to DEA's domestic efforts, we have redirected the focus of our Mobile Enforcement Teams (METs). DEA created the MET Program in 1995 to enhance our ability to attack violent drug trafficking organizations. MET was established on the premise that a skilled and trained team of investigators targeting violent drug gangs would be a tremendous resource for local law enforcement. MET teams are deployed on a temporary basis (averaging 6 months per deployment) at the request of state and local law enforcement officials to assist the disruption or dismantlement of violent drug trafficking organizations and gangs.

Beginning in March 2005, DEA redirected its METs to prioritize deployments to assist with methamphetamine investigations. This shift was due to the rise in meth drug trafficking organizations and the violence associated with them. Currently, these teams focus on targeting methamphetamine Priority Target Organizations (PTOs) and clandestine laboratory operators in areas of the United States that have a limited DEA presence.

The significant reduction in the number of domestic small toxic labs this year, due in large part to recent legislation restricting access to methamphetamine precursor chemicals, will allow DEA's Clandestine Laboratory Enforcement Teams (CLETs) to expand their efforts beyond dismantling methamphetamine labs to also include the targeting of Mexican methamphetamine trafficking organizations. These DEA clandestine lab teams will use their lab expertise to trace precursor chemicals and seize finished methamphetamine and drug proceeds from drug trafficking organizations in the U.S. and Mexico. These teams also will work to identify and dismantle U.S.-based methamphetamine transportation and distribution cells.

Other domestic initiatives will include a national listing on the DEA Website of the addresses of properties in which methamphetamine labs or chemical dumpsites have been found. The registry will provide owners or renters with notice that a property may once have been used to produce methamphetamine and that there may be potential toxic hazards within the property.

DEA's longstanding enforcement efforts against methamphetamine include utilizing the Consolidated Priority Organization Targets (CPOTs) List, the PTO program, and the Organized Crime Drug Enforcement Task Force (OCDETF) program. These programs all provide assistance in identifying and targeting the most significant methamphetamine trafficking organizations, with the intent to disrupt and dismantle the organizations.

The FY 2006 CPOTs list has identified 8 of the 46 designated organizations as being engaged in methamphetamine trafficking. At the end of the second quarter of FY 2006, DEA had 149 active PTO investigations linked to those 8 CPOTs, of which 28 were active PTO investigations with methamphetamine as the primary type of drug. Since the inception of the PTO program in 2001, the DEA has either disrupted or dismantled in excess of 460 PTOs where methamphetamine was the primary drug involved.

To further coordinate and focus our methamphetamine and precursor chemical initiatives, the FY 2006 Department of Justice (DOJ) Appropriations Act directs the Attorney General to establish a Methamphetamine Task Force (MTF) within DEA. The purpose of the Task Force is to improve and target the Federal government's policies with respect to the production and trafficking of methamphetamine. The MTF is comprised of three DEA Special Agents, two Diversion Investigators (DIs), three Attorneys, and one Program Analyst. These are veteran personnel with extensive experience and knowledge in the field who will collect and analyze investigative and intelligence information from numerous sources. Their analysis will focus on trends in chemical trafficking and manufacturing methods, changes in trafficking routes and patterns, and regional abuse and distribution patterns. They also will analyze and monitor foreign and domestic precursor sources and trafficking trends, as well as methods of financing. In addition, the MTF will be involved in tracking sources of chemicals and equipment, as well as methods of procurement and clandestine laboratory cleanup issues. Another aspect of the MTF's duties will involve the proposal of various recommendations addressing issues that are identified from their analysis. These recommendations will be forwarded to the National Synthetic Drugs Interagency Working Group for review and action.

In addition, the Combat Methamphetamine Epidemic Act of 2005 provides effective new tools to use in the battle against methamphetamine. The ability of pseudoephedrine to be sold on the spot market will be effectively taken away. These transactions, which were not regulated under the prior law, will be treated as new imports or exports and, therefore, subject to 15 day advance notification during which DEA will verify the legitimacy of the transaction. In addition, DOJ has the authority to establish production and import quotas for ephedrine, pseudoephedrine, and phenylpropanolamine. These quotas will allow for greater control of precursors that are imported into the United States.

Partnership with State and Local Law Enforcement

DEA has long prided itself on the outstanding relationship it has developed with its federal, state, and local counterparts. Whether on individual cases, through the High Intensity Drug Trafficking Area (HIDTA) program, or in formal DEA task force settings, many of the investigations we are working with our counterparts are among the best in the agency. With respect to our formalized state and local task force program it is important to note that DEA's successful enforcement efforts across the United States are not only led by DEA Special Agents but also by Task Force Officers (TFOs) from state and local agencies who are assigned to DEA offices. These TFOs are deputized by the DEA and have the same authority as DEA Special Agents. TFOs assigned to DEA offices throughout the country work alongside our Special Agents, DIs, and Intelligence Research Specialists with the same goal: to target the most significant drug trafficking organizations that can be identified in their areas of responsibility. Working in a task force setting brings together the expertise of the individual investigators and agencies and serves as a force multiplier, by which law enforcement can better attack the drug threats, to include methamphetamine, facing our nation. Many of these TFOs are members of our CLETs.

DEA continues to take a very aggressive role in training our drug law enforcement counterparts with respect to methamphetamine investigations. To expand and improve our efforts, DEA is establishing a new state-of-the-art clandestine lab training facility at the DEA Academy in Quantico, Virginia. The construction of this facility is expected to begin in the fall of 2006. Once the facility is operational, DEA will continue to train state and local officers, as well as foreign law enforcement officials, on the latest safety techniques and the latest techniques in detecting and investigating clandestine methamphetamine labs.

In addition, DEA continues its work to ensure that only legitimate businesses with adequate chemical controls are licensed to handle bulk pseudoephedrine and ephedrine in the United States, primarily through the efforts of our DIs. DIs are specialists in working with legitimate businesses to ensure compliance with the laws and regulations that govern the manufacture, sale, and transport of pharmaceuticals and other controlled chemicals. The investigative work done by these DIs, through their knowledge of pharmaceuticals and chemicals, plays a critical role in preventing the diversion of List I chemicals and pharmaceutical controlled substances. In the past 7 years, over 2,000 chemical registrants have been denied, surrendered, or withdrawn their registrations or applications as a result of DEA investigations. Between 2001 and 2004, DIs physically inspected more than half of the 3,000 chemical registrants at their places of business. We investigated the adequacy of their security safeguards to prevent the diversion of chemicals to the illicit market and audited their recordkeeping to ensure compliance with federal regulations.

International Initiatives

The manufacture and use of methamphetamine is not a problem confined to the United States but one that has spread to many regions of the world. In fact, the International Narcotics Control Board (INCB) noted in its 2005 report *Precursors and Chemicals Frequently Used in the Illicit Manufacture of Narcotic Drugs and Psychotropic Substances* that the illicit manufacture of methamphetamine is spreading throughout the world at an alarming rate.

Specifically, the INCB report stated that the illicit manufacture of amphetamine-type stimulants (ATS)*, and of methamphetamine in particular, is spreading in North America and South-East Asia, but also increasingly to other areas such as Africa, Eastern Europe, and Oceania. There are an estimated 26.2 million ATS users in the world, compared to an estimated 13.7 million cocaine users and 10.6 million heroin users. The report further stated that the spread of methamphetamine is due to the simple manufacturing process and the availability of the required precursors.

From DEA's perspective, increased international cooperation is essential to our continued efforts to combat methamphetamine. Some of the most significant and successful international efforts to combat methamphetamine involve a series of enforcement initiatives worked jointly between law enforcement in the United States and Canada from the late 1990s into 2003. These enforcement initiatives, known as Operations MOUNTAIN EXPRESS I, II, and III and Operation NORTHERN STAR, were principally responsible for the significant reduction in the amount of pseudoephedrine entering the United States for use in super labs. In turn, most of the super labs and the pseudoephedrine needed for them moved from the United States to Mexico.

DEA is the lead agency in working with our Mexican counterparts to combat methamphetamine. Since 2001, DEA with support from the Department of State and other U.S. law enforcement agencies has provided or sponsored training on numerous occasions for our Mexican counterparts in the areas of clandestine laboratories, chemical training, and related prosecutions. Training has been provided both to officials who regulate precursor chemicals and pharmaceuticals at the state and Federal level within Mexico, as well as agents from the Agencia Federal de Investigaciones (AFI) and a number of prosecutors within the Mexican Organized Crime Unit (SIEDO). The combined numbers of students who have received training through these cooperative efforts exceed 450.

Mexico has independently implemented several controls on pseudoephedrine in cooperation with industry and is considering others. Those implemented now, or planned soon, include: (1) limiting retail sales to pharmacies; (2) limiting sale quantities to 3 boxes of 60 milligram or more combination pseudoephedrine products; and (3) distributors voluntarily agreeing to limit sales to customers with appropriate government registrations (pharmacies) and with legitimate commercial needs. Mexico also imposed recently a policy limiting imports of pseudoephedrine and ephedrine to manufacturers only. Wholesale distributors are barred from importing raw material pseudoephedrine and ephedrine, and importers are limited to shipments of no more than 3 metric tons at a time. In addition, the United States and Mexico have jointly obtained a commitment from Hong Kong not to ship chemicals to the United

* In Europe and Asia the term "amphetamine-type stimulants" is used rather than a specific reference to methamphetamine. The term ATS includes the following: amphetamine, methamphetamine, and MDMA (Ecstasy), and its analogues. This term also is used by the United Nations.

States, Mexico, or Panama until receiving an import permit, or equivalent documentation, and to pre-notify the receiving country before shipment. Combined with other controls that the Government of Mexico has put in place, this agreement has significantly reduced the number of suspect shipments of methamphetamine precursor chemicals from Hong Kong to Mexico.

Very recently, Mexico began imposing import quotas tied to estimates of legitimate national needs, which are based on extrapolations from a large population sample. A study conducted by The Federal Commission for the Protection against Sanitary Risk (COFEPRIS) estimated that there was an excess of imports of pseudoephedrine products of approximately 60 to 100 metric tons in 2004. The Government of Mexico reported that its efforts to control methamphetamine precursor chemicals reduced imports in 2005 by 40 percent to 130 metric tons from its peak of 220 metric tons in 2004. DEA has been advised that it is the Government of Mexico's intention to reduce further pseudoephedrine and ephedrine importation permits to 70 metric tons in total for 2006. Mexican officials have further advised that this 70-ton limit also applies to combination products containing pseudoephedrine and/or ephedrine.

An example of Mexico's interdiction efforts concerning pseudoephedrine occurred during December 2005, when approximately 3.2 metric tons (approximately 5.1 million pseudoephedrine combination tablets) of pseudoephedrine were seized by Mexican authorities in the Port of Manzanillo, Mexico. The tablets were concealed within a shipment of electric fans, which were packaged in approximately 1,260 boxes. During the follow-up joint investigation conducted by DEA and Hong Kong Customs and Excise Department, officials disclosed that the shipment originated in mainland China and transited one of the mainland China/Hong Kong border crossings before being subsequently loaded on a marine vessel en route to Mexico.

Additional steps are also being taken by the United States and Mexico. At the May 2006 National Methamphetamine and Chemicals Initiative (NMCI) Strategy Conference in Dallas, Attorney General Gonzales announced important new anti-methamphetamine domestic initiatives, as well as new partnerships between the United States and Mexico in fighting methamphetamine trafficking. Joined by Mexican Attorney General Daniel Cabeza De Vaca, Attorney General Gonzales unveiled DOJ-led initiatives to improve enforcement, increase law enforcement training, improve information-sharing, and increase public awareness.

Among the United States/Mexico partnership efforts is an agreement between DEA and the Mexican government to establish specialized methamphetamine enforcement teams on either side of the border. In Mexico, these teams will focus on investigating and targeting the most wanted Mexican methamphetamine drug trafficking organizations, while DEA-led efforts on the United States side will focus on the methamphetamine traffickers and organizations transporting and distributing the finished methamphetamine being produced in Mexico. Other initiatives that are part of the United States/Mexico partnership include:

- A new DEA, U.S. Immigration and Customs Enforcement (ICE) and Customs and Border Protection effort to focus on ports of entry with the intent of targeting suspicious cargo that is likely to be related to methamphetamine trafficking organizations;
- A Bi-national Law Enforcement Working Group that will focus on methamphetamine production and trafficking from both an enforcement and intelligence perspective;

- A DEA and Mexican National Conference for Information, Analysis and Planning in Order to Fight Crime effort to further share intelligence information and continue to develop stronger working relationships. Such collaborative efforts will focus on investigating large-scale methamphetamine trafficking organizations that are operating in Mexico and the United States.

- A jointly developed DEA and Mexican police Most Wanted List of chemical and methamphetamine trafficking organizations that will focus bilateral law enforcement efforts on the biggest threats;

- An agreement between the DEA Office of Diversion Control and Mexico's chemical regulatory agency, COFEPRIS, to a personnel exchange in which chemical regulatory experts from within each agency will be embedded within the other's agency for a specific period to observe, learn best practices, and then implement joint strategies complimentary to both regulatory agencies;

- Eight DEA trucks used in clandestine lab enforcement operations that have been refurbished by the Department of State and donated to Mexico to be used by the above referenced specialized Mexican enforcement teams; and

- In conjunction with the Department of State's (DOS) Bureau for International Narcotics and Law Enforcement Affairs, DEA will provide training for nearly 1,000 Mexican police officials to focus on a variety of investigative, enforcement, and regulatory methods related to methamphetamine trafficking.

Another important aspect of our international efforts to combat this drug has been the assignment of DIs to a number of our foreign offices. The DIs coordinate with foreign host country counterparts to establish effective systems of chemical controls and ensure customers in foreign countries receiving U.S. exports of pharmaceutically controlled substances are in fact, legitimate companies.

In addition to these efforts with Mexico, the DEA, operating under the auspices of the INCB's Project Prism, hosted a meeting in February in Hong Kong for law enforcement and regulatory officials of producing countries of ephedrine/pseudoephedrine and 3-4 methylenedioxyphenyl-2-proponone. The objective of this meeting was to develop and enhance systems for voluntary cooperation in data collection and the exchange in law enforcement channels of information on pharmaceutical preparations containing ephedrine and pseudoephedrine, as well as bulk precursor chemicals. This was the first time that almost all of the countries that produce these chemicals and those countries affected by methamphetamine have sat down together to discuss this problem.

While there were some differences of opinion as to the manner and channels in which information regarding the licit trade in these substances should be exchanged, it was important to bring precursor-chemical-producing nations and nations in which illicit drug manufacturing occurs together for candid discussions. The communication that occurred between countries attending the open forum meeting was encouraging. DEA, in cooperation with the Department of State (DOS), will continue discussions with all involved countries. The discussions will seek to determine the worldwide production of these chemicals to further identify producers and distributors, to gain better insight as to what form (bulk versus tablets) the chemicals are manufactured and distributed at various stages, and to learn where the chemicals are destined.

The Hong Kong meeting also helped to lay a foundation for discussions and negotiations between concerned governments, which led to the passage of a resolution at the 49th Commission on Narcotic Drugs in Vienna, Austria in March of this year. The resolution, entitled "Strengthening

Systems for Control of Precursor Chemicals Used in the Manufacture of Synthetic Drugs," involves the synthetic drug precursors previously mentioned, as well as preparations containing these substances and phenyl-2-propanone (P2P).

The resolution calls on all nations who are signatories to the various United Nations' conventions dealing with drugs and precursor chemicals to provide to the INCB annual estimates of their legitimate requirements for these substances and preparations containing these substances. The resolution also calls for nations to ensure that their imports of these substances are commensurate with their respective nation's legitimate needs and urges them to continue to provide to the INCB, subject to their national legislation and taking care not to impede legitimate international commerce, information on all shipments of these drugs and precursor chemicals. The resolution further requests countries to permit the INCB to share the shipment information on these consignments with concerned law enforcement and regulatory authorities to prevent or interdict diverted shipments. While we consider this resolution an important first step, our ability to obtain additional information from the INCB is contingent upon nations providing the information requested pursuant to the resolution.

Most recently, the Combat Methamphetamine Epidemic Act of 2005 will expand the notice of importation to include all information known to the importer on the chain of distribution. If it is determined that an importer is refusing to cooperate in providing such information or DEA has concerns about the downstream customers, the DEA may issue an order prohibiting the importation of Scheduled Listed Chemical Products (SLCP). Further, the Act requires the DOS to identify the five largest exporting countries and the five largest importing countries with the highest diversion of SLCPs and provide an economic analysis of worldwide production as compared to legitimate demand.

FOLLOWING THE MONEY

The Office of National Drug Control Policy estimates that Americans spend approximately $65 billion per year on illegal drugs. With only approximately $1 billion seized per year, domestically, by all Federal agencies combined, no one can claim to have discovered the "holy grail" of drug financial investigations. DEA's revenue denied program comprises a global accounting of DEA's efforts to bankrupt DTOs, especially those with international DTOs that target our communities with their poison. DEA is an agency with global reach, with 86 offices in 62 countries. DEA's financial enforcement strategy is "mission driven" in that we are focused on the flow of money back to the international sources of supply, since this is the very money that is destined to finance the next cycle of illegal drugs that will target our consumer market here in the United States. This is also the money that allows the international DTO's to continue to operate. It is important to us at DEA to carry the fight to the doorstep of those DTOs that spread their poison in the United States and drain billions of dollars each year from our economy.

There is little doubt that the sole reason people sell drugs is for the money. Money serves as both the motivating force and the lifeblood of DTOs. Therefore, attacking the financial infrastructure of DTOs has to play a key role in any viable drug enforcement strategy. DEA's objective with financial investigations is to identify and halt the use of drug proceeds that finance the continued operations of DTOs.

Financial Investigations Strategy

Since the major DTOs involved in methamphetamine production are also involved in the smuggling of marijuana, heroin, and cocaine, it is virtually impossible to differentiate the source of the drug money by the type of drug. In the case of methamphetamine, payments to sources of supply are almost exclusively in the form of currency. Thus, financial investigations relating to the movement of funds to Mexico are not classified or segregated by any particular type of drug. However, illicit drug proceeds can be categorized based on how they are used by the DTOs. Drug proceeds are used to pay sources of supply, to support the infrastructure of the organization, and to acquire personal assets. The "cash on hand" left over can be considered as either part of the organization's working capital or personal wealth.

To significantly reduce the supply of illegal drugs, DEA must focus our efforts on the drug proceeds used to pay the sources of drug supply. Denying the sources of supply revenue from the distribution of drugs will hamper their capability to acquire or produce additional drugs and support their organizations. The higher in the drug distribution chain we can deny the revenue flow, the greater effect this denial will have on the entire distribution network.

Payments to sources of drug supply flow almost exclusively in the form of currency. This currency is handled and transported covertly, just like the drugs that generated it. Thus, the investigation of this component of drug proceeds is a "contraband" investigation, as opposed to an "asset tracing" investigation, which are more traditional money laundering investigations that other agencies are better equipped and more experienced in dealing with than the DEA. DEA, on the other hand, is the best equipped and trained agency to carry out "contraband" investigations. DEA, on the other hand, is well-equipped and trained to carry out "contraband" investigations. Accordingly, DEA "financial investigations" focus on identifying and interdicting those drug proceeds flowing back to the source of drug supply.

In this type of money flow investigation, the financial transactions are also overt acts in the drug conspiracy and, oftentimes, provide the best evidence in linking local drug organizations to their sources of drug supply. Since drug money flows toward the "command and control" of the DTO, as opposed to away from "command and control" like drugs, a money flow investigation enables an investigator to work his/her way up the distribution chain, which is the primary objective of all drug investigations. To ensure maximum effectiveness, DEA money flow investigations are designed to be compatible with, not competitive with, the long-term asset-tracing type investigations that have traditionally been the norm. In fact, whenever DEA is involved in a long-term, asset-tracing type investigation, there is always an agency such as the Internal Revenue Service (IRS) involved as well.

A 2005 DEA study determined that during 2003 and 2004 there were excess U.S. dollars present in Mexico that could not be accounted for from legitimate sources totaling at least $9.2 billion and $10.2 billion, respectively. It is estimated that the four major drugs that are smuggled into the United States from Mexico (i.e. methamphetamine, heroin, cocaine, and marijuana.) generate as much as $22 billion per year for the sources of supply.

DEA has identified the following as the major money laundering threats relating to movement of drug proceeds to Mexico:

- Bulk currency smuggling to include the transportation organizations that service the Mexican DTOs.
- Mexican currency exchange houses, referred to as Casas de Cambio and Centros Cambiario.
- The remission of drug proceeds through U.S. based money remitters.

To address these threats, DEA has formulated a strategy that encompasses intelligence-based enforcement, as well as domestic and international collaborative efforts to target the movement of bulk currency and ultimately attack the command and control targets in the United States and Mexico. By working closely with our Federal, state, and local law enforcement counterparts in the United States and our counterparts in Mexico, we exploit the intelligence from bulk currency interdictions to identify, target, and ultimately, prosecute the command and control targets on either side of the border.

DEA also works closely with the Treasury Department, Financial Crimes Enforcement Network (FinCEN) and the Office of Foreign Assets Control (OFAC) to identify opportunities to apply regulatory sanctions and freezing orders against these Mexican DTOs. Through enforcement operations, analytical analysis of the Bank Secrecy Act, and other financial records, we identify the movement of drug funds. We also target rogue remitter agencies and agents who are complicit in the movement of drug money to Mexico, through criminal enforcement and asset forfeiture.

To carry out our strategy, DEA, through the Office of Financial Operations, has instituted a number of national initiatives, that target bulk currency smuggling and the remission of drug money through U.S. wire remitters.

In October 2004, DEA instituted the Bulk Currency Initiative. The Bulk Currency Initiative is an information sharing vehicle by which our state and local counterparts can share the information they obtain from making a currency seizure, whether it be along the nation's highways or in operation at an airport. Information obtained by DEA in this manner many times can be tied to other investigations throughout the world. The currency seizure itself then becomes an overt act in the drug conspiracy investigation and often helps to identify other co-conspirators within a DTO that were previously unknown. This initiative resulted in an increase in DEA's currency seizures for FY 2005 of over $80 million, from $259 million to $339.6 million, an increase of 31 percent. This initiative continues, and DEA hopes to see similar results for this fiscal year.

To coordinate multi-jurisdictional bulk currency investigations, DEA's Special Operations Division (SOD) instituted the Money Trail Initiative. In the first year and a half, the Money Trail Initiative was responsible for the dismantlement of six national organizations involved in the transportation of bulk currency drug proceeds from various points in the United States to Mexico. As of July 2006, this initiative has resulted in the arrest of 418 defendants and the seizure of $65.4 million in United States currency, $14.5 million in assets, 59.6 metric tons of marijuana, 9.7 metric tons of cocaine, 126.7 kilograms of methamphetamine, 9 kilograms of heroin, 249 vehicles, and 77 weapons. One of these SOD investigations, Operation Choque, resulted in the identification and arrest of Mexican CPOTs Oscar, Miguel, and Luis Arriola-Marquez, and the dismantlement of their organization, which, based on ledgers seized by Mexican authorities, was responsible for the smuggling of at least 14,000 kilos of cocaine into the United States and the smuggling of $240 million out of the United States. Based on information supplied by DEA, Mexican authorities have seized over $18 million of the Arriola-Marquez Organization's assets.

Domestic efforts

DEA has 24 Financial Investigation Teams (FITs). These teams are located in each of its 21 domestic field divisions, as well as in our Bogotá and Bangkok Country Offices. Each domestic field division has one FIT located in the same city as its division office, with the exception of the Miami Field Division, whose FIT is located in Ft. Lauderdale, Florida, and the Chicago Field Division, which has two FITs based in Chicago.

The FITs are tasked with carrying out DEA's national financial initiatives, providing guidance to other DEA personnel in financial investigations, conducting the more sophisticated financial investigations, and serving as DEA's local point of contact with the financial community. Administrator Tandy has mandated that all DEA investigations include a financial investigation. The FITs are not expected to conduct all DEA financial investigations. However, they do provide guidance, when needed, to other DEA investigators on their financial investigations.

DEA has assigned 159 Special Agents, 8 Intelligence Research Analysts, and 3 DIs to the FIT Teams, which averages 7 Special Agents per FIT. With the exception of the Washington D.C. and San Francisco Field Divisions, each FIT is multi-agency, with participation requested and encouraged from Federal, state and local agencies. Current participation by outside agencies is as follows:

- IRS-Criminal Investigation: 12 full time and 4 part time Special Agents
- ICE: 4 full time and 2 part time Special Agents
- FBI: 1 full time Special Agent
- U.S. Postal Inspection Service: 2 part time Postal Inspectors
- National Guard: 3 full time Analysts
- Financial Investigative Contractors: 24 full time and 5 part time
- State & local Police Officers: 63 full time and 5 part time

The Special Agents, Postal Inspectors and Police Officers from these outside agencies conduct drug-related financial investigations jointly with their DEA counterparts. This team effort brings the specialized expertise and jurisdictions of their parent agencies to the table, where all participants have the same access to the DEA databases as their DEA counterparts.

In addition to the FITs, DEA has a number of Special Agent personnel assigned to liaison positions within the Intelligence Community, Department of Defense and the Executive Office of the President (ONDCP) who enhance our ability to conduct financial investigations. These Special Agents have sign-on authority to the databases maintained by these agencies that they need to perform their liaison duties. In addition, DEA has a limited number of Special Agents assigned to other law enforcement agencies. These agents have direct sign-on authority to the databases of the agencies to which they are assigned. One example of this is the ICE-led El Dorado Task Force in New York, where DEA has a full enforcement group assigned.

International Challenges

Within the United States, regulators and law enforcement have a fairly accurate overview of financial transactions. Particularly after the additional tools provided by the USA PATRIOT Act came into force, law enforcement generally has access to the information it needs to identify and thwart significant money laundering efforts within the United States. However, this same transparency is not present in many other countries, including Mexico. Accordingly, DEA believes that most drug proceeds are now smuggled out of the United States to Mexico in bulk, rather than inserted into the financial system within the United States.

Because of the lack of transparency of their financial system, the Mexican financial services industry continues to be a facilitator for drug money movement. Although it is a sophisticated financial sector, obtaining financial information from the Mexican financial services industry remains difficult.

However, based on intelligence information from various DEA, ICE, and other United States law enforcement operations, we do know that once bulk currency is delivered to its intended recipients in Mexico, it can take a number of paths. Most commonly, bulk currency is deposited into the Mexican banking system through casas de cambio, centros cambiarios and banks, and then repatriated to the U.S. banking system through correspondent banking and bank note sales to United States institutions. While some of the bulk cash can be used to purchase precursors and equipment for methamphetamine manufacture, it also can be infused into the financial system through Mexican front companies or used to purchase real estate, businesses and other luxury assets in Mexico. In some instances, the bulk cash is converted to larger denominated United States dollars at casas de cambio or centros cambiarios for further smuggling to Colombia or for further smuggling to Panama for delivery to the Panama Free Trade Zone to purchase commodities on behalf of Colombian businesses. The combination of widespread corruption within Mexico, coupled with insufficient regulatory and criminal enforcement, makes disguising and moving drug proceeds in Mexico a relatively safe and simple task.

As part of our strategy to employ regulatory measures against money laundering systems that facilitate drug money laundering, DEA works closely with the FinCEN and other law enforcement agencies. DEA provided information to support the issuance of FinCEN's April 2006 Advisory to all United States financial institutions on the smuggling of bulk cash and the role of Mexican casas de cambio in the repatriation of those drug dollars into the United States banking system. DEA enjoys a very close working relationship with the OFAC. Much of the information used by OFAC to support its designations under the Kingpin and Specially Designated Narcotics Trafficker authorities is provided by DEA.

CONCLUSION

DEA continues to fight methamphetamine on all fronts, by targeting both the trafficking organizations and the financial proceeds they generate. As the international threat of methamphetamine spreads, cooperative efforts among agencies and nations become even more vital. Cooperative efforts and initiatives to combat methamphetamine production and control chemical shipments on an international scale are critical to DEA's ability to combat methamphetamine trafficking in the United States.

The *Synthetics Drug Control Strategy* provides DEA and contributing agencies a framework to continue the ongoing efforts and chart new strategies to achieve domestic and international progress against methamphetamine and other synthetic drug trafficking and abuse. DEA's core competency, the disruption and dismantlement of drug trafficking organizations impacting the United States, is an integral component to *Synthetics Drug Control Strategy*.

Thank you for the opportunity to appear before you today to discuss this important issue. I will be happy to answer any questions that you may have.

Written Testimony of Lieutenant Daniel L. Springer
Commander – Missouri River Drug Task Force
Gallatin County Sheriff's Office

Before the Senate Committee on Finance
Hearing on "Breaking the Methamphetamine Supply Chain:
Law Enforcement Challenges"
September 12, 2006

Good morning Mr. Chairman, Senator Baucus, and members of the Committee. It is my great pleasure to be here today.

In 1992 the Missouri River Drug Task Force (MRDTF) was established in Montana as a regionally-proactive enforcement response designed to aggressively combat the increasing effects of dangerous drug use and distribution occurring within seven specific jurisdictions of concern. The Missouri River Drug Task Force has nine full-time investigators and covers an area of 17,000 square miles. Massachusetts and Connecticut combined, does not equal the size of our jurisdiction.

Financial allocations received from the "Byrne Memorial Grant" served as the fiscal catalyst behind the jurisdictional alignment. Operating beneath this collaborative investigative premise, MRDTF investigations, in conjunction with State and Local authorities, DEA, ICE, ATF, IRS and the National Park Service have been instrumental in the identification, disruption, and dismantling of Drug Trafficking Organizations (DTO) engaged in the distribution of dangerous drugs within Montana, Idaho, Washington, Oregon, California, and Utah.

Narcotic Officers across the country are facing multiple challenges regarding methamphetamine. The largest challenge is the fight itself. We are working with decreased funding, limited resources, a growing epidemic and vicious drug related crimes. Forty-two percent of Law Enforcement agencies recognize methamphetamine as the number one drug concern within their jurisdiction. There is no close second.

When I started as a patrol deputy ten years ago it was extremely rare to find even personal-use methamphetamine on the street. Today, it is not only common--it is the norm--and often in larger quantities than personal use. Methamphetamine hit our area like a freight train and we have seen nothing but a steady increase in the supply and the demand over the past ten years. If your area has not been hit by this epidemic, be very thankful; but prepare yourselves for something that you have never seen before.

The MRDTF has seen a consistent rise in drug activity throughout our jurisdiction over the past ten years. With this increase in drug activity, there has been an increase in crime. However, the primary funding source of the MRDTF, the Byrne Memorial Grant, has decreased by 62 % over the past five years.

Due to significant cuts in federal funding, the number of investigators needed to combat this epidemic has stagnated to a point where we are just maintaining rather than conducting pro-active, hard-hitting investigations.

The advantage of the Byrne Memorial Grant has been the ability to use the money in multiple ways. The Byrne Grants allow us to use the money for salaries, overtime, vehicles, drug "buy" money, informant payments, support staff salaries and many other areas. I would ask for a consistent and stable form of funding that does not keep agencies hanging in the balance from year to year. A funding source of this nature would allow for extended planning and extended expectations.

The Montana State Legislature has recently passed pre-cursor laws limiting access to items used in the making of methamphetamine. These laws have apparently been highly successful and we have seen a dramatic decrease in the number of "mom and pop" methamphetamine labs. However, we have seen a dramatic increase in the importation of methamphetamine. The methamphetamine imported to Montana is primarily coming from Washington, Oregon, Idaho, and Utah and eventually Mexico. The Super Labs of Mexico are supplying the majority of the methamphetamine within the United States and the factories used to make pseudoephedrine are shipping it to Mexico in mass quantities.

Directly linking methamphetamine to other crimes is not easy to do. Very few defendants admit to committing the crime, let alone admit to committing that crime while using meth or in an attempt to purchase meth. One thing we do know is that methamphetamine is no longer the "cheap" drug used by those who can't afford other drugs. In our area, the price of methamphetamine is currently twice the price of cocaine. With the increase in price, and the addictive nature of this drug, the pursuit of methamphetamine has increasingly become a criminal motive for violent and weapons-related criminal acts. The increasing frequency of burglaries, thefts, robberies, and assaults each serve to reflect the devastating social effects of methamphetamine on our local communities.

Through my very small window of the world, I see individuals getting killed over drugs. I see people losing family members to drugs; I see families and friends being torn apart due to drugs; and I see the productive citizens of our communities becoming victims of crimes due to drugs. I see the enormous toll that methamphetamine takes on an individual both mentally and physically in a very short period of time.

Money alone cannot solve the methamphetamine issue in Montana. However, without a sustainable source of financial support, the success and momentum of these historically complex and effective efforts will inevitably falter.

Local enforcement efforts are arguably the first and last line of defense in the war on methamphetamine. And while our communities cannot afford to lose the battle, the MRDTF cannot afford to wage the war alone.

Senate Finance Committee Hearing
Questions Submitted for the Record From Lt. Dan Springer
Breaking the Methamphetamine Supply Chain: Law Enforcement Challenges
September 12, 2006

Question 1:

Given your limited resources, have you been able to take any other approaches to combating the meth epidemic besides Task Forces?

Answer:

Senator Baucus' office has recently assisted the Missouri River Drug Task Force in contacting the Internal Revenue Service with the hope that their criminal investigators would be available during appropriate investigations. The IRS has responded positively and we have already built a good working relationship with the local investigators. We have partnered with the Drug Enforcement Agency and are looking at ways to have a larger DEA presence within the Missouri River Drug Task Force. The Missouri River Drug Task Force has supported and assisted with legislative measures too limit the access to ingredients used in making methamphetamine. The Missouri River Drug Task Force has met with the US Attorney's office in Montana multiple times and has continued to build positive relationships with their office. The Montana State Department of Criminal Investigations has created a fusion center with the hope that all agencies will share intelligence information. In the last year, our task force has been sharing any and all appropriate information in an attempt to conduct intelligence based narcotics investigations.

Question 2:

Without challenging the security of classified information, can you please describe some inexpensive steps that you have taken?

Answer:

The Missouri River Drug Task Force has taken steps beyond enforcement of the law in order to combat the methamphetamine epidemic. The task force gives over 60 drug awareness talks per year to community organizations. These organizations range from school age parents, College courses, community groups, (lion's club, Rotary etc.). We have recently been assisting the local Department of Public Health and Human Resources with their Drug Endangered Children protocols. The Missouri River Drug Task Force has used forfeiture accounts to pay for our local Drug Treatment Court officials to attend national seminars.

Testimony
of
Crow Tribal Chairman, Carl Venne
Before the United States Senate Finance Committee

Senate Finance Committee Hearing on Methamphetamine Law Enforcement / Money Laundering

September 12, 2006

Good Morning, Honorable members Committee Members. I bring you greetings from Crow Country. My name is Carl Venne and I serve as Chairman of the great Crow Tribe of Indians, the Apsaalooka Nation. I was elected as Crow Tribal Chairman in November 2002 and I serve as an Advisory Council Member of the Montana Meth Project. I have more than three decades of experience serving in various tribal government roles. The majority of my professional experience has been as a police officer and law enforcement official, after obtaining a degree in law enforcement from the University of Minnesota at St. Paul.

The Apsaalooka Nation, often referred to as the Crow Reservation, is located in south-central Montana with the Wyoming state line as the southern border. Crow County includes over 2.5 million acres with its northwestern boundary approximately ten (10) miles from Billings, the largest city in the State of Montana. The Department of Interior Bureau of Indian Affairs ("BIA") Law Enforcement is responsible for covering 184 interstate miles and 3,500 road miles.

The Crow (Apsáalooke) Tribe of Indians has a membership of approximately 11,000, of whom 7,900 reside on the Crow Indian Reservation. Eighty-five percent speak Crow as their first language. The tribe calls itself "Apsaalooke," which means "children of the large-beaked bird." The Crow people, throughout the periods of various social change, have found strength and stability through cultural preservation. However, this strength and stability of the proud Crow people has met a new and dangerous enemy.

Crystal Methamphetamine ("Meth") has become the number one threat to our Tribal communities. As Native Americans, we honor our families, culture, and clan system and traditional values, but our greatest resource is our children. The Crow children affected by this devastating drug hold the future of our Crow Nation. These children are crying for help, but we cannot always hear their cry. With this in mind, the Crow Tribe has declared War on Meth. Meth has violated our communities destroying lives, affecting school systems, undermining social values, affecting employers, taxing the health care system, and taxing the law enforcement and social workers. There is no entity or organization on the Crow Reservation that is exempt from the devastating destruction of Meth. The Crow Tribal Rural Domestic Violence Program reported that from January 2005 to 2006, 76 adults and 127 children were referred, and of these numbers, 75% of the referrals were meth related.

Within the last 10 years, meth has flourished on the Crow reservation like a plague. Devastatingly, our Crow people have created a Crow language term to identify meth, "Baãchialiche", which means white stuff due to its abundance in our Reservation culture. Meth has no discrimination to age, educational status, religion, or financial status. Instead, meth uses an individual's weaknesses and strengths to maintain a presence within our communities. Using the strength of our family values, many non-Crow's marry a Crow woman, which guarantees the individual a bond with the family and communities. Drug distributors have found a loop that allows them unlimited trafficking access on the Crow Reservation as well as other Tribal communities. The easy accessibility of transporting drugs through Interstate-90 and US Highway 212 has made the Crow and Northern Cheyenne Reservation easy targets for drug trafficking. The BIA Law Enforcement has responded to 23,995 calls for service to I-90, 95% were drug or alcohol related.

The consequence of this drug has been the death of many young adults. In 2005, there were five suicides on the Crow Reservation all were related to meth use. In 2006 on the Northern Cheyenne Reservation, there were three suicides in on week all of which were related to meth use. On average there is an average of 1 – 2 suicide attempts a week on the Crow Reservation. The Crow people cannot wait for another organization to fix the Meth Epidemic that exists on our reservation, but we know we cannot fight this fight alone. The government, state and local agencies must combined efforts to fight the War on Meth. One recovering addict stated. "The worst part of using is coming down, life is not worth living for when you are in this zone, if you can image the worst feeling in the world that is how you feel, not even the smile of your own child can make you happy".

The meth dealers use the jurisdiction to their advantage. They move frequently on and off the reservation, from the reservation to reservation border towns and local cities. Big Horn County has not provided any relief to the drug problem on and near the reservation. The BIA Law Enforcement resources, which has jurisdiction on the reservation are spread thin. In 2005, the Crow BIA Law Enforcement covered 2.5 acres of land with 10 police officers and 1 guard. The total Indian Country law enforcement in Montana serviced 63,592 people with 138 sworn police officers at a ratio of 2.17 officers per 1,000 people covering 9.5 million acres of reservation land. The challenges we face on the Crow Reservation are not having adequate personnel to address the drug problems that exist on the reservation. Because of the staff shortage the BIA Law Enforcement are reactive rather than being proactive. The local Law Enforcement is not able to apply their attention in even a moderate scale to the drug problem. The Crow Tribe funded a special agent position that works directly with the BIA Law Enforcement, FBI, and DEA, but this too is not enough.

To obtain adequate resource the local, city, and federal law enforcement must maintain better communication. FBI and DEA need to address all levels of distribution, not only the high level distributors, but also the low level street distributors that have a major impact on reservation communities and boarder towns. A liaison between all entities would improve the relationship and allow for better data sharing and information. Address jurisdictional barriers with border towns that have not joined the Safe Trails Task Force. Other needed resources;

- More Officers
- Training for officers in drug interdiction
- Surveillance equipment
- Vehicles
- Additional funding and resources for prevention activities
- Alternative Sentencing and Family Court
- Reservation boundary boarder control

On August 22, 2006 six government entities signed an agreement to form a drug task force that would focus on southeastern Montana's Indian Reservations. The Crow/Northern Cheyenne Safe Trails Task Force has formulized key players that will work fulltime on addressing drug trafficking on the Crow and Northern Cheyenne Indian Reservations. The organizations that participated in the signing ceremony include the Crow Tribe, Northern Cheyenne Tribe, Drug Enforcement Agency, Federal Bureau of Indian Affairs, Bureau of Indian Affairs Office of Law Enforcement and Security, Colstrip Police Department. Each of the agencies has equal voice in the operation of the task force. Each agency will bring different resources to the table and the task force will be cross deputized to avoid jurisdictional barriers.

There are currently no mechanisms in place to share data and information from federal to local law enforcement entities. This has created a communication barrier, which also hinders the law enforcement's ability to track suspected drug dealers that travel from reservation to reservation. To improve the overall relation between all law enforcement agencies, there needs to be a data base to assist in tracking the drug dealers that are living on the reservation.

Again, I thank you for the opportunity to provide testimony before this honorable committee on a matter of critical importance to the Crow nation and to many other Native American communities. I believe the attention you have given this powerful enemy is a first step toward its defeat. Thank you.

In: Methamphetamine: Background, Controls and Issues ISBN: 978-1-60692-548-5
Editor: Andrea S. Sandoval

Chapter 7

INTERNATIONAL METH TRAFFICKING

Karen P. Tandy

INTRODUCTION

Chairman Hagel, Chairman Coleman, Senator Sarbanes, Senator Dodd, and distinguished members of the Senate Foreign Relations Committee, on behalf of the Drug Enforcement Administration (DEA), I appreciate your invitation to testify today regarding DEA's efforts to combat the international trafficking of methamphetamine.

OVERVIEW

Methamphetamine poses a unique and significant threat to the United States. Methamphetamine is unique in that it is a synthetic drug, it is not dependent on cultivation of a crop, its production requires no specialized skill or training, and its precursor chemicals have historically been easy to obtain and inexpensive to purchase. These factors have contributed to methamphetamine's rapid sweep across our nation. This drug is a threat because it is powerfully addictive to those who use it, and because it can cause harm even to those who are not involved in its use or distribution. Those who suffer the "second hand" effects of methamphetamine include the victims of methamphetamine-related crimes, innocent children whose homes have been turned into clandestine lab sites, law enforcement officers that work with the hazardous materials found at lab sites, and the environment from the five to six pounds of toxic waste produced for every pound of methamphetamine cooked. Methamphetamine has not only left a mark on the United States, but continues to be a significant problem in Asia and is increasingly becoming a problem in other parts of the world.

Methamphetamine also presents a dual threat to law enforcement authorities. They must simultaneously combat both small toxic labs (STLs), which have spread across much of our nation and "super labs," which are primarily controlled by Mexican drug trafficking organizations and are supplying the majority of the methamphetamine consumed in this country. The critical tool in combating both of these types of labs is the control of methamphetamine's primary precursor chemicals: ephedrine, pseudoephedrine, and phenylpropanolamine[1].

In response to the threat posed by methamphetamine, the DEA continues to aggressively combat this drug through our domestic and international enforcement efforts. Domestically, law enforcement efforts have been aided by State and Federal legislation placing restrictions on the sale of methamphetamine's precursor chemicals. Of note, the recent passage of the re-authorization of the USA PATRIOT Act (particularly Title VII, the "Combat Methamphetamine Epidemic Act of 2005") has provided important additional tools to enhance law enforcement efforts both domestically and internationally.

The DEA, through our law enforcement partnerships across the country and around the world, has initiated successful investigations that have disrupted and dismantled significant methamphetamine trafficking organizations. We also have taken an active role in fighting the diversion of methamphetamine's key ingredients, ephedrine and pseudoephedrine. These efforts, through both enforcement and international agreements, have resulted in a substantial reduction in the amount of precursor chemicals entering the United States. However, with this success, we have seen an increase in the flow of these precursor chemicals to Mexico, and an increase in the trafficking of finished meth across the Southwest border into the United States.

In addition, the Department of Justice, with the help of federal, State, and local law enforcement, has been committed to prosecuting methamphetamine traffickers. Over the past five years, data shows there has been an increase in the number of methamphetamine defendants charged by U.S. Attorneys' offices and sentenced by U.S. District Courts. U.S. Attorney case data shows a 34 percent increase[2] in the number of defendants charged over the past five years. Data from the Sentencing Commission also shows a similar significant increase, finding a 42 percent increase[3] in the number of defendants sentenced over the past five years.

METHAMPHETAMINE – THREAT ASSESSMENT

Methamphetamine consumed in the United States originates from two general sources, controlled by two distinct groups. Most of the methamphetamine consumed in the United States is produced by Mexico-based and California-based Mexican traffickers. These drug trafficking organizations control "super labs" (a laboratory capable of producing 10 pounds or more of methamphetamine within a single production cycle), and have distribution networks throughout the United States, as well as access to drug transportation routes to smuggle the methamphetamine from Mexico into the United States. Current drug lab seizure data suggests that roughly 80 percent of the methamphetamine used in the United States comes from these larger labs, which are increasingly found in Mexico.

These same Mexican criminal organizations control most mid-level and retail methamphetamine distribution in the Pacific, Southwest, and west-central regions of the United States, as well as much of the distribution in the Great Lakes and Southeast regions.

The second source for methamphetamine used in this country comes from small toxic labs (STLs). These STLs produce relatively small amounts of methamphetamine and are generally not affiliated with major trafficking organizations. Currently, DEA estimates that STLs are responsible for approximately 20 percent of the methamphetamine consumed in this country. Initially found only in most Western States, over the past 10 years there has been an eastward expansion of STLs across the United States. A number of factors have served as catalysts for the spread, including the presence of "recipes" easily accessible over the Internet, ingredients needed to produce methamphetamine which were available in many over-the-counter cold medications and common household products found at retail stores, coupled with the relatively simple process involved to manufacture methamphetamine. Today, thanks in large part to the legislative restrictions placed on the sales of methamphetamine precursor chemicals, the DEA expects to see a significant decrease in the number of STLs found this year.

The manufacture and use of methamphetamine is not a problem confined to the United States, but one that has spread to many regions of the world. In fact, the International Narcotics Control Board (INCB) noted in its 2005 report "Precursors and Chemicals Frequently Used in the Illicit Manufacture of Narcotic Drugs and Psychotropic Substances," that the illicit manufacture of methamphetamine is spreading throughout the world at an alarming rate. Globally, the number of users of amphetamine-type stimulants – a majority of which use methamphetamine - outnumber cocaine and heroin users combined.

Specifically, the INCB indicated that the illicit manufacture of amphetamine-type stimulants (ATS)[4], and of methamphetamine in particular, is spreading in North America and South-East Asia, but also increasingly to other areas such as Africa, Eastern Europe, and Oceania. There are an estimated 26.2 million ATS users in the world, compared to an estimated 13.7 million cocaine users and 10.6 heroin users. The report further stated that the spread of methamphetamine is due to the simple manufacturing process and the availability of the required precursors.

THE DEA'S ENFORCEMENT EFFORTS

The DEA believes that international cooperation is the key in combating methamphetamine. Some of the most significant and successful international efforts to combat methamphetamine involve a series of enforcement initiatives worked jointly between law enforcement in the United States and Canada from the late 1990s into 2003. These enforcement initiatives, known as Operations MOUNTAIN EXPRESS I, II and III and Operation NORTHERN STAR, were principally responsible for the significant reduction in the amount of pseudoephedrine entering the United States for use in Mexican-controlled super labs. In turn, most of the super labs and the pseudoephedrine needed for them moved from the United States to Mexico.

DEA's longstanding enforcement efforts against methamphetamine include utilizing the Consolidated Priority Organization Targets (CPOTs) List, the Priority Target Organization (PTO) program, and the Organized Crime Drug Enforcement Task Force (OCDETF) program. The programs all provide assistance in identifying and targeting the most significant methamphetamine trafficking organizations, with the intent to disrupt and dismantle the organizations.

The FY 2006 CPOT list has identified 8 of the 46 designated organizations as being engaged in methamphetamine trafficking, 7 of these 8 are Mexican CPOT targets. At the end of the second quarter of FY 2006, the DEA had 149 active PTO investigations linked to those 7 CPOTs, of which 28 were active PTO investigations with methamphetamine as the primary type of drug. Since the inception of the PTO program in 2001, the DEA has either disrupted or dismantled more than 460 PTOs, where methamphetamine was the primary drug involved.

To enhance our international efforts to combat this drug, DEA has assigned Diversion Investigators (DIs) to a number of our foreign offices. These DIs, through their knowledge of pharmaceuticals and chemicals, play a critical role in preventing the diversion of List I chemicals which are used in the manufacture of methamphetamine and of pharmaceutical controlled substances. The DIs coordinate with foreign host country counterparts to establish effective systems of chemical controls and to ensure that customers in foreign countries receiving U.S. exports of pharmaceutically controlled substances are in fact legitimate companies. Foreign-based Diversion Investigators were intricately involved in two DEA operations in Hong Kong and Mexico run under the auspices of ***Project Prism*** that resulted in significant seizures of pseudoephedrine.

In addition to these DEA-specific activities, the DEA works internationally though a variety of existing international efforts. *Project Prism* is an international initiative aimed at assisting governments in developing and implementing operating procedures to control and more effectively monitor trade in ATS precursors to prevent their diversion. There are currently 95 countries and 5 international organizations participating in this initiative. Since March 2004, *Project Prism* has used pre-export notifications to monitor shipments of ephedrine, pseudoephedrine, pharmaceutical preparations containing ephedrine or pseudoephedrine, phenyl-2-propanone, and 3 ,4-methylenedioxyphenyl-2- propanone. Under *Project Prism* (through the end of 2005), over 5 metric tons of 60 milligram tablets of pseudoephedrine were seized in the United States, Mexico, and Panama. These pseudoephedrine tablets could have produced over 3 metric tons of methamphetamine (at a 60 percent conversion rate).

The FY 2006 Department of Justice Appropriations Act directs the Attorney General to establish a Methamphetamine Task Force (MTF) within DEA. The purpose of the Task Force is to improve and target the Federal government's policies on production and trafficking of methamphetamine. The MTF is comprised of three DEA Special Agents, two Diversion Investigators, three attorneys, and one Program Analyst. These are veteran personnel with extensive experience and knowledge in the field who will collect and analyze investigative and intelligence information from numerous sources. Their analysis will focus on trends in chemical trafficking and manufacturing methods, changes in trafficking routes and patterns, and regional abuse and distribution patterns. While DEA continues to aggressively target the flow of foreign and domestic precursor sources and smuggling efforts, to include methods of financing, the MTF will review DEA enforcement efforts with an eye toward identifying new trends. In addition, the MTF will be involved in chemical and equipment sources, methods of procurement, and clandestine laboratory cleanup issues. Another aspect of the MTF's duties will be making recommendations addressing issues that are identified from their analysis. These recommendations ultimately will be forwarded to the National Synthetic Drugs Interagency Working Group for review and action.

The DEA also continues its work to ensure that only legitimate businesses with adequate chemical controls are licensed to handle bulk pseudoephedrine and ephedrine in the United

States. In the past seven years, over 2,000 chemical registrants have been denied, surrendered, or withdrawn their registrations or applications as a result of DEA investigations. We investigated the adequacy of their security safeguards to prevent the diversion of chemicals to the illicit market, and audited their recordkeeping to ensure compliance with federal regulations. In addition to an initial on-site inspection, DEA Diversion Investigators, between 2001 and 2005, have physically re-inspected nearly seventy-five percent of the 3,000 chemical registrants at their place of business.

THE INTERNATIONAL CONTROL OF PRECURSOR CHEMICALS

With the increase in the diversion of precursor chemicals and the corresponding need for closer monitoring of chemical shipments, certain foreign governments in chemical source countries require a permit or written authorization from an importing country's government stating the legitimacy of the transaction. Under Federal law, the DEA must be notified only if an ephedrine or pseudoephedrine product is destined for, or will transit through, the United States. But the legal and regulatory tools to limit imports and after-import distribution were relatively insufficient. Moreover, the prevailing interpretation of the 1988 United Nation's Convention that controls chemicals exempts most finished pharmaceutical products containing pseudoephedrine in combination with other ingredients by allowing them to be shipped in international commerce without pre-notification—a loophole that continues to be exploited by drug traffickers. These pharmaceutical preparations contain pseudoephedrine and are used in the manufacture of methamphetamine. Since modification of the 1988 UN Convention is unrealistic, the United States, along with a number of our counterparts, has been working to gain international support for voluntary international cooperation to pre-notify shipments of these products. These efforts are being pursued by the U.S. through the drug control commission of the Organization of American States ("CICAD"), through the UN Commission on Narcotic Drugs, and bilaterally with selected nations.

Until passage of the Combat Methamphetamine Epidemic Act of 2005, U.S. law did not involve a permit-based system. Any company that imported or exported ephedrine, pseudoephedrine or phenylpropanolamine was required to notify the DEA of the transaction. This was not a permit for the transaction but rather a declaration that the transaction would take place. In other countries, companies must obtain a permit before importing or exporting regulated chemicals.

The 1988 U.N. Convention recommended that countries implement a permit system for chemical imports and exports, (Paragraph 8(b)(iii)), and some countries (e.g. Germany, China, and India) have implemented this system. Other countries consider chemicals such as pseudoephedrine to be pharmaceutical drugs and therefore issue permits for their import and export.

The Combat Methamphetamine Epidemic Act makes it unlawful to import into the United States ephedrine, pseudoephedrine, and phenylpropanolamine except as DEA, by delegation, finds to be necessary to provide for medical, scientific, or other legitimate purposes. DEA is working to implement this system through the promulgation of regulations. This system, in conjunction with a system of quotas for ephedrine, pseudoephedrine, and phenylpropanolamine also established by the Combat Methamphetamine Epidemic Act of

2005, will provide greater control over the importation and distribution of these three chemicals.

INTERNATIONAL COOPERATION

International cooperation is key in combating methamphetamine and its precursor chemicals.[5] The DEA has had the lead for the United States in working with our Mexican counterparts to combat methamphetamine. This cooperative effort extends into several areas of support. Since 2001, the DEA has provided training to our Mexican counterparts regarding clandestine laboratories, chemical training, and prosecution. Training has been provided to officials who regulate precursor chemicals and pharmaceuticals at the state and federal level within Mexico, as well as agents from the Agencia Federal de Investigaciones (AFI) and a number of prosecutors within the Mexican Organized Crime Unit (SIEDO). Over 450 students have received training through this cooperative effort.

In addition, the United States and Mexico have jointly obtained a commitment from Hong Kong not to ship chemicals to the United States, Mexico, or Panama until receiving an import permit or equivalent documentation and giving prior notification to the receiving country before shipment. If suspect shipments can be identified before they arrive in Mexico, it is easier for law enforcement to take effective action by either attempting to seize the shipment or by conducting a controlled delivery of the chemicals in order to identify the traffickers and the shipments ultimate destination.

Mexico has independently implemented several important voluntary controls on pseudoephedrine in cooperation with the industry, and is considering others. Those implemented now, or planned soon, include (1) limiting retail sales to pharmacies; (2) limiting sales quantities to three boxes of approximately 9 grams total; and (3) distributors voluntarily agreeing to limit sales to customers with appropriate government registrations (pharmacies) and with legitimate commercial needs.

Additionally, Mexico recently imposed a policy limiting imports of pseudoephedrine and ephedrine to manufacturers only, and limits importers to shipments of no more than 3 metric tons at a time. Wholesale distributors are barred from importing raw material pseudoephedrine and ephedrine. These importation restrictions have been coupled with recently imposed import quotas tied to estimates of national needs, which are based on extrapolations from a large population sample. Through a study, The Federal Commission for the Protection against Sanitary Risk (COFEPRIS) revealed that there is an excess of imports of pseudoephedrine products of approximately 60 to 100 metric tons. This study showed that the highest peak of respiratory diseases in Mexico was registered in 1999 with 29 million cases. That year, pseudoephedrine imports accounted for approximately 55,000 kilograms. In 2003, there was a slight decrease of reported respiratory diseases to approximately 27 million cases; however pseudoephedrine imports increased to 159,000 kilograms. Equally, in 2004 there were 28 million respiratory cases compared with 216,000 kilograms of pseudoephedrine imported. COFEPRIS determined that these imports were not related to the epidemiological index. The DEA has been advised that it is the Government of Mexico's intention to reduce pseudoephedrine and ephedrine importation permits to 70 tons, in 2006. These permits are to be split evenly among the Mexican-based pharmaceutical manufacturing companies. This is a significant reduction from the 2005 pseudoephedrine and ephedrine importation levels. Mexican officials have further advised that this 70 ton limit also applies to combination products containing pseudoephedrine and/or ephedrine.

Mexico's efforts to control methamphetamine precursor chemicals have not been limited to regulatory actions. An example of Mexico's pseudoephedrine interdiction efforts occurred during December 2005, when approximately 3.2 metric tons (approx. 5.1 million pseudoephedrine combination tablets) of pseudoephedrine were seized by Mexican authorities in the Port of Manzanillo, Mexico. The tablets were concealed within a shipment of electric fans, which were packaged in approximately 1,260 boxes. During the follow-up joint investigation conducted by DEA and the Hong Kong Customs and Excise Department, officials disclosed that the shipment of electric fans containing the tablets originated in mainland China and transited one of the mainland China/Hong Kong border crossings before being loaded on a marine vessel en route to Mexico.

In addition to these efforts with Mexico, the DEA, operating under the auspices of ***Project Prism,*** hosted a meeting in February in Hong Kong for law enforcement and regulatory officials from countries that produce ATS precursor chemicals. The purpose of this meeting was to develop and enhance systems for voluntary cooperation in data collection to build a consensus towards exchange of information on pharmaceutical preparations containing ephedrine and pseudoephedrine as well as bulk precursors. This was the first time that almost all of the countries that produce these chemicals and those countries affected by methamphetamine have sat down together to discuss this problem.

While there were some differences of opinion as to the manner and channels in which information regarding the licit trade in these substances should be exchanged, the communication that occurred between countries attending the open forum meeting was encouraging. Although we were disappointed that China chose not to send a delegation, the DEA, in cooperation with the Department of State, will continue discussions with all involved countries to determine the worldwide production of these chemicals, identify producers and distributors, gain better insight as to what form (bulk versus. tablets) the chemicals are manufactured and distributed at various stages, and learn where the chemicals are destined. In fact, during the week of June 5, a contingent from China came to DEA headquarters and met with high level officials in part, to discuss the many aspects involved in the importation of these precursor chemicals.

The Hong Kong meeting also helped to lay a foundation for the discussions and negotiation among concerned governments which led to the passage of a resolution at the 49th Commission on Narcotic Drugs (CND) in Vienna, Austria, in March of this year. The resolution, entitled "Strengthening Systems for Control of Precursor Chemicals Used in the Manufacture of Synthetic Drugs," involves the methamphetamine precursors previously mentioned, as well as preparations containing these substances, and phenyl-2-propanone (P2P) as well.

The resolution, which was adopted by the CND on March 15, 2006, calls on UN member states to provide to the International Narcotics Control Board (INCB) annual estimates of their legitimate requirements for these substances, and preparations containing these substances, and to ensure that its imports of these substances are commensurate with their respective nation's legitimate needs. It is anticipated that the legitimate requirements estimates provided to the INCB will be published in their annual precursor report, the next of which is scheduled to be released in March 2007.

The resolution also urges countries to continue to provide to the INCB, subject to their national legislation and taking care not to impede legitimate international commerce, information on all shipments of these substances, to include pharmaceutical preparations. Finally, the resolution requests countries grant permission to the INCB to share the shipment information on these consignments with concerned law enforcement and regulatory authorities to prevent or interdict diverted shipments. At present, DEA, as a member of the *Project Prism* task force, is working with the task force to come up with an initial initiative to address some of our specific concerns regarding the flow of these important precursors to the Western hemisphere.

While this resolution is an important first step, it will take several years to be fully implemented. Its success will depend upon our ability to obtain additional information from the INCB, which is contingent upon nations providing the information requested pursuant to the resolution.

Recent Developments

At the National Methamphetamine and Chemicals Initiative (NMCI) Strategy Conference in Dallas last month, Attorney General Gonzales announced important new anti-methamphetamine domestic initiatives as well as new partnerships between the U.S. and Mexico in fighting methamphetamine trafficking. Joined by Mexican Attorney General Daniel Cabeza De Vaca, Attorney General Gonzales unveiled several Department of Justice-led initiatives aimed at improved enforcement, increased law enforcement training, improved information-sharing, and increasing public awareness.

Among the U.S./Mexico partnership efforts is an agreement between DEA and the Government of Mexico to establish specialized methamphetamine enforcement teams on both sides of the border. In Mexico, these teams will focus on investigating and targeting the most wanted Mexican methamphetamine drug trafficking organizations, while DEA-led efforts on the U.S. side will focus on the methamphetamine traffickers and organizations transporting and distributing the methamphetamine that was produced in Mexico.

Other initiatives that are part of the U.S./Mexico partnership include:

A new DEA and U. S. Customs and Border Protection Service effort to focus on ports of interest within the United States and target suspicious cargo that is likely to be related to methamphetamine trafficking organizations;

A bi-national Law Enforcement Working Group that will focus on methamphetamine production and trafficking from both an enforcement and intelligence perspective;

A DEA and Mexican CENAPI effort to further share intelligence information and continue to develop stronger working relationships. Such collaborative efforts will focus on investigating large-scale meth trafficking organizations that are operating in Mexico and the United States.

A "Most Wanted Methamphetamine and Chemical Drug Trafficking Organization List" jointly developed by DEA and Mexican police. The list will focus bilateral law enforcement efforts on the most significant threats;

An agreement between the DEA Office of Diversion Control and Mexico's chemical regulatory agency, COFEPRIS, to a personnel exchange in which chemical regulatory experts from within each agency will be embedded within the other's agency for a specific period to observe, learn best practices, and then implement joint strategies complimentary to both regulatory agencies;

The transfer of eight DEA trucks used in clandestine lab enforcement operations that have been refurbished and donated to Mexico to be used by specialized Mexican methamphetamine enforcement teams; and

A new DEA-led training effort for nearly 1,000 Mexican police officials to focus on a variety of investigative, enforcement, and regulatory methods related to methamphetamine trafficking which is being funded by the Department of State's (DOS) Bureau for International Narcotics and Law Enforcement Affairs (INL).

Domestically, as part of this announcement, the DEA is expanding the primary focus of our clandestine lab enforcement teams. The significant reduction in the number of domestic small toxic labs this year, due in large part to recent legislation restricting access to methamphetamine precursor chemicals, will allow these teams to expand their efforts beyond dismantling methamphetamine labs to also include the targeting Mexican methamphetamine trafficking organizations. These DEA clandestine lab teams will use their lab expertise to trace chemicals, finished methamphetamine, and drug proceeds to drug trafficking organizations in the U.S. and Mexico. These teams also will work to identify and dismantle U.S.-based methamphetamine transportation and distribution cells.

Other DEA domestic initiatives include creating a national listing on the DEA Web site of the addresses of properties in which methamphetamine labs or chemical dumpsites have been found. The registry will provide information for owners or renters that a property has been used to produce methamphetamine, as a public service alert that there may be potential toxic hazards within the property, if not rendered safe by clean-up efforts.

In addition, a new clandestine lab training facility at the DEA Academy in Quantico, Virginia, will be established in the fall of 2006. At this facility, DEA will train US and foreign law enforcement officials on the latest techniques in clandestine lab detection, enforcement, and safety in a state-of-the- art facility.

As stated by Attorney General Gonzales at the NMCI conference last month, "These initiatives represent a policy of true mutual cooperation that will put methamphetamine use and all its horrors firmly on the road to extinction. If we work together, sharing resources and intelligence, the law enforcement agencies of both the U.S. and Mexico will be able to better attack the meth problem at every stage in the production and distribution chain."

New Tools in the Fight Against Methamphetamine

Many states have enacted various types of legislation to control the sale of pseudoephedrine. With the recent passage of the Combat Methamphetamine Epidemic Elimination Act of 2005, the combination of State and federal legislation has begun to have some effect. Although the overall number of STLs in the United States is decreasing, the demand for methamphetamine has not diminished. DEA will continue to use the additional tools we have been given to address both domestic and international components in this battle.

In an effort to provide further information to America's youth about the dangers of methamphetamine, the DEA developed and launched a website entitled "justthinktwice.com." This website is devoted to and designed by teenagers to give them the hard facts about methamphetamine and other illicit drugs. Through this website, the DEA is telling teens to "think twice" about what they hear from friends, popular culture, and adults who advocate drug legalization. Information is also provided regarding the harm drugs cause to their health, their families, the environment, and to innocent bystanders.

Internationally, the Combat Methamphetamine Epidemic Act of 2005 will expand the notice of importation to include all information known to the importer on the chain of distribution. If it is determined that the importer is refusing to cooperate in providing such information, or DEA has concerns about the downstream customer, the DEA may issue an order prohibiting the importation of Scheduled Listed Chemical Products (SLCP). Further, the Act requires the DOS to identify the five largest exporting countries and the five largest importing countries with the highest diversion of SLCPs and provide an economic analysis of worldwide production as compared to legitimate demand. Combined with the other measures of the Act which provide for the domestic regulation of precursor chemicals, the Combat Methamphetamine Epidemic Act of 2005 provides effective new tools to use in the battle against methamphetamine.

CONCLUSION

The DEA continues to fight methamphetamine on all fronts. Our enforcement efforts are focused on disrupting and dismantling the highest level methamphetamine trafficking organizations operating on both a domestic and international level. DEA enforcement and diversion initiatives involve not just the "finished product," but also the precursor chemicals necessary to produce this poison. To further enhance our efforts, the DEA has initiated an internal methamphetamine task force, which will help coordinate our overall efforts to combat this drug.

As the international threat of methamphetamine spreads, cooperative efforts among nations become vital. Cooperative efforts and initiatives to combat methamphetamine production and control chemical shipments on an international scale are critical to DEA's ability to combat methamphetamine trafficking in the U.S.

Thank you for the opportunity to appear before you today to discuss this important issue. I will be happy to answer any questions that you may have.

End Notes

[1] Phenylpropanolamine is a precursor chemical for amphetamine, rather than methamphetamine, although the production process is essentially identical.

[2] There were 5,120 defendants charged in FY 2005, compared to 3,815 defendants charged in FY 2001.

[3] There were 4,839 defendants sentenced in FY 2005 (including both Pre-Booker and Post-Booker cases), compared to 3,414 defendants sentenced in FY 2001.

[4] In Europe and Asia the term "amphetamine-type stimulants" is used rather than a specific reference to methamphetamine. The term ATS includes the following: amphetamine, methamphetamine, and MDMA (Ecstasy), and its analogues. This term is also used by the United Nations

[5] One of the most significant and successful international efforts to combat methamphetamine's precursor chemicals involved a series of enforcement initiatives worked jointly between law enforcement in the United States and Canada from the late 1990s into 2003. These enforcement initiatives, known as Operations Mountain Express I, II and III and Operation Northern Star, were principally responsible for the significant reduction in the amount of pseudoephedrine entering the United States for use in Mexican controlled super labs. In turn, most of these super labs and the pseudoephedrine required for the labs to produce methamphetamine moved from the United States to Mexico.

In: Methamphetamine: Background, Controls and Issues
Editor: Andrea S. Sandoval
ISBN: 978-1-60692-548-5

Chapter 8

EFFORTS TO CONTROL THE INTERNATIONAL PRODUCTION AND TRAFFICKING OF METHAMPHETAMINE

Anne W. Patterson

Chairman Hagel, Chairman Coleman, Senator Sarbanes, Senator Dodd, and other distinguished Members, thank you for the opportunity to discuss the Department of State's efforts to curb the international production and trafficking of methamphetamine. I appreciate your continuing interest in this growing challenge and thank you for holding a hearing on such an important and timely subject.

Methamphetamine abuse continues to be an enormous problem in this country. Current data on drug and laboratory seizures suggest that roughly 80 percent of the methamphetamine used in the United States comes from larger laboratories, which are increasingly found in Mexico. As we have reported in the annual *International Narcotics Control Strategy Report* (INCSR), methamphetamine abuse is a growing problem throughout the world. According to the UN Office on Drugs and Crime's (UNODC) latest statistics, approximately 35 million people in the world use amphetamine- type stimulants (ATS),[1] including methamphetamine and ecstasy.

Synthetic drugs such as methamphetamine and ecstasy present a unique challenge to our international drug control policy. These drugs are relatively easy and inexpensive to produce, offer enormous profit margins, and often do not have the same social stigma associated with the use of other drugs. Unlike drugs derived from organic materials, such as cocaine or heroin, their production is not limited to a specific geographic region. Therefore, we must remain vigilant to ensure that progress in one area is not offset by setbacks in others.

In order to address international methamphetamine production and trafficking, the Department of State plays an integral role in the Administration's *Synthetic Drug Control Strategy*. We emphasize two key areas: (1) seeking greater international control and transparency in the production, sale, and transportation of methamphetamine's precursor chemicals and the pharmaceutical preparations containing them; and (2) significantly expanding our support and cooperation with the Government of Mexico on precursor control and other methamphetamine specific initiatives.

INTERNATIONAL PRECURSOR CHEMICAL CONTROL

Most of the methamphetamine consumed in the United States – somewhere between 75 and 85 percent – is produced with chemicals that are diverted from the legitimate flow of international commerce. Therefore, a central focus of the Administration's strategy is to encourage transparency in the international trade in methamphetamine's precursor chemicals and the pharmaceutical preparations containing them.

The most comprehensive agreement on international chemical control is the 1988 UN *Convention Against Illicit Traffic in Narcotic Drugs and Psychotropic Substances*. While the Convention covers methamphetamine's precursor chemicals such as ephedrine and pseudoephedrine, it exempts finished pharmaceutical preparations containing them. This situation allows criminal organizations to circumvent the Convention by purchasing uncontrolled pharmaceutical preparations on the international market, instead of the regulated bulk precursor chemicals. Furthermore, many countries have simply been reluctant to share information regarding their trade in these substances, because much of the data is commercially sensitive. Complicating matters further, in some countries, these chemicals are regulated by health officials, rather than law enforcement agencies.

Given these challenges, we have found that seeking voluntary cooperation, based on mutual benefit, is the best way to obtain information on the trade in precursor chemicals beyond what is required by the Convention. The U.S. Drug Enforcement Administration (DEA) has been successful in this regard. DEA works with its international drug law enforcement and regulatory partners to target organizations involved in the trafficking of these essential precursor chemicals. By promoting voluntary cooperation between law enforcement entities, pursuant to joint investigations, DEA has been able to monitor some suspect shipments to detect and prevent the diversion of chemicals for illicit uses.

DEA also works with foreign law enforcement and regulatory counterparts through *Project Prism*, an international initiative supported by the International Narcotics Control Board (INCB). *Project Prism* brings together relevant institutions and experts from Member States in order to assist governments in developing and implementing operating procedures to control and more effectively monitor the trade in precursor chemicals. *Project Prism* also collects information on pre-export notifications to monitor shipments of the essential precursor chemicals used to produce methamphetamine and other synthetic drugs.

Beyond these established mechanisms to ensure that chemical imports are inline with legitimate requirements, the Department of State, DEA, and the Office of National Drug Control Policy (ONDCP) are working to elevate the threat of methamphetamine in international fora and in bilateral relations. In March, a U.S. sponsored resolution entitled *Strengthening Systems for Control of Precursor Chemicals Used in the Manufacture of Synthetic Drugs* was adopted by consensus at the 49th UN Commission on Narcotic Drugs (CND).[2] This resolution specifically requests countries to provide the INCB with annual estimates of their legitimate requirements for PMK (a precursor for ecstasy), pseudoephedrine, ephedrine, and phenyl-2-propanone (P2P), as well as the pharmaceutical preparations containing these substances. The resolution also requests countries to permit the INCB to share such information with concerned law enforcement and regulatory agencies. In addition, the INCB has since agreed to publish the data collected on legitimate requirements, which will allow governments to track any spikes in imports, a possible signal of illegal diversion.

The resolution also urges countries to continue to provide to the INCB – subject to their national legislation and taking care not to impede legitimate international commerce – information on all shipments of these substances, including pharmaceutical preparations containing them. Finally, the resolution requests that countries grant permission to the INCB to share the shipment information on these consignments with concerned law enforcement and regulatory authorities to prevent or interdict diverted shipments.

To promote the full implementation of this resolution, the Department of State intends to contribute $700,000 in FY 2006 funds, double our FY 2005 contribution, to help fund the INCB's activities. While we consider the adoption of our CND resolution an important first step, we will continue to encourage countries to actively provide information to the INCB and support its expanding role. The Department of State, DEA, and ONDCP will also work to identify new mechanisms that might promote the further exchange of information and expertise pertinent to the control of methamphetamine and other synthetics.

Finally, the Department of State also works through the Inter- American Drug Abuse Control Commission (CICAD), to evaluate the use of precursor chemicals and assist countries in strengthening controls. Many nations in the Western Hemisphere still lack the capacity to distinguish between the legitimate international trade in precursor chemicals and pharmaceuticals, and any excess production that is being diverted for illicit use. Therefore, the United States, through its work with CICAD, has assisted in the development of model regulations, information-sharing mechanisms, and guides and reference tools for the control of chemicals.

Cooperation with Mexico

Early in my tenure I visited Mexico and met with many officials who were increasingly concerned about Mexico's own problem with methamphetamine abuse and addiction. Methamphetamine is a common challenge, as the drug is now harming communities in Mexico along traditional drug trafficking routes, which is an inevitable part of the drug business.

It is likely that methamphetamine production has steadily migrated into Mexico, because production in the United States and Canada has declined due to stricter regulations and enhanced law enforcement efforts. Today, Mexican drug trafficking organizations now produce and traffic a large percentage of the methamphetamine consumed in the United States. They also control super labs, a laboratory capable of producing 10 pounds or more of methamphetamine within a single production cycle, located throughout Mexico and California. These same Mexican criminal organizations control most mid-level and retail methamphetamine distribution in the Pacific, Southwest, and west-central regions of the United States, as well as much of the distribution in the Great Lakes and Southeast regions. It is also likely that these organizations are capitalizing on their huge resources and existing smuggling and distribution networks to traffic methamphetamine into the United States. However, Mexico is increasingly aware of its own methamphetamine problem and is beginning to make progress in limiting imports of the essential chemicals used to produce methamphetamine.

Between 2002 and 2004, Mexico saw a remarkable 140 percent increase in its imports of pseudoephedrine and ephedrine, indicating a strong likelihood of illegal diversion. Recognizing that these imports far exceeded legitimate demand, Mexico enacted a series of regulations and policies to restrict imports and better regulate the sale of precursor chemicals. For instance, between 2004 and 2005, the Mexican government banned pseudoephedrine imports of over three tons and restricted the importation of pseudoephedrine to only drug companies. In order to further prevent the illegal diversion of these chemicals, Mexico restricted the sale of pseudoephedrine-based products to only licensed pharmacies, restricted the amount that can be purchased by an individual, and instituted a policy that requires all shipments of pseudoephedrine to be transported in police- escorted armored vehicles equipped with GPS tracking systems. In 2005, the result of these import restrictions and domestic regulations was a 40 percent reduction of legitimate imports and this year the Government of Mexico is committed to reducing imports even further. However, the threat of illegal smuggling of precursor chemicals and pharmaceutical preparations from third countries into Mexico will continue to be a challenge.

To counter illegal smuggling and methamphetamine production, the State Department works closely with the Government of Mexico on a wide range of counterdrug, law enforcement, and border security initiatives, and provides assistance and training that specifically targets methamphetamine.

For instance, we are supporting the enhancement of a Sensitive Investigations Unit dedicated to targeting criminal groups involved in methamphetamine production and trafficking. Working with DEA we are assisting in the establishment of specialized Mexican Clandestine Laboratory Response Teams to target organizations involved in the operation of clandestine methamphetamine labs and are providing training for a select group of Mexican authorities to improve prosecutions in chemical control and synthetic drug cases. In cooperation with DEA, we provided Mexico with a new mobile laboratory vehicle equipped with specialized equipment to safely locate and dismantle methamphetamine labs. We have also refurbished and donated eight additional used laboratory vehicles to Mexican law enforcement.

In addition, the Department continues to provide basic training and technical assistance to Mexican chemical control agencies in order to promote comprehensive chemical control projects. Together with UNODC, we have also supported a national computer data system that permits the Government of Mexico to monitor the importation and movement of chemicals used for methamphetamine production at 17 sites throughout the country.

Along with these methamphetamine-specific initiatives, we will continue ongoing programs that directly confront methamphetamine trafficking, including: targeting international crime along our common border, enhancing Mexican law enforcement's ability to disrupt the international drug trade, and continuing cooperation and coordination between the law enforcement agencies of our two countries.

Currently, the Interagency is in the process of finalizing the implementation strategy for the *National Southwest Border*

Counternarcotics Strategy that has identified key strategic objectives and provide specific recommendations to address the illicit narcotics threat and significantly improve overall interdiction efforts along the Southwest Border. This strategy reflects the Department of State's long-range objective to strengthen the Government of Mexico's law enforcement capacity.

East and South East Asia

While most of the Department of State's efforts to curb methamphetamine production, trafficking, and abuse concentrate on international precursor chemical control and cooperation with Mexico, we also have smaller programs in Asia, where 60 percent of the world's ATS users live (most of whom are methamphetamine users in East and South- East Asia). The scope of the problem in Asia is quite troubling. For example, methamphetamine is by far the most commonly abused drug in Thailand. Japan has an estimated 600,000 addicts and between one and three million "casual" users nationwide. And in the Philippines, statistics from rehabilitation centers show that 84 percent of patients list methamphetamine as their drug of choice.

While the United States is not the destination market for these narcotics, Asia produces the majority of the world's ATS to feed growing demand in Oceana and East and South East Asia. To help stem production, trafficking, and abuse in East and South East Asia, the Department of State has supported bilateral and multilateral efforts. We have provided funding to the ASEAN and China Cooperative Operations in Response to Dangerous Drugs (ACCORD) program to combat drug production, trafficking, and abuse, with a particular focus on ATS. We have also provided funding to Indonesia and the Philippines for DEA law enforcement training, including: basic drug investigations, chemical control, and clandestine laboratory training. Finally, the Department of State has provided support for demand reduction and treatment programs in Laos, Thailand, Vietnam, Cambodia, and elsewhere in Southeast Asia. Demand reduction programs like these and others have been proven highly effective throughout the world and can be implemented through correctional systems, schools, religious institutions, or even civil society groups.

Implementing the International Provisions of the Combat Methamphetamine Epidemic Act

The Department of State has begun taking steps to implement the international provisions of the Combat Methamphetamine Epidemic Act (CMEA). Beginning on March 1, 2007, our annual INCSR will include a new section reporting on the top five exporters of methamphetamine's precursor chemicals and pharmaceutical preparations containing them, as well as the top five importers of these chemicals with the highest rates of diversion. After this chapter is issued, the President will then determine if the identified countries are "cooperating fully" with the United States or taking adequate measures on their own to address the production and trafficking of illegal drugs. Shortly after the INCSR is submitted to Congress, the Department of State will then issue a separate report on the countries that were not "certified" by the President. This additional report will address steps being taken by the country (or countries) to prevent the diversion of precursor chemicals and pharmaceutical preparations. The CMEA also requires a report on the total worldwide production as compared to the legitimate demand for these chemicals. In addition, we are complying with the CMEA by continuing our bilateral partnership with Mexico and will be reporting on our cooperation on chemical control and law enforcement activities with the Government of Mexico.

Currently, the Department has established an interagency International Chemical Assessment Work Group composed of experts from the Department of State, ONDCP, DEA, the Department of Justice, the U.S. Trade Representative, the intelligence community, and other relevant agencies to develop a methodology for how countries will be evaluated in accordance with the CMEA. Based on this group's recommendations, the Department of State will develop guidance for our overseas Embassies on how to best report on the information required by the CMEA. This process will augment any commercial data that is publicly available to determine the top five exporters and top five importers with the highest rate of diversion.

CONCLUSION

I would like to close by thanking Congress for its leadership on this issue. The CMEA has provided the Administration with new tools and has focused our efforts on this important issue. I look forward to continue working with Congress, the U.S. law enforcement community, and global partners in meeting and countering this common threat. Thank you for the opportunity to testify today and I look forward to answering your questions.

End Notes

[1] ATS generally refers to amphetamine, methamphetamine, and MDMA (ecstasy), and its analogues.

[2] The UN Commission on Narcotic Drugs is the central policy-making body within the United Nations system dealing with drug-related matters.

In: Methamphetamine: Background, Controls and Issues ISBN: 978-1-60692-548-5
Editor: Andrea S. Sandoval

Chapter 9

TESTIMONY BY THE HONORABLE JOHN P. WALTERS, DIRECTOR, OFFICE OF NATIONAL DRUG CONTROL POLICY, BEFORE THE SUBCOMMITTEE ON INTERNATIONAL ECONOMIC POLICY, EXPORT AND TRADE PROMOTIONS

INTRODUCTION

Chairman Hagel, Chairman Coleman, Senator Sarbanes, Senator Dodd, and distinguished Members of the Subcommittees: thank you for the opportunity to appear before you today to discuss such an important issue and to address our international efforts against methamphetamine and its precursors.

Since the early 1990s, and especially over the last few years, the illicit use of synthetic drugs has become a severe and troubling problem, at both the international and national levels. The most devastating of these synthetic drugs for the United States has been methamphetamine.

In response to these developments, in October 2004, the United States Government released the *National Synthetic Drugs Action Plan*, the first comprehensive national plan to address the problems of synthetic and pharmaceutical drug trafficking and abuse. The *Action Plan* outlined current Federal and state efforts in the areas of prevention, treatment, regulation, and law enforcement and made concrete recommendations for enhancing government efforts to reduce synthetic drug abuse.

On June 1, building on these earlier efforts ONDCP, DOJ, DHS and HHS released the *Synthetic Drug Control Strategy*. The *Synthetics Strategy*, a companion document to the President's *National Drug Control Strategy*, details plans for unprecedented cooperation with Mexico and other international partners to drastically reduce the flow into the United States of both methamphetamine and the precursor chemicals used to produce the drug. The *Synthetics Strategy* calls for 15 percent reductions in methamphetamine use and prescription drug abuse over the next three years and a 25 percent reduction in domestic meth labs.

The *Synthetics Strategy* outlines a three-tiered approach to the United States' international efforts: improving intelligence and information on the global market for precursor chemicals; effective implementation of the Combat Meth Act, signed into law by President Bush this March, which sets a national standard for restricting the retail sale of precursor chemicals within the United States; and strengthening law enforcement and border control activities, particularly with Mexico.

The Spread of Meth & Latest Trend Data

In the past decade and a half, methamphetamine use has spread eastward across the United States. Between 1992 and 2003, the treatment admission rate for methamphetamine and amphetamine increased from 10 to 57 admissions per 100,000 population aged 12 or older (an increase of over 470 percent). Additionally, between 2001 and 2004, the positive drug-testing rates among the general United States workforce for methamphetamine/ amphetamine increased from 0.29 percent to 0.52 percent of all tests (an increase of 79 percent). However, this trend reversed in 2005 when the incidence of methamphetamine/amphetamine positive drug-testing rates declined 8% to 0.48 percent. The news is even more encouraging when we look only at methamphetamine, which we can do for the first time thanks to a new analysis of the testing results by Quest Diagnostics. The incidence of methamphetamine positives dropped from 0.3 3% in 2004 to 0.26% in 2005 and down further, to 0.18%, for the first five months of 2006, a 45 percent reduction over two years and significant downward trend.

There is additional good news when we look closely at the data for youth drug use. Methamphetamine use rates have dropped by almost one-third among 8th , 10th and 12th graders combined since 2001. The Center for Disease Control's Youth Risk Behavior Survey found a 3 6.7% decline in lifetime youth meth use since 2001. There is much additional work to do to fight the threat of methamphetamine, both at home and abroad, but the latest information we have received is good news for Americans.

United States' Response

In response to the increased threat from methamphetamine, United States law enforcement agencies have increased their efforts both domestically and internationally to stem the flow of methamphetamine and the precursors that are used to produce it. States have also taken decisive action with dramatic results.

Within the past two years, 39 states have imposed new regulations on the retail sale of the methamphetamine precursor pseudoephedrine (P SE) and preparations that contain pseudoephedrine. These restrictions vary from state to state in their severity and content, as the severity and nature of the meth problem itself differs significantly among different states. States with the strictest pseudoephedrine laws have seen significant reductions in the seizure of small toxic labs. For example, 1,063 lab incidents occurred in Oklahoma in 2003. After instituting strict laws controlling pseudoephedrine in March 2004, lab seizures in Oklahoma dropped by 37.3 percent to 667 lab incidents in 2004. Only 218 labs were reported seized in Oklahoma during 2005, a dramatic decline of 67.3% from the previous year. As more states have adopted similar restrictions, and as states and the federal government have taken other actions to combat use of the drug, the United States has seen national declines in the number of super labs and total labs seized. In fact, the total number of lab incidents in the United States declined from 17,675 in 2004 to 12,213 in 2005. This substantial 30.9% decline is the result of the hard work by state, local, and federal law enforcement officers across this country, as well as enactment and effective implementation of new laws controlling precursors enacted by 39 states.

Congress has also taken decisive steps to combat methamphetamine production and precursor diversion through the passage of the Combat Meth Act. This legislation is an important and positive step forward and has provided many useful tools both domestically and internationally.

Many of the restrictions on consumer retail sales of products containing pseudoephedrine have been in effect for over two months with remainder of the restrictions taking effect 30 September 2006. The reduction of domestic methamphetamine production has been achieved by controlling the precursors used to make the drug and when the Combat Meth Act is fully implemented we expect this national trend to continue. Concerning national demand for legitimate products containing pseudoephedrine, ephedrine, and phenylpropanolamine, the Drug Enforcement Administration is gathering and analyzing information regarding the licit national demand for these products, so that the agency may meet its obligation under the Combat Meth Act to set manufacturing quotas. We expect the retail sales restrictions and the ceiling on pseudoephedrine imports to have a significant positive affect on the domestic diversion of pseudoephedrine.

The Combat Meth Act also contains mechanisms to assist in reducing international diversion of methamphetamine precursors. The Department of State will identify the top five exporters and the top five importers of ephedrine, pseudoephedrine, and phenylpropanolmine, (which are the precursors for methamphetamine/amphetamine), with the highest rate of diversion for illicit uses. The State Department will publish the list of those countries in the annual International Narcotics Control Strategy Report that will be released no later than March 1, 2007. The President will determine whether the identified countries are "cooperating fully" with the United States or taking adequate measures on their own to address the production and trafficking of illegal drugs. The Department of State has formed an interagency working group to develop and implement a workable methodology that will be used to identify the top five countries in each category. The Administration is committed to using the new tools provided by the Combat Meth Act effectively to foster better international controls on methamphetamine precursors.

Reducing precursor diversion and decreasing the number of domestic labs not only reduces methamphetamine production and the environmental damage caused by the production process, but also reduces the threat that these labs pose to our citizens. Methamphetamine production and use exact a huge toll on families and particularly children. Methamphetamine production can occur in homes and apartments where children live, exposing them to a variety of toxic and noxious substances. The research of current and future health risks of such exposure is ongoing, but it appears that the consequences to the health of the meth-exposed child are severe. Children of methamphetamine users are also exposed to the numerous social and developmental problems that result from their parent's abuse problem. While under the influence of methamphetamine, these parents do not care for themselves, let alone their children. While on a multi-day methamphetamine binge, these parents have no interest in the needs of a child; they are simply focused on their high. When the binge ends they sleep for days at a time, while their children continue to be without parental care.

In October 2003, the Office of National Drug Control Policy launched a national Drug-Endangered-Children initiative to assist with coordination among existing state programs that help rehabilitate children who have been affected by methamphetamine. The results of this initiative have been promising with the number of affected children, as reported by the National Drug-Endangered-Children Program, dropping from 3,708 in 2003, to 3,104 in 2004 and for 2005 there were 1,660 affected children reported. Although this trend is promising we must continue our efforts.

The United States has had domestic success fighting the spread of methamphetamine production by controlling the precursors. We can achieve this impact globally by working cooperatively with our international partners. Disrupting the methamphetamine market will continue to rely on our ability to work together to reduce the flow of methamphetamine and prevent the diversion of its precursors – principally pseudoephedrine, ephedrine, and pharmaceutical preparations that include these chemicals.

International Efforts

In targeting international methamphetamine production, the Department of Justice, primarily acting through the Drug Enforcement Administration, is the lead U.S. government agency. Recently, its attention has been focused primarily on Mexico—a major producer or transshipment point for much of the methamphetamine entering America.

Over the past few years, rising seizures at the U. S. Southwest border indicate increasing production of methamphetamine within Mexico, as do reports of additional methamphetamine lab seizures within Mexico, and reports from state and local law enforcement throughout the United States concerning the influx of out-of-state methamphetamine within their jurisdictions.

The increase in Southwest Border seizures of methamphetamine from 2001 to 2004 has been significant with 1,170 kilograms in 2001; 1,130 kilograms in 2002; 1,790 kilograms in 2003; and, 2,320 kilograms in 2004.

Because the U.S. government's counterdrug, counterterror, and immigration enforcement missions are interrelated, improved counterdrug efforts will also enhance border security. In February 2005, the President's Homeland Security Advisor directed the development of a strategy to address the drug threat to the Southwest Border. Interagency efforts, at this time, are culminating in a coordinated *National Southwest Border Counternarcotics Strategy* that will identify key strategic objectives and provide specific recommendations to address the illicit narcotics threat and significantly improve overall interdiction efforts along the Southwest Border.

Although this is a significant and growing threat, Mexico has taken some important steps. Through its Federal Commission for the Protection Against Sanitary Risks (COFEPRIS), the government of Mexico is implementing several important wholesale and retail controls on pseudoephedrine in cooperation with the pharmaceutical industry and is considering others. Mexican pharmacies are moving pseudoephedrine combination products behind the counter and limiting retail sales to 9 grams. In addition, Mexico recently imposed a policy limiting imports of pseudoephedrine and ephedrine to manufacturers only. Wholesale distributors are barred from importing raw pseudoephedrine and ephedrine. Furthermore, importers can import shipments of no more than 3,000 kilograms at a time. Mexico also has begun imposing import quotas tied to estimates of licit national need after a study revealed that imports far exceeded this amount. As a result, Mexico's PSE imports have dropped from 216 metric tons in 2004 (COFEPRIS), to 132.5 metric tons in 2005 (COFEPRIS), with a goal of 70 metric tons for 2006 (COFEPRIS).

With United States support, Mexico is training and equipping methamphetamine-focused law enforcement teams to combat the spread of methamphetamine production in Mexico. DEA is providing laboratory investigation and processing training for Mexican law enforcement elements, enabling them to identify and destroy methamphetamine labs. Additionally, Mexican authorities have seized more than 55 million methamphetamine precursor pills since December 2000.

Canada, like Mexico, is aiding in the fight against trafficking and diversion. Canada has taken numerous steps over the past few years to prevent the diversion of pseudoephedrine and ephedrine through increased control of imports and exports. From 2000 to 2004, lawful pseudoephedrine imports into Canada fell from just over 500 to less than 50 metric tons. Additionally, from 2003 to 2004, lawful ephedrine imports fell from 19 to 7 metric tons, and overall pseudoephedrine and methamphetamine seizures of shipments into the United States have dropped over the past year. These reduced precursor imports into Canada resulted in sharp declines in the amounts of pseudoephedrine and ephedrine diverted into the United States for the manufacture of methamphetamine. The number of Superlabs in the United States detected by law enforcement fell from 143 in 2002 and 130 in 2003 to just 55 in 2004 and seizures of pseudoephedrine at our northern border are now down by 92 percent.

In addition to working with Mexico and Canada on this issue, the United States continues to work with the primary producing and exporting countries for bulk ephedrine and pseudoephedrine—China, Germany, and India. In addition to working with each of these nations multi-laterally, which I will address when discussing the recently adopted U.S. sponsored resolution at the Commission on Narcotic Drugs (CND), DEA continues to actively work cooperatively with each of these nations on precursor chemical investigation and regulatory issues. To accomplish this task, DEA has assigned chemical Diversion Investigators to their country offices in each of these nations to address this important issue.

The United States and Mexico are also working to gain broader international support for pre-notification of international shipments of combination tablets containing pseudoephedrine through multilateral bodies such as the Organization of American States and the Project Prism initiative facilitated by the United Nations International Narcotics Control Board. Extending these pre-export notifications (PENs) to pharmaceutical preparations that contain pseudoephedrine and ephedrine are critical to controlling the diversion of precursors. Under the 1988 UN Convention on Psychotropic Substances, signatory countries are only required to provide PENs on bulk pseudoephedrine, bulk ephedrine, and single-entity tablets containing these substances; pharmaceutical preparations (combination products) are exempt. Additionally, unlike the United States, many nations have not suffered the significant costs associated with Small Toxic Labs. Many countries are either unaware that diverted pharmaceutical preparations containing pseudoephedrine or ephedrine are often used as the main precursor for methamphetamine production (and how easily they can be converted into methamphetamine), or face continued challenges in stopping this diversion.

Multi-faceted Approach

ONDCP, the DEA, and the Department of State are working with the major PSE and Ephedrine producing/exporting countries of China, Germany, and India on a multi-faceted approach:

(1) I am meeting with the ambassadors from these countries to discuss Amphetamine-Type Stimulants (ATS) and precursor control/diversion issues. To date, I have met with the Chinese Ambassador to the United States, Zhou Wenzhong, the Deputy Chief of Mission of the Indian Embassy, Ambassador R.S. Jassal and the Head of the European Union's Delegation to the United States, John Bruton. The meetings were very positive and productive; all expressed their desire to work with the United States on solutions to this problem.

(2) In late February 2006, DEA hosted a meeting in Hong Kong with Law Enforcement Officials from India, Germany, and several major PSE and ephedrine importing countries to discuss PSE and ephedrine diversion control issues. There was an overall agreement that more must be done internationally to control diversion and it was a significant first step in the process.

(3) In March 2006, at the 49th United Nations Commission on Narcotic Drugs (CND) in Vienna, Member States adopted a U.S. sponsored resolution on synthetics drugs. The resolution:

  (a) Requests that countries estimate their licit need for PSE and ephedrine (in addition to precursor chemicals for ecstasy) as well as the pharmaceutical preparations containing them. By knowing countries' licit requirements, the resolution aims to reduce surpluses and potential diversion of the precursors.
  (b) Requests exporting countries to verify the authenticity of each export shipment.
  (c) Urges exporting countries to provide to the International Narcotics Control Board information on all shipments of pseudoephedrine, ephedrine, licit pharmaceutical preparations containing these substances, and other chemicals.
  (d) Requests member states to allow the International Narcotics Control Board to share shipment information with concerned countries' law enforcement and regulatory authorities to prevent or interdict diverted shipments. The intent is to prevent diversion while not impeding legitimate international commerce.
  (e) Requests countries to ensure that the quantity of imports is commensurate with their legitimate requirements

Implementation of the resolution will mean that each country that exports or imports methamphetamine precursors will be pressured to take concrete actions. Our government will be working through our Embassies to encourage countries to move quickly to meet their new obligations. In addition we will continue to provide assistance, through the State Department, to the INCB to facilitate their administration of these new measures.

CONCLUSION

The United States has had significant success fighting the spread of methamphetamine production by controlling precursor chemicals domestically. This type of impact can be achieved globally if nations combat the problem cooperatively. Disrupting the methamphetamine market will depends on our ability to work together to prevent the diversion of its precursors – principally pseudoephedrine, ephedrine, and pharmaceutical preparations that include these chemicals used in manufacturing the drug and then to crimp the flow of manufactured methamphetamine coming into the United States.

Thank you again for the opportunity to testify on this important topic, and I welcome any questions the Subcommittees may have regarding methamphetamine, and the Administration's efforts to reduce its use, production, trafficking, and the diversion of its precursors.

In: Methamphetamine: Background, Controls and Issues ISBN: 978-1-60692-548-5
Editor: Andrea S. Sandoval

Chapter 10

REMARKS PREPARED FOR DELIVERY BY ATTORNEY GENERAL MICHAEL B. MUKASEY AT THE NATIONAL METHAMPHETAMINE CHEMICALS INITIATIVE CONFERENCE-ST. LOUIS, MISSOURI-MAY 7, 2008

Good morning. Thank you Director Walters. And thanks to all of you for inviting me to join you today.

The National Methamphetamine Chemicals Initiative is known for promoting a culture of collaboration. That's exactly the approach we need for this challenge – as for so many others we face in law enforcement. Collaboration – between one city and another, one state and another, one country and another – is vital to what we do; and all of you are vital to getting it done.

Given the need for collaboration, it is gratifying to see the wide mix of people here – prosecutors, investigators, and local, state, and federal officials, as well as representatives from other nations. I am especially pleased to welcome my colleague, Attorney General Eduardo Medina Mora of Mexico, and our other partners from around the world.

Those in this audience are well aware that methamphetamine is an extremely addictive and destructive drug. It does fearsome damage to the user. It wreaks havoc on families, and it puts children in danger – especially when parents decide to cook meth in their home. It devastates neighborhoods. The volatility of the manufacturing process can endanger entire city blocks around a clandestine lab.

The good news is, thanks to the work of people like you, we're making great strides in our battle against meth. Sustained and aggressive law enforcement efforts, as well as laws controlling access to over-the-counter medicines containing precursor chemicals, have led to dramatic decreases in domestic production in the United States. Since 2003, for example, the number of meth labs seized in the United States has decreased by 72 percent. By all indications, that reflects a real reduction in the number of labs out there.

The reduction in domestic labs means fewer drug-endangered children and fewer meth-related toxic dump sites in our country. It means fewer neighborhoods devastated by meth use or endangered by meth production. And, as you are all aware, it means fewer casualties among law enforcement officers and other first responders. In an especially good sign, from

2003 to 2007, the number of state and local police officers injured in connection with meth investigations dropped by close to 80 percent.

As we all know, however, criminals change their methods in response to law enforcement tactics. The crackdown on domestic labs and the tightening of controls on over-the-counter drugs containing precursor chemicals led, in large part, to an increase in the production of meth in other countries. That, in turn, has called for new enforcement tactics and increased international cooperation.

Mexico in particular has responded to that call and is a resolute ally in the fight against the meth threat. Through the brave leadership of President Calderon and Attorney General Medina Mora, Mexico has responded to the threat with its own increased restrictions on precursor chemicals and aggressive enforcement action against the manufacturers and traffickers of meth.

Mexico has seized labs, including superlabs, and has hit the traffickers where it really hurts: in their pocketbooks. Most prominent, of course, was the seizure last year by Mexican law enforcement of more than $205 million dollars from the Mexico City residence of a man charged in connection with the manufacture and sale of precursor chemicals. That remains the single largest drug-related cash seizure in world history, and by itself, appears to have put a large dent in the illicit chemicals trade and the related meth trade.

All the data indicate that these efforts – here and abroad – are working. There has been almost a 50% decrease in methamphetamine seizures across our Southwest Border. The price per gram of meth has increased dramatically nationwide – over 84% last year alone. The purity of the meth we are seizing is decreasing – over 25% in that same period. In cities throughout our country, there have been prolonged shortages of meth. And the number of people testing positive for meth in workplace drug screenings has declined more than 50% in the past two years.

We have had great successes in combating the meth problem. But we cannot let our successes diminish our efforts because the threat posed by meth is still too great, and meth producers and smugglers continue to adapt in response to what we do.

For example, in response to increased restrictions on the sale of over-the-counter medicines containing precursor chemicals, it appears that manufacturers are increasingly relying on so-called "smurfers" – that is, people who make repeated retail purchases of these medicines in quantities just below the legal threshold.

And as countries like Mexico have tightened their own controls and increased law enforcement efforts, traffickers have begun to migrate to more hospitable locations. We're already seeing alternative production methods, substitute chemicals, and more use of exotic chemical source, production, and transit countries.

Just as they react to what we do, we must react to each new shift in tactics by meth producers and smugglers. Today, I'd like to focus on four of the tools we are using to do just that.

First, the Department of Justice has many and varied enforcement structures that we can, and do, use to disrupt meth drug trafficking organizations.

Our Organized Crime and Drug Enforcement Task Forces leverage the expertise of state, local, and federal law enforcement to target and disrupt methamphetamine organizations.

These task forces also oversee the Department's Consolidated Priority Organization Target strategy, and lead the development of our list of the most prolific drug organizations. Notably, 12 of the 53 groups currently on that list are involved with meth, including, for the first time, a pseudoephedrine trafficking organization. These are significant targets, and we're going after them aggressively.

The inter-agency Special Operations Division, led by the DEA, brings together agents and analysts from 14 different agencies with attorneys from the Department's Criminal Division. They coordinate large cases that cross district and national borders, and we've had great success with this approach.

A recent example of this kind of coordination is the interestingly named Operation Funk 49. In that case, a tip from a meth user on the streets of San Diego led initially to large-scale San Diego distributors. From there, the investigation spread to North Carolina, Georgia, and other parts of California, and finally into Mexico. The result was more than 200 arrests nationwide, the seizure of more than 800 pounds of meth (and a lot of cocaine as well), the recovery of 75 weapons, and the forfeiture of over $27 million in U.S. currency.

Second, in order to disrupt the evolving meth supply chain, we are continuing to work with our international partners – not only Mexico, but also other countries, including China, Germany and India, that serve as primary sources of precursor chemicals; and countries in Central and South America, Africa and the Middle East that now serve as the primary transshipment points for those chemicals.

International efforts to monitor and control the lawful trade in precursor chemicals are especially important, because such a large proportion of the chemicals used unlawfully to manufacture meth originates in that trade. The International Narcotics Control Board, for example, works directly with regulatory and law enforcement authorities from major source and recipient nations to identify suspect shipments and, once they are identified, to share that information promptly with the affected countries. In addition, to help monitor the international trade in key chemical precursors, over 100 countries and jurisdictions have shared with the Board estimates of their national needs for certain chemicals, and we are working to increase that number.

The promise of this sort of international collaboration is illustrated well by voluntary international efforts like Operation Crystal Flow, which focused on the trade in precursor chemicals to the Americas, Africa, and West Asia. The six-month operation produced notifications that resulted in the cancellation, seizure, or suspension of 53 tons of precursor chemicals – a quantity capable of producing about 48 tons of meth, with a street value in this country of over $4 billion.

Third, the Department continues to educate prosecutors and agents on how best to bring methamphetamine cases, and to assist other countries in their efforts to do the same. We offer advanced training at our National Advocacy Center in South Carolina. And we have provided significant training resources to our international partners. Through the DEA and the State Department, for example, we have helped train over 4000 Mexican law enforcement officials on meth- related subjects, including clandestine meth lab investigations and response techniques.

We are also taking steps through this training to foster the kind of international collaboration that is crucial. Thus, for example, I'm pleased to announce that we will be inviting representatives from Mexico to participate as both students and presenters at a National Advocacy Center training conference on methamphetamine this September. We intend to bring together those Mexican representatives with prosecutors and agents from our Southwest Border districts to strengthen our joint enforcement efforts.

The United States and Mexico have also joined forces to provide training to Central American law enforcement agencies, as we expect meth traffickers to target that region as they're pushed out of our countries. Prosecutors, police, and regulatory officials have done assessments and provided training in every country in Central America over the last two years. We hope to continue and expand this effort in the hemisphere. Finally, at the Department we have a responsibility not only to uphold and enforce the law, but also to help shape it. Over the last 15 years, we've worked extensively with Congress to pass laws that strengthen our hand.

The Combat Methamphetamine Epidemic Act, which took effect in 2006, put products that contain the key ingredients behind the counter at retail stores, limited retail sales, and regulated the much-abused "spot market." State legislatures have passed their own measures to combat meth manufacturing and to make it more difficult for manufacturers to obtain precursor ingredients.

Groups like this one were crucial in highlighting the need for these reforms. We will continue to rely on your ideas, comments and analyses as we consider whether the law strikes the right balance and try to identify and close gaps that meth manufacturers and traffickers exploit.

So, while there are many reasons to celebrate our successes in combating methamphetamine, there's still much to be done. We are also trying to draw lessons from our successes in fighting meth that we can apply to other pressing problems. In that connection, it is especially important that you are expanding your focus to the diversion of pharmaceutical controlled substances.

The increased abuse of legally produced drugs is deeply disturbing. Too many young people mistakenly view these drugs as safe for recreational use simply because they're legally produced and available by prescription. And the ease with which both adults and children can order these pills over the Internet is alarming. To help address this issue, the Administration has worked diligently with Senators Feinstein and Sessions to craft legislation to reduce the illegal trafficking of controlled substances over the Internet. That bill, the Ryan Haight Online Pharmacy Consumer Protection Act, passed the Senate unanimously last month, and is now pending before the House. We look forward to working with the full Congress to enact this important legislation to provide law enforcement and prosecutors with the additional tools they need.

As with meth, the Department is dedicated to addressing these problems. And we are all too glad to have the assistance of the National Methamphetamine Chemicals Initiative, which has always been at the cutting edge of these issues.

So, thank you for your efforts and for your dedication to these causes, which are of overriding importance to our nation. And thank you for your time this morning.

CHAPTER SOURCES

The following chapters have been previously published:

Chapter 1 – This is an edited, excerpted and augmented edition of a United States Congressional Research Service publication, Report Order Code RL33857, dated January 24, 2007.

Chapter 2 – This is an edited, excerpted and augmented edition of a United States Congressional Research Service publication, Report Order Code RS22325, dated March 18, 2008.

Chapter 3 – This is an edited, excerpted and augmented edition of a United States Department of Justice, National Drug Intelligence Center, publication, Product No. 2006-Q0317-004, dated November 2006.

Chapter 4 – This is an edited, excerpted and augmented edition of a United States Derpartment of State, Bureau of International Narcotics and Law Enforcement Affairs, Memorandum for the Secretary of State, dated March 1, 2007.

Chapter 5 – This is an edited, excerpted and augmented edition of an Executive Office of the President of the United States Progress Report, dated November 30, 2006.

Chapter 6 – These remarks were delivered as Statement at the Hearing before the Committee on Finance, U.S. Senate, dated September 12, 2006.

Chapter 7 – These remarks were delivered as Statement of Karen P. Tandy, Administrator, Drug Enforcement Administration, U.S. Department of Justice, before the Subcommittee on International Economic Policym Export and Trade Promotion, and Subcommittee on Western Hemisphere, Peace Corps and Narcotics Affairs, Committee on Foreign Relations, U.S. Senate, dated June 21, 2006.

Chapter 8 – These remarks were delivered as Statement of Anne W. Patterson, Assistant Secretary, Bureau of International Narcotics and Law Enforcement Affairs, U.S. Department of State, before the Subcommittee on International Economic Policym Export and Trade Promotion, and Subcommittee on Western Hemisphere, Peace Corps and Narcotics Affairs, Committee on Foreign Relations, U.S. Senate, dated June 21, 2006.

Chapter 9 – These remarks were delivered as Statement of the Honorable John P. Walters, Director, Office of National Drug Control Policy, before the Subcommittee on International Economic Policym Export and Trade Promotion, and Subcommittee on Western Hemisphere, Peace Corps and Narcotics Affairs, Committee on Foreign Relations, U.S. Senate, dated June 21, 2006.

Chapter 10 – These remarks were prepared to be delivered by Attorney General Michael B. Mukasey at the National Methamphetamine Chemicals Initiative Conference, dated May 7, 2008.

INDEX

D

E

F

G

H

I

J

K

L

M

N

O

P